Antibiotic Basics for Clinicians:

The ABCs of Choosing the Right Antibacterial Agent

SECOND EDITION

Antibiotic Basics for Clinicians:

The ABCs of Choosing the Right Antibacterial Agent

SECOND EDITION

Alan R. Hauser, MD, PhD

Departments of Microbiology/Immunology and Medicine
Northwestern University, Chicago, Illinois

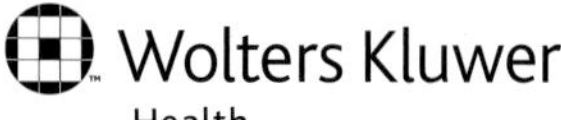

Lippincott Williams & Wilkins

Philadelphia • Baltimore • New York • London
Buenos Aires • Hong Kong • Sydney • Tokyo

Acquisitions Editor: Susan Rhyner
Development Editor: Kathleen Scogna
Production Manager: Steve Boehm
Marketing Manager: Joy Fisher-Williams
Designer: Stephen Druding
Compositor: Absolute Service, Inc.

Second Edition

351 West Camden Street
Baltimore, MD 21201

Two Commerce Square
2001 Market Street
Philadelphia, PA 19103

Printed in People's Republic of China

9 8 7 6

Library of Congress Cataloging-in-Publication Data

Hauser, Alan R., 1959-
Antibiotic basics for clinicians : the ABCs of choosing the right antibacterial agent / Alan R. Hauser. — 2nd ed.
p. ; cm.
Includes bibliographical references and index.
ISBN 978-1-4511-1221-4
I. Title.
[DNLM: 1. Bacterial Infections—drug therapy—Examination Questions. 2. Bacterial Infections—drug therapy—Outlines. 3. Anti-Bacterial Agents—therapeutic use—Examination Questions. 4. Anti-Bacterial Agents—therapeutic use—Outlines. WC 18.2]

615.3'29—dc23

2011037815

DISCLAIMER

Care has been taken to confirm the accuracy of the information present and to describe generally accepted practices. However, the authors, editors, and publisher are not responsible for errors or omissions or for any consequences from application of the information in this book and make no warranty, expressed or implied, with respect to the currency, completeness, or accuracy of the contents of the publication. Application of this information in a particular situation remains the professional responsibility of the practitioner; the clinical treatments described and recommended may not be considered absolute and universal recommendations.

The authors, editors, and publisher have exerted every effort to ensure that drug selection and dosage set forth in this text are in accordance with the current recommendations and practice at the time of publication. However, in view of ongoing research, changes in government regulations, and the constant flow of information relating to drug therapy and drug reactions, the reader is urged to check the package insert for each drug for any change in indications and dosage and for added warnings and precautions. This is particularly important when the recommended agent is a new or infrequently employed drug.

Some drugs and medical devices presented in this publication have Food and Drug Administration (FDA) clearance for limited use in restricted research settings. It is the responsibility of the health care provider to ascertain the FDA status of each drug or device planned for use in their clinical practice.

To purchase additional copies of this book, call our customer service department at (800) 638-3030 or fax orders to (301) 223-2320. International customers should call (301) 223-2300.

Visit Lippincott Williams & Wilkins on the Internet: http://www.lww.com. Lippincott Williams & Wilkins customer service representatives are available from 8:30 am to 6:00 pm, EST.

CCS0416

Dedicated to Anne, Grace, and John

PREFACE

Which is more difficult: learning a large body of information or applying the newly learned information? Although the answer is debatable, it is clear that health care professionals must do both. Most health care training programs consist of an initial phase of classroom lectures and small group sessions in which the intricacies of cranial nerves, the Krebs cycle, and renal physiology are mastered. Following this phase, trainees suddenly are immersed in the real world of patients who present with complaints of a cough, a painful lower back, or a fever. As an infectious disease subspecialist, I have often seen this culture shock expressed as the blank look of a medical student when asked, "So, what antibiotic should we start this patient on?" Obviously, a basic understanding of the principles of pharmacology and microbiology is insufficient for most trainees when suddenly faced with the complexities of an infected patient.

This book is meant to be a guide to antibiotics not only for students studying to be physicians, nurse practitioners, physician assistants, pharmacologists, or medical technologists, but will also prove useful for residents, fellows, and practicing clinicians. It is designed to serve as a bridge between the book knowledge acquired during the initial phase of training and the reflexive prescribing habits of experienced practitioners. Just as the initial bewildering complexities of electrocardiograms and chest radiographs disappear when the first principles underlying these tests are appreciated and understood, so too do the difficulties of antibiotic selection. By supplying the rationale behind antibiotic selection for many common bacterial pathogens and infectious disease presentations, much of the memorization (and magic and mystery) that usually accompanies proper prescribing of antibiotics is eliminated. Where memorization is unavoidable, learning aids are presented that will make the process as painless as possible.

This book can be easily read and comprehended in 1 or 2 weeks by a busy student or practitioner. As a result, it is not a comprehensive guide to the antibiotic metropolis but merely an outline of the major thoroughfares of antibiotic therapy so that readers can more easily fill in the residential streets and alleys as they gain experience. In terms of the war analogy used throughout the book, the emphasis is on strategy, not tactics. Thus, only commonly used antibiotics are mentioned, and some oversimplification and omissions are unavoidable. It is hoped that the reader will be able to master the major concepts and rules so that with subsequent clinical exposure and practice, the nuances and exceptions to these rules may be assimilated.

The scope of this volume is limited to antibacterial agents, arguably the most complex and frequently encountered antibiotics that must be mastered by health care practitioners. Future volumes will address antiviral, antifungal, and antiparasitic agents.

The second edition of this book has been updated and expanded to include newer antibiotics that have become available during the past 3 years. In addition, several older antibiotics that have enjoyed renewed popularity (e.g., colistin and nitrofurantoin) are now also discussed. Emerging resistant organisms such as community-acquired methicillin-resistant *Staphylococcus aureus* and *Klebsiella pneumoniae* carbapenemase-producing bacteria have been incorporated. Likewise, sections have been updated to reflect recent changes in treatment guidelines, such as those pertaining to *Clostridium difficile* colitis and urinary tract infections.

After completing this book, it is hoped that the reader will view antibiotics as valuable friends in the fight against infectious diseases and not as incomprehensible foes blocking his or her progress toward clinical competency. In addition, the reader will obtain a foundation that can be built upon throughout his or her career, as new antibiotics become available.

I am indebted to many people who have contributed in large and small ways to this book but would especially like to acknowledge a few individuals. Many thanks to Mike Postelnick, Kristin Darin, and Marc Scheetz for advice and for reviewing portions of this book; Andy Rabin for providing quotes from the medieval literature; and Joe Welch for invaluable advice. Thank you to Kathleen Scogna, Michael Brown, and Steve Boehm at Lippincott Williams & Wilkins for their assistance, patience, and advice throughout the process of putting together the second edition of this book. I am grateful to the intelligent and inquisitive medical students at Northwestern University who asked the many questions that inspired this book. And finally, I wish to thank my wife, Anne, who made this whole project possible.

CONTENTS

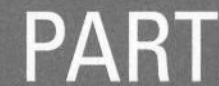

PART I

Bacterial Basics

"Know the enemy and know yourself; in a hundred battles you will never be in peril."

—The Art of War, Sun Tzu

Pathogenic bacteria are both wonderful and horrible little creatures that self-replicate and survive in the rather harsh and hostile environment of the human body. In many ways, they are quite different from us, a characteristic that has been exploited by the developers of antimicrobial agents that specifically target these differences. To understand how antibiotics inhibit or kill bacteria, we must first understand the structure and function of these tiny pathogens.

Three aspects of bacteria must be understood to appreciate how antibiotics target and hinder them: the bacterial cell envelope, biosynthetic processes within bacteria, and bacterial replication. Whereas the bacterial cell envelope is a unique structure not present in human cells, bacterial protein production and DNA replication are processes analogous to those used by human cells but which differ from these human pathways in the components utilized to accomplish them. Each of these three characteristics will be discussed in detail in the following chapters.

ADDITIONAL READINGS

Jorgensen JH, Ferraro MJ. Antimicrobial susceptibility testing: a review of general principles and contemporary practices. *Clin Infect Dis*. 2009;49:1749–1755.

Murray PR, Rosenthal KS, Pfaller MA. *Medical Microbiology*. 5th ed. Philadelphia, PA: Elsevier; 2005.

Neidhardt FC. Bacterial processes. In: Ryan KJ, Ray CG, eds. *Sherris Medical Microbiology: An Introduction to Infectious Disease*. 4th ed. New York, NY: McGraw-Hill; 2004:27–51.

Wang JC. DNA topoisomerases. *Annu Rev Biochem*. 1985;54:665–697.

CHAPTER 1

Cell Envelope

"While styles of armor varied and changed from one decade to the next, the basics were a suit of plate armor consisting of a chest piece, a skirt of linked hoops, and arm and leg pieces, all worn over a hauberk or shirt of chain mail and a leather or padded tunic, or a tight-fitting surcoat. . . . Chain mail covered the neck, elbows, and other joints; gauntlets of linked plates protected the hands."

—A DISTANT MIRROR, BARBARA W. TUCHMAN

The **cell envelope** is a protective layer of armor that surrounds the bacterium and allows it to survive in diverse and extreme environments. The cell envelopes of some bacteria consist of a **cytoplasmic membrane** surrounded by a tough and rigid mesh called a cell wall (Fig. 1-1); these bacteria are referred to as **gram-positive** bacteria. In contrast, the cell envelope of a **gram-negative** bacterium consists of a cytoplasmic membrane surrounded by a thin cell wall that is itself surrounded by a second lipid membrane called the **outer membrane**. The outer membrane contains large amounts of **lipopolysaccharide (LPS)**, a molecule that is very toxic to humans. The space between the outer membrane and the cytoplasmic membrane, which contains the cell wall, is called the **periplasmic space** or the **periplasm**. Whether a bacterium is gram-positive or gram-negative can usually be determined by a technique called Gram staining, which colors gram-positive bacteria blue or purple and gram-negative bacteria pink. Gram staining is often the first step used by a hospital microbiology laboratory in identifying an unknown bacterium from a clinical specimen.

As in human cells, the cytoplasmic membrane prevents ions from flowing into or out of the cell itself and maintains the cytoplasm and bacterial components in a defined space. The cell wall is a tough layer that gives a bacterium its characteristic shape and protects it from mechanical and osmotic stresses. In gram-negative bacteria, the outer membrane acts as an additional protective barrier and prevents many substances from penetrating into the bacterium. This layer, however, does contain channels called **porins** that allow some compounds such as molecules used in metabolism by the bacterium to pass through.

Since human cells do not possess a cell wall, this structure is an ideal target for antimicrobial agents. To appreciate how these agents work, we must first understand the structure of the cell wall. This complex assembly is made up of a substance called **peptidoglycan**, which itself consists of long sugar polymers. The polymers are repeats of two sugars: *N*-acetylglucosamine and *N*-acetylmuramic acid (Fig. 1-2). If the cell wall were to consist of these polymers alone, it would be quite weak. However, peptide side chains extend from the sugars in the polymers and form cross-links, one peptide to another. These cross-links greatly strengthen the cell wall, just as cross-linking of metal loops strengthened the chain mail armor used by medieval knights.

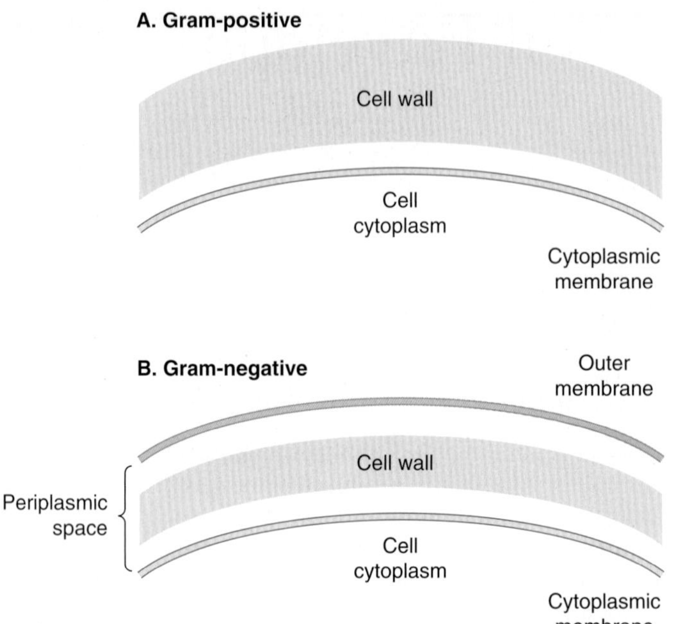

FIGURE 1-1. Structure of the bacterial cell envelope. **A.** Gram-positive. **B.** Gram-negative.

The cross-linking of peptidoglycan is mediated by bacterial enzymes called **penicillin-binding proteins (PBPs)**. (The reason for this nomenclature will become apparent in later chapters.) These enzymes recognize the terminal two amino acids of the peptide side chains, which are usually D-alanine–D-alanine, and either directly cross-link them to a second peptide side chain or indirectly cross-link them by forming a bridge of glycine residues between the two peptide side chains.

The formation of a tough cross-linked cell wall allows bacteria to maintain a characteristic shape. For example, some bacteria are rod shaped and referred to as **bacilli**. **Cocci** are spherical in shape. **Coccobacilli** have a morphology that is intermediate between that of bacilli and cocci. Finally, **spirochetes** have a corkscrew shape.

QUESTIONS (answers to questions are found in Appendix 9)

1. The bacterial cell wall is composed of ________________.

2. ________________ are enzymes that cross-link peptidoglycan polymers.

3. ________________ are rod-shaped bacteria.

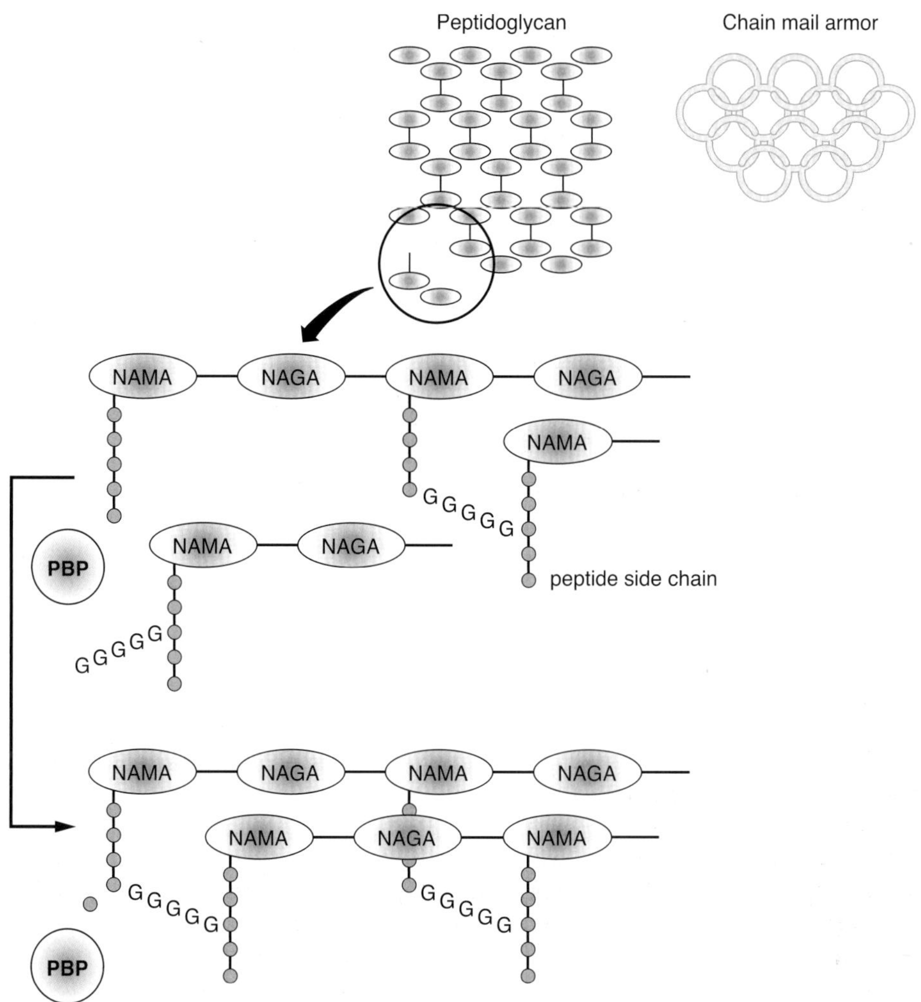

FIGURE 1-2. Structure of peptidoglycan. Peptidoglycan synthesis requires cross-linking of disaccharide polymers by penicillin-binding proteins (PBPs). NAMA, N-acetylmuramic acid; NAGA, N-acetylglucosamine; GGG, glycine bridge.

CHAPTER 2

Protein Production

"Plunder fertile country to supply the army with plentiful provisions."

—THE ART OF WAR, SUN TZU

Like all invading armies, bacteria causing an infection need to be resupplied. They require the proper resources to allow for replacement of old worn-out parts and for building new bacteria. Bacteria acquire these resources from the "country" they are invading, which is the human body. Among the most abundant of the synthesized replacement parts are proteins. The synthesis of these proteins is accomplished using the same general processes that are utilized by human cells (Fig. 2-1). First, a number of raw materials or building blocks, such as RNAs, amino acids, and energy-containing nucleoside triphosphates, must be acquired and available within the bacterium. If this condition is met, template bacterial genes are transcribed into RNA by special bacterial enzymes. RNA is then translated into protein. Since some of the bacterial components essential for these processes differ significantly from their human cell counterparts, protein production in bacteria is amenable to inhibition by antibiotics.

RAW MATERIALS

The process of synthesizing new proteins requires abundant amounts of building blocks as well as energy. For example, it is estimated that the energy of three or four nucleoside triphosphates (e.g., adenosine triphosphate [ATP] or guanosine triphosphate [GTP]) is required to add a single amino acid to a growing protein. The bacterium generates these raw materials and energy by taking up fuel sources such as glucose from the environment and processing them through metabolic pathways that harness their energy and generate intermediate compounds.

These metabolic pathways are quite complex and differ significantly between bacteria and human cells. They can be effectively used to divide bacteria into two categories: **aerobes** and **anaerobes**. Aerobic bacteria use oxygen from their environment in the process of metabolism, whereas anaerobic bacteria do not. In fact, strict anaerobes are killed by oxygen because they lack enzymes that detoxify some of the harmful byproducts of oxygen, such as hydrogen peroxide and superoxide radicals. *Mycobacterium tuberculosis* is an example of a strict aerobic bacterium; strict anaerobic bacteria include *Clostridium difficile* and *Bacteroides fragilis*. Many bacteria have metabolic pathways that allow them to utilize oxygen when it is present but to function as anaerobes when it is absent. These bacteria are said to be **facultative** with respect to oxygen use and obviously survive fine in the presence or absence of oxygen. Examples of such facultative bacteria include *Escherichia coli* and *Staphylococcus aureus*. Other bacteria grow best in the presence of small amounts of oxygen, less than would be found in air. These bacteria are said to be **microaerophilic**. *Campylobacter jejuni* is an example of a microaerophilic bacterium.

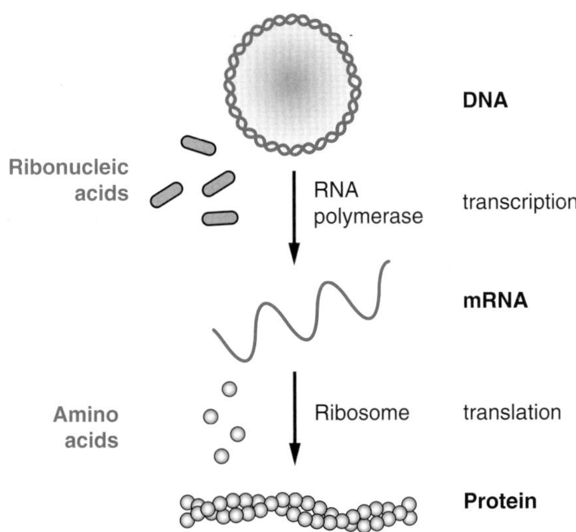

FIGURE 2-1. An overview of the process by which proteins are produced within bacteria.

The energy available in the fuel consumed by bacteria is harnessed and stored in the form of nucleoside triphosphates and, in some cases, in the generation of a proton gradient between the interior and exterior of the cell. The potential energy stored in this gradient is referred to as the **proton motive force**. As protons flow down this gradient (from outside the bacterium to inside the bacterium) and through the cytoplasmic membrane, this energy is utilized to power important processes such as the active transport of nutrients into the cell and the generation of ATP.

TRANSCRIPTION

Transcription is the process by which the information in the DNA of a bacterial gene is used to synthesize an RNA molecule referred to as **messenger RNA (mRNA)**. As in human cells, the enzyme complex **RNA polymerase** is used by bacteria to accomplish this. RNA polymerase binds to DNA and uses this template to sequentially add ribonucleic acids to a corresponding molecule of mRNA. This process is quite efficient; under ideal conditions, bacterial RNA polymerase can make mRNA at a rate of 55 nucleotides per second.

Although both molecules perform similar functions, bacterial RNA polymerase is quite distinct from eukaryotic RNA polymerase. (Eukaryotes, unlike bacteria, are organisms that contain nuclei and other membrane-bound organelles within their cells. Examples include animals, plants, fungi, and protozoa.) Structurally, bacterial RNA polymerase consists of five subunits and has overall dimensions of approximately $90 \times 90 \times 160$ angstroms, whereas yeast RNA polymerase has many more subunits and has dimensions of $140 \times 136 \times 110$ angstroms. Functional differences also exist. For example, whereas bacterial RNA polymerase by itself is sufficient to initiate transcription, eukaryotic RNA polymerase requires the help of additional transcription factors. The importance of transcription to the health of the bacterium and the differences between bacterial and eukaryotic RNA polymerases make this enzyme complex an ideal target for antimicrobial compounds.

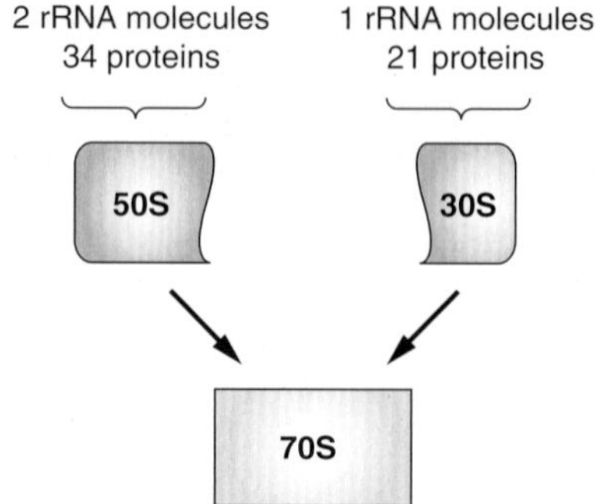

FIGURE 2-2. Structure of the bacterial ribosome.

TRANSLATION

In both eukaryotes and bacteria, macromolecular structures called **ribosomes** do the work of synthesizing proteins from the information present in mRNA, a process called **translation**. These large complexes are composed of both **ribosomal RNA (rRNA)** and proteins. Bacterial ribosomes, however, differ significantly from their eukaryotic counterparts. The **70S bacterial ribosome** is made of a **50S subunit** and a **30S subunit** (Fig. 2-2). ("S" stands for Svedberg units, which are a measure of the rate of sedimentation in an ultracentrifuge. Svedberg units, thus, reflect the size of a complex but are not additive.) These subunits themselves are complex structures. For example, the 50S subunit is made of 2 rRNA molecules and 34 proteins, whereas the 30S subunit consists of 1 rRNA molecule and 21 proteins. In contrast, the eukaryotic ribosome is 80S in size and consists of a 60S subunit and a 40S subunit. Each of these, in turn, is made of multiple rRNA molecules and proteins.

The complete ribosome functions together with another type of RNA, **transfer RNA (tRNA)**, to manufacture new proteins. The ribosome binds to and reads the mRNA template and appropriately incorporates amino acids delivered by the tRNA into the nascent protein based on the information in this template. The importance of translation is indicated by the fact that half of all RNA synthesis in rapidly growing bacteria is devoted to rRNA and tRNA. The essential role played by protein synthesis in bacterial growth and the dissimilarity between the bacterial ribosome and the human ribosome make the former an attractive antibiotic target. Indeed, numerous classes of antimicrobial agents act by binding to and inhibiting the bacterial ribosome.

QUESTIONS

1. ________________ bacteria are those that grow in the absence of oxygen.
2. ________________ is an enzyme complex that makes mRNA from a DNA template.
3. The 70S bacterial ribosome consists of ________________ and ________________ subunits, which themselves consist of ________________ and ________________.

CHAPTER 3

Reproduction

"We think we have now allotted to the superiority in numbers the importance which belongs to it; it is to be regarded as the fundamental idea, always to be aimed at before all and as far as possible."

—On War, Carl Von Clausewitz

In the battle between bacteria and the human immune response, numbers are key. Bacteria are continuously multiplying in an attempt to overwhelm the host's defensive capabilities, and immune factors are constantly attempting to eradicate the invaders. It is this balance that is often tipped in favor of the human immune response by antibiotics.

An illustrative example of the importance of bacterial multiplication in infection is shigellosis. This form of infectious diarrhea is caused by the bacterium *Shigella* and can occur following ingestion of as few as 200 organisms. Yet, over a short period, these 200 organisms lead to diarrhea in which billions of bacteria are expelled every day in the feces. Obviously, rapid bacterial multiplication is essential for this disease.

Bacterial multiplication occurs by binary fission, the process by which a parent bacterium divides to form two identical daughter cells. This requires the synthesis of numerous biomolecules essential for construction of the daughter cells. Nearly all bacteria have a single circular chromosome, the replication of which is an integral part of cell division. Replication occurs when bacterial enzymes use the existing chromosome as a template for synthesis of a second identical chromosome. To accomplish this, a ready supply of deoxynucleotides must be available for incorporation into the nascent DNA molecule. This process is more complicated than one might suspect, and other enzymes are also required to regulate the conformation of the DNA to allow for optimal replication of the chromosome. These complex processes afford several opportunities for antimicrobial agents to inhibit bacterial growth.

SYNTHESIS OF DEOXYNUCLEOTIDES

An abundant supply of deoxyadenosine triphosphate (dATP), deoxyguanosine triphosphate (dGTP), deoxycytidine triphosphate (dCTP), and deoxythymidine triphosphate (dTTP) is essential for the production of DNA molecules during DNA replication. Bacteria use several synthetic pathways to manufacture these DNA building blocks. **Tetrahydrofolate (THF)** is an essential cofactor for several of these pathways and is synthesized as follows (Fig. 3-1): The enzyme dihydropteroate synthase uses dihydropterin pyrophosphate and *para*-aminobenzoate (PABA) to generate dihydropteroate, which is subsequently converted to dihydrofolate. Dihydrofolate reductase then converts dihydrofolate into THF. THF is required for the ultimate synthesis of several nucleotides. Although humans readily absorb folate, a precursor of THF, from their diet, most bacteria are unable to do so and must synthesize this cofactor. This synthetic pathway is thus an attractive target for antimicrobial compounds.

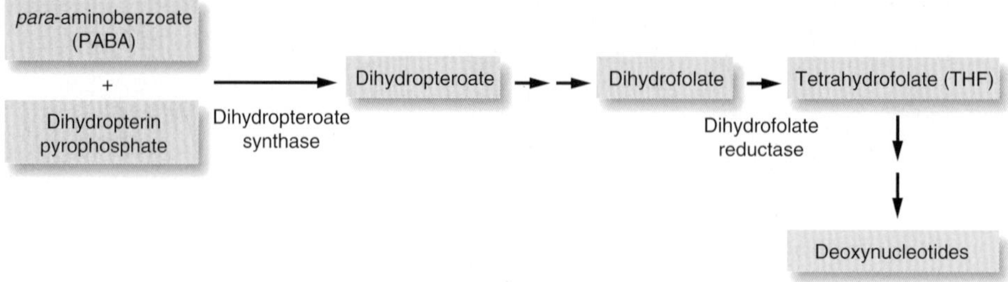

FIGURE 3-1. Bacterial synthesis of tetrahydrofolate.

DNA SYNTHETIC ENZYMES

The enzyme **DNA polymerase** is responsible for replicating the bacterial chromosome, but other enzymes are also required for this process. One example is the **topoisomerases** that regulate **supercoiling**, or twisting of the DNA. To understand supercoiling, one must appreciate the consequences of having a chromosome composed of helical DNA. The double helix structure of DNA dictates that in a relaxed state, it will contain 10 nucleotide pairs per each helical turn. However, by twisting one end of the DNA while holding the other end fixed, one can increase or decrease the number of nucleotide pairs per helical turn, say to 11 or 9 (Fig. 3-2). This results in additional stress on the DNA molecule, which is accommodated by the formation of supercoils. When there is an increase in the number of nucleotide pairs per helical turn, the supercoiling is said to be positive. When there is a decrease, the supercoiling is said to be negative. An analogous process occurs in bacteria. Because parts of the chromosome are "fixed" due to associations with large protein complexes, twists that occur in one portion cannot freely dissipate but accumulate and form supercoils. So where do the twists come from? RNA polymerase is a large molecule that is unable to spin freely while it moves along the bacterial chromosome during transcription. Thus, as RNA polymerase forges its way along the chromosome, separating the DNA strands as it goes, positive supercoiling occurs in front of the enzyme, whereas negative supercoils accumulate behind it. In theory, excess supercoiling could present a barrier to DNA replication and transcription.

To visualize supercoiling, hold a coiled telephone cord tightly with your left hand at a point about a foot from receiver. Now with your right hand, grab the cord at the same point and "strain" the cord through your fingers, moving your hand toward the telephone receiver. In this example, the cord is the helical chromosomal DNA and your right hand is the RNA polymerase moving along the chromosome. Note how supercoils accumulate in the cord ahead of your hand. Now, let the telephone receiver dangle in the air. The weight of the receiver removes the supercoils from the cord, forcing the cord to take on an overly twisted conformation. But the receiver is now no longer fixed, so it can spin freely to relieve this stress.

A second consequence of the circular nature of the bacterial chromosome is that following completion of replication, the two daughter chromosomes will frequently be interlinked (Fig. 3-3). This obviously presents an obstacle for the dividing bacterium while it tries to segregate one chromosome to each of the daughter cells.

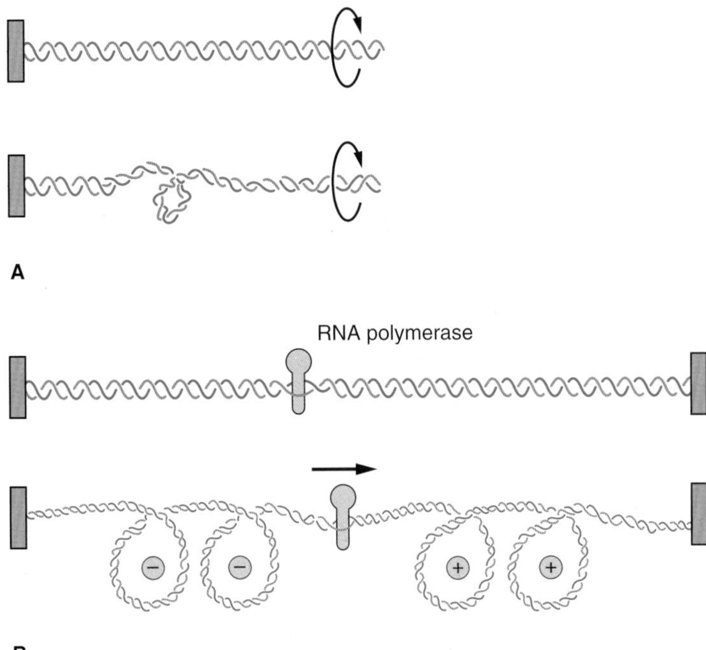

FIGURE 3-2. Supercoiling of the double helical structure of DNA. **A.** Twisting of DNA results in formation of supercoils. **B.** During transcription, the movement of RNA polymerase along the chromosome results in the accumulation of positive supercoils ahead of the enzyme and negative supercoils behind it. (Adapted with permission from Alberts B, Johnson A, Lewis J, et al. *Molecular Biology of the Cell*. New York, NY: Garland Science; 2002:314.)

Bacteria overcome both these problems by producing topoisomerases, enzymes that remove or add supercoiling to DNA. They do this by binding to the DNA, cutting one or both strands of the DNA, passing either a single strand of DNA or double-stranded DNA through the break, and then relegating the DNA. The passage of one or two strands of DNA through the break in essence removes or adds one or two supercoils to the chromosome. It may also unlink two interlocked chromosomes following replication. In this way, bacteria are able to regulate the degree of supercoiling in their chromosomes and allow for separation of chromosomes following DNA replication.

QUESTIONS

1. Tetrahydrofolate is required for several pathways involving the synthesis of ________________.
2. The chromosomes of most bacteria are ________________.
3. ________________ are enzymes that regulate DNA supercoiling.

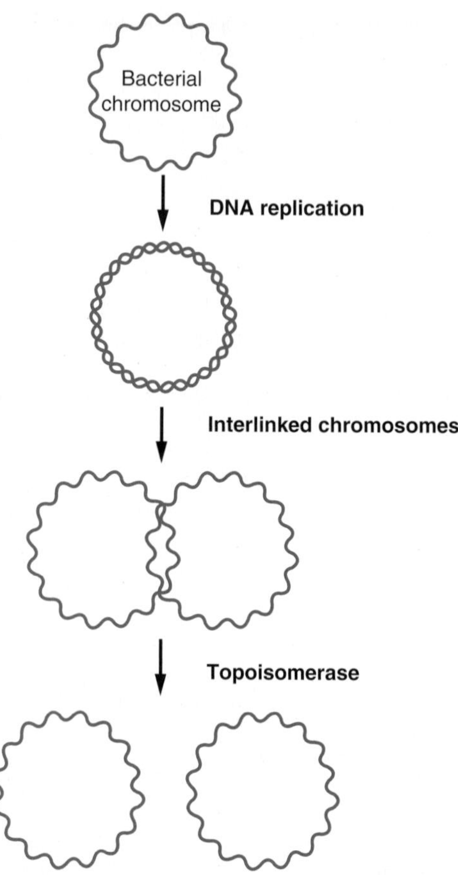

FIGURE 3-3. Replication of the bacterial chromosome. A consequence of the circular nature of the bacterial chromosome is that replicated chromosomes are interlinked, requiring topoisomerase for appropriate segregation.

CHAPTER 4

Measuring Susceptibility to Antibiotics

"The best form of defense is attack."

—On War, Carl von Clausewitz

We have now discussed three processes of bacteria that are both essential for their survival and distinct from corresponding human cell processes: generation of the cell envelope, production of bacterial proteins, and replication of the bacterial chromosome. Each of these processes provides multiple targets for antibiotics that inhibit bacteria. Antibiotics can be divided into two classes: Those antibiotics that kill bacteria are called **bactericidal**, and those that merely suppress bacterial growth are called **bacteriostatic**. Bacteriostatic antibiotics rely on the immune system to eradicate the nonmultiplying bacteria from the patient.

The susceptibility of a bacterial isolate to a given antibiotic is quantified by the **minimum inhibitory concentration** (**MIC**) and the **minimum bactericidal concentration** (**MBC**). As its name implies, the MIC measures the minimum concentration of antibiotic that is still able to suppress growth of the bacterial isolate. Likewise, the MBC is the minimum concentration of antibiotic that results in killing of the bacterial isolate.

In practice, several assays have been developed to measure whether any given bacterial isolate is susceptible or resistant to a particular antibiotic. In the **Kirby-Bauer method**, antibiotic-impregnated wafers are dropped onto agar plates streaked with bacteria. The antibiotics diffuse from the wafers, establishing a gradient with lower concentrations occurring further from the wafer. Bacterial growth will be suppressed in a zone surrounding the wafer, and measurement of the diameter of the zone can be used to determine whether the bacterial strain is susceptible or resistant to the antibiotic. **Etests** operate on a similar principle except that an elongated strip is used instead of a wafer. The strip is impregnated with a decreasing gradient of antibiotic concentrations along its length. When it is dropped onto the agar plate that has been streaked with a lawn of bacteria, the bacteria will grow right up to the end of the strip where little antibiotic is present but will be unable to grow near the end of the strip that contains high concentrations of antibiotics. The spot where the bacterial lawn first touches the strip is used to estimate the MIC, a process facilitated by MIC designations marked onto the strip itself. **Broth dilution methods** operate on a similar principle except that the antibiotic dilutions are created in wells of liquid media rather than in agar. In these assays, the well with the greatest dilution of antibiotic that still does not support the growth of the bacterium identifies the MIC. Today, the microbiology laboratories of most large hospitals rely on machines that utilize these principles to automatically test hundreds of bacterial isolates.

In the following section, we will discuss the individual antibiotics that bind to essential bacterial targets as well as the protective mechanisms that have evolved within bacteria to thwart their action.

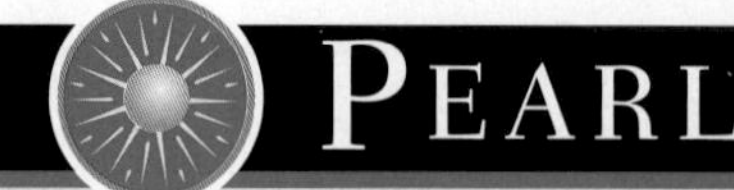

The immune system appears to be relatively ineffective in the eradication of bacteria in certain types of infections, such as meningitis and endocarditis. In these infections, bactericidal antibiotics should be used instead of bacteriostatic antibiotics.

QUESTIONS

1. ________________ antibiotics kill rather than inhibit the growth of bacteria.
2. The ________________ method of measuring antibiotic susceptibility utilizes antibiotic impregnated wafers dropped onto an agar plate streaked with a lawn of bacteria.
3. The ________________ method of measuring antibiotic susceptibility utilizes serial dilutions of antibiotics in liquid media.

PART II

Antibacterial Agents

"The warrior, in accordance with his aims, maintains various weapons and knows their characteristics and uses them well."

—The Book of Five Rings, Miyamoto Musashi

To protect the human body from the onslaught of bacterial pathogens, a large number of antimicrobial compounds have been developed that target points of vulnerability within these invaders. These agents can be grouped into three broad categories based on their mechanism of action: (1) those that target the bacterial cell envelope, (2) those that block the production of new proteins, and (3) those that target DNA or DNA replication.

We will now discuss the individual antimicrobial agents. For each, a summary of its antimicrobial spectrum is given in the form of traffic signs. For this purpose, bacteria are broadly grouped into four categories: aerobic gram-positive bacteria, aerobic gram-negative bacteria, anaerobic bacteria, and atypical bacteria. The activity of an antibiotic against a particular category of bacteria is represented by a "walk" sign (active), a "caution" sign (sometimes active), or a "stop" sign (not active). Thus, in the example shown in the second figure, one should **go** ahead and use the antibiotic to treat an infection caused by gram-positive bacteria, **stop** if considering using the antibiotic to treat an infection caused by gram-negative bacteria, and proceed with **caution** if treating an infection caused by anaerobic or atypical bacteria. Note that these are only general indications of the antibiotic's activity against these classes of bacteria. There are almost certainly exceptions, and many other factors, such as the antibiotic's ability to achieve high concentrations at the site of the infection, whether it kills or merely inhibits the bacteria, contraindications to the drug, and the patient's antibiotic history, must be taken into account when actually choosing an appropriate agent. Nonetheless, the traffic sign representation will be useful as a first step in learning the antimicrobial spectra of individual antibiotics.

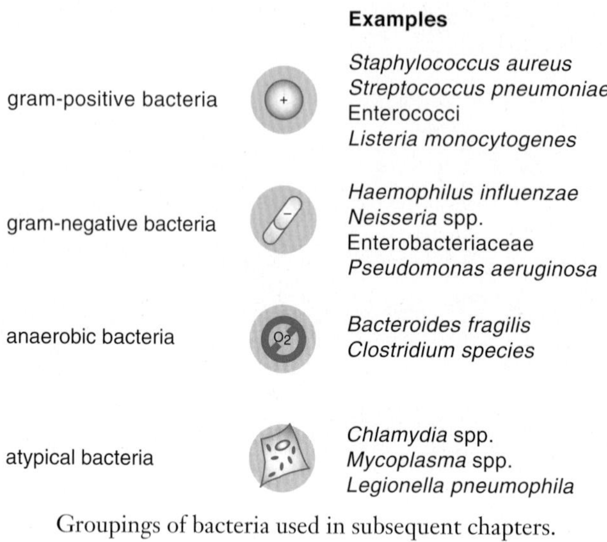

Groupings of bacteria used in subsequent chapters.

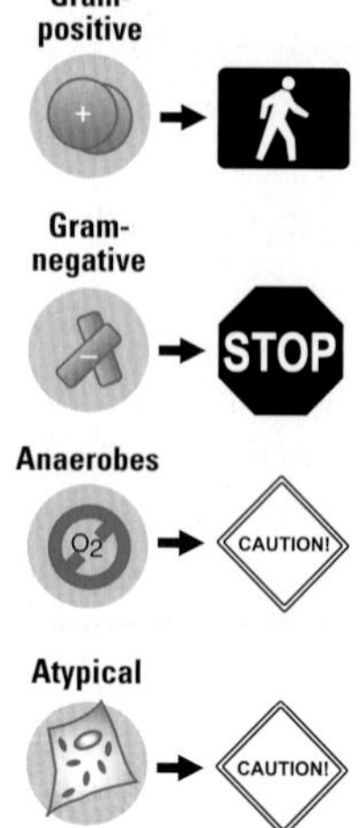

Traffic sign representation of antimicrobial spectrum of activity.

ADDITIONAL READINGS

For excellent overviews of antibiotics, please see these references:

Mandell GL, Bennett JE, Dolin R. *Mandell, Douglas, and Bennett's Principles and Practice of Infectious Diseases*. 6th ed. Philadelphia, PA: Elsevier; 2005.

Mascaretti OA. *Bacteria versus Antibacterial Agents: An Integrated Approach*. Washington, DC: ASM Press; 2003.

Thompson RL, Wright AJ. Symposium on antimicrobial agents, parts I–XVII. *Mayo Clin Proc.* 1998–2000:73–75.

Walsh C. *Antibiotics: Actions, Origins, Resistance*. Washington, DC: ASM Press; 2003.

CHAPTER 5

Antibiotics that Target the Cell Envelope

"Though the knights, secure in their heavy armour, had no scruples in riding down and killing the leather-clad foot-soldier, it is entertaining to read of the fierce outcry they made when the foot-soldier retaliated with steel crossbow. . . . The knights called Heaven to witness that it was not honourable warfare to employ such weapons in battle, the fact being that they realized that armour was no longer the protection to their persons which it was before the days of heavy crossbows. . . ."

—The Crossbow, Sir Ralph Payne-Gallwey

If the cell envelope is the bacterium's armor, then β-lactam antibiotics, glycopeptides, daptomycin, and colistin are the crossbows capable of piercing it. These antimicrobial agents attack the protective cell envelope, turning it into a liability for bacterium. In the following sections, we will discuss how these antibiotics kill bacteria, the types of bacteria they are active against, and their toxicities.

β-Lactam Antibiotics

The exciting story of β-lactam antibiotics began in 1928, when Alexander Fleming noticed that a mold contaminating one of his cultures prevented the growth of bacteria. Because the mold was of the genus *Penicillium*, Fleming named the antibacterial substance "penicillin," the first of a long line of β-lactam agents. Characterization of this compound progressed rapidly, and, by 1941, clinical trials were being performed with remarkable success on patients.

The essential core of penicillin is a four-member ring called a **β-lactam ring** (Fig. 5-1). Modifications of this basic structure have led to the development of several useful antibacterial compounds, each with its own characteristic spectrum of activity and pharmacokinetic properties. These include the **penicillins**, **cephalosporins**, **carbapenems**, and **monobactams** (Table 5-1). It is important to remember, however, that the antibacterial activity of each β-lactam compound is based on the same basic mechanism (Fig. 5-2). Although somewhat of an oversimplification, β-lactam antibiotics can be viewed as inhibitors of penicillin-binding proteins (PBPs) that normally assemble the peptidoglycan layer surrounding most bacteria. It has been hypothesized that the β-lactam ring mimics the D-alanyl–D-alanine portion of the peptide side chain that is normally bound by PBPs. PBPs thus interact with the β-lactam ring and are not available for synthesis of new peptidoglycan (Fig. 5-3). The disruption of the peptidoglycan layer leads to lysis of the bacterium.

As is the case with all antibiotics, resistance to β-lactams can be divided into two main categories: intrinsic and acquired. **Intrinsic resistance** refers to a resistance mechanism that is intrinsic to the structure or physiology of the bacterial species. For example, the porins in the outer membrane of all *Pseudomonas aeruginosa* strains do not allow passage of ampicillin to the periplasmic space, and all strains of *P. aeruginosa* are therefore resistant to this antibiotic. In contrast, **acquired resistance** occurs when a bacterium that was previously sensitive to an antibiotic acquires a mutation or exogenous genetic material that allows it to now resist the activity of that antibiotic. For example, most strains of *P. aeruginosa* are susceptible to the carbapenem imipenem, which gains access to the PBPs of this organism by passing through a specific protein channel found in the outer membrane. However, following exposure to imipenem, spontaneous mutations may occur that result in loss of production of this channel. This, in turn, causes acquired resistance to imipenem. Practically speaking, intrinsic resistance usually implies that all strains of a bacterial species are resistant to a given antibiotic, whereas acquired resistance affects only some strains of a bacterial species.

Resistance usually results from failure of an agent to avoid one of six potential **P**itfalls in the process by which β-lactam antibiotics cause bacterial pathogens to perish (Fig. 5-4). These are the six **P**s: (1) **P**enetration—β-lactams penetrate poorly into the intracellular compartment of human cells, so bacteria that reside in this compartment

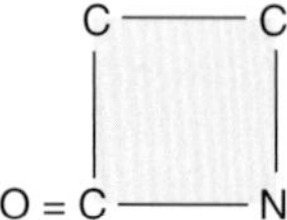

FIGURE 5-1. The structure of the β-lactam ring.

Table 5-1	β-Lactam Antibiotics
Penicillins	
Cephalosporins	
Carbapenems	
Monobactams	

are not exposed to them. A β-lactam antibiotic cannot kill a bacterium if it cannot get to it. (2) **P**orins—if a β-lactam antibiotic does reach the bacterium, it must gain access to its targets, the PBPs. In gram-positive bacteria, this is not difficult because the PBPs and the peptidoglycan layer are relatively exposed, but in gram-negative bacteria, they are surrounded by the protective outer membrane. β-lactams must breach this membrane by diffusing through porins, which are protein channels in the outer

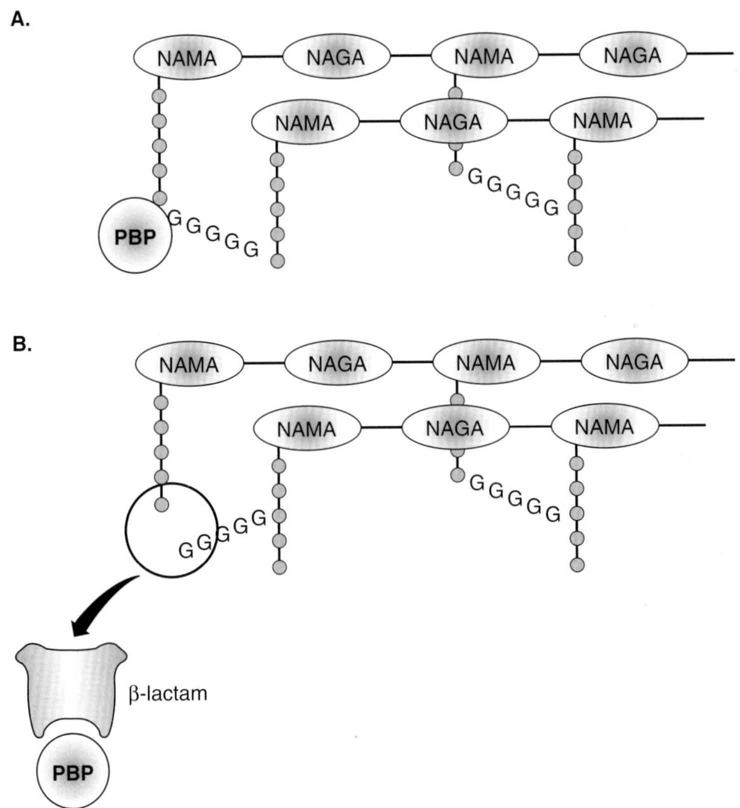

FIGURE 5-2. Mechanism of action of β-lactam antibiotics. **A.** Normally, a new subunit of *N*-acetylmuramic acid (NAMA) and *N*-acetylglucosamine (NAGA) disaccharide with an attached peptide side chain is linked to an existing peptidoglycan polymer. This may occur by covalent attachment of a glycine (G) bridge from one peptide side chain to another through the enzymatic action of a PBP. **B.** In the presence of a β-lactam antibiotic, this process is disrupted. The β-lactam antibiotic binds the PBP and prevents it from cross-linking the glycine bridge to the peptide side chain, thus blocking incorporation of the disaccharide subunit into the existing peptidoglycan polymer.

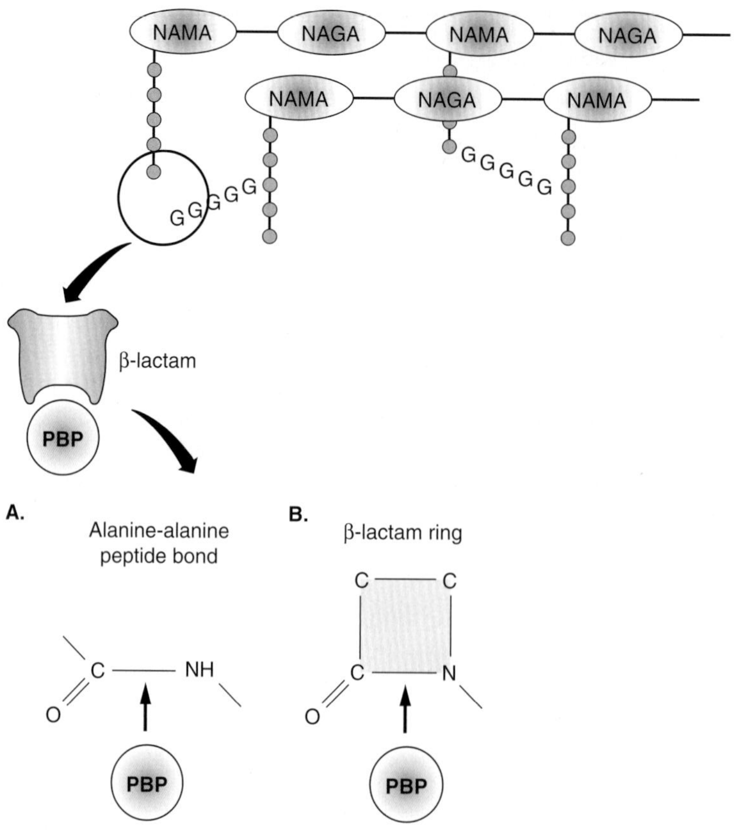

FIGURE 5-3. Mechanism of penicillin-binding protein (PBP) inhibition by β-lactam antibiotics. **A.** PBPs recognize and catalyze the peptide bond between two alanine subunits of the peptidoglycan peptide side chain. **B.** The β-lactam ring mimics this peptide bond. Thus, the PBPs attempt to catalyze the β-lactam ring, resulting in inactivation of the PBPs.

membrane. Many gram-negative bacteria have porins that do not allow passage of certain β-lactams to the periplasmic space. (3) **P**umps—some bacteria produce **efflux pumps**, which are protein complexes that transport antibiotics that have entered the periplasmic space back out to the environment. These pumps prevent antibiotics from accumulating within the periplasm to concentrations sufficient for antibacterial activity. (4) **P**enicillinases (really β-lactamases, but that does not start with P)—many bacteria, both gram-positive and gram-negative, make **β-lactamases**, enzymes that degrade β-lactams before they reach the PBPs. (5) **PBP**s—some bacteria produce PBPs that do not bind β-lactams with high affinity. In these bacteria, β-lactams reach their targets, the PBPs, but cannot inactivate them. (6) **P**eptidoglycan is absent—there are a few bacteria that do not make peptidoglycan and that therefore are not affected by β-lactams. To be effective, β-lactam agents must successfully navigate around each of these potential pitfalls. It is important to note that β-lactam antibiotics are a heterogeneous group of compounds; some may be blocked at certain steps through which others may proceed without difficulty.

One point about β-lactamases: They come in many flavors—that is to say that some are specific for a few β-lactam antibiotics, whereas others have activity against

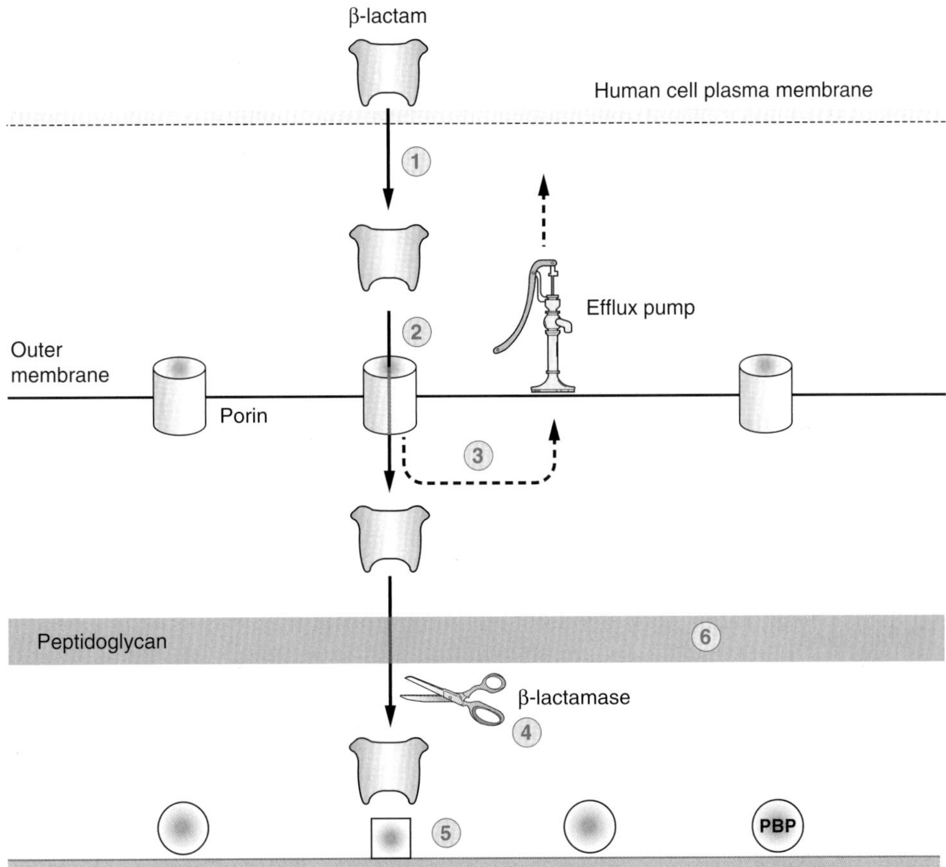

FIGURE 5-4. Six Ps by which the action of β-lactams may be blocked: (1) penetration, (2) porins, (3) pumps, (4) penicillinases (β-lactamases), (5) penicillin-binding proteins (PBPs), and (6) peptidoglycan.

HISTORY

By chance, Alexander Fleming took a 2-week vacation immediately after inoculation of his soon-to-be contaminated agar plates. Since he knew he would not be able to examine the plates for 2 weeks, he incubated them at room temperature instead of 37° C to slow the growth rate of the bacteria. His vacation changed the course of human events. Penicillium grows at room temperature but not 37°C—had Fleming not taken a vacation, he never would have observed the bactericidal effects of the mold. So, vacations truly do make one more productive at work.

Friedman M, Friedman GW. *Medicine's Ten Greatest Discoveries.* New Haven, CT: Yale University Press; 1998.

nearly all β-lactam agents. For example, the β-lactamase of *Staphylococcus aureus* is relatively specific for some of the penicillins, whereas the extended-spectrum β-lactamases made by some strains of *Escherichia coli* and *Klebsiella* spp. (abbreviation for the plural of species) degrade nearly all penicillins, cephalosporins, and monobactams. Different species or strains of bacteria produce different types of β-lactamases that confer upon them unique antibiotic resistance patterns. Thus, generalizations about β-lactamases and their effects on specific antibiotics must be made with caution.

Despite their many limitations, β-lactam antibiotics remain some of the most powerful and broad-spectrum antibiotics available today. They comprise a significant proportion of the total antibiotics prescribed every year.

Questions

1. All β-lactam antibiotics act by preventing proper construction of the bacterial ______________ layer.
2. The four major classes of β-lactam antibiotics are ______________, ______________, ______________, and ______________.
3. All β-lactam antibiotics exert their action by binding to ______________.
4. ______________ are enzymes that cleave β-lactam antibiotics, thus inactivating them.

Penicillins

The penicillins each consist of a thiazolidine ring attached to a β-lactam ring that is itself modified by a variable side chain ("R" in Fig. 5-5). Whereas the thiazolidine–β-lactam ring is required for antibacterial activity, the side chain has been manipulated to yield many penicillin derivatives that have altered pharmacologic properties and antibacterial spectra of activity.

As a result of modifications to the R side chain, penicillins come in several classes: the **natural penicillins**, the **antistaphylococcal penicillins**, the **aminopenicillins**, and the **extended-spectrum penicillins** (Table 5-2). In addition, some of the penicillins have been combined with **β-lactamase inhibitors**, which markedly expand the number of bacterial species that are susceptible to these compounds. The members of each class share similar pharmacokinetic properties and spectra of activity but may be quite distinct from members of other classes.

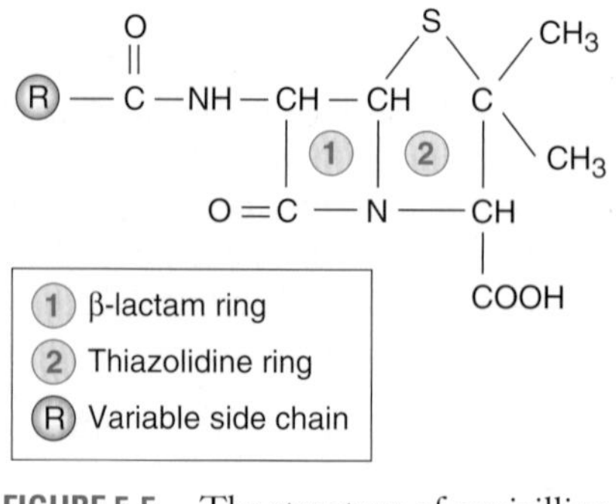

1 β-lactam ring
2 Thiazolidine ring
R Variable side chain

FIGURE 5-5. The structure of penicillins.

Table 5-2 The Penicillins

Category	Parenteral Agents	Oral Agents
Natural penicillins	Penicillin G	Penicillin V
Antistaphylococcal penicillins	Nafcillin, oxacillin	Dicloxacillin
Aminopenicillins	Ampicillin	Amoxicillin, ampicillin
Aminopenicillins + β-lactamase inhibitors	Ampicillin-sulbactam	Amoxicillin-clavulanate
Extended-spectrum penicillins	Piperacillin, ticarcillin	
Extended-spectrum penicillins + β-lactamase inhibitors	Piperacillin-tazobactam, ticarcillin-clavulanate	

NATURAL PENICILLINS

The natural penicillins, **penicillin G** and **penicillin V**, are the great grandparents of the penicillin antibiotic family but still have much to say about the treatment of antibacterial infections. They are called *natural* penicillins because they can be purified directly from cultures of *Penicillium* mold. The R side chain of penicillin G is shown in Figure 5-6 and consists of a hydrophobic benzene ring.

Since nearly all bacteria have cell walls composed of peptidoglycan, it is not surprising that the natural penicillins are active against some species of gram-positive, gram-negative, and anaerobic bacteria, as well as some spirochetes. Despite this broad range of activity, most bacteria are either intrinsically resistant or have now acquired resistance to the natural penicillins. Understanding the reasons for this can help one remember which species remain susceptible. In turn, the bacterial spectra of the natural penicillins can be used as a foundation for remembering the spectra of the other classes of penicillins. The six **P**s explain resistance to the natural penicillins: (1) **P**enetration—natural penicillins, like most β-lactams, penetrate poorly into the intracellular compartment of human cells, so bacteria that for the most part reside in this compartment, such as *Rickettsia* and *Legionella*, are protected from them. (2) **P**orins—Some gram-negative bacteria, such as *E. coli*, *Proteus mirabilis*, *Salmonella enterica*, and *Shigella* spp., have porins in their outer membranes that do not allow passage of the hydrophobic natural penicillins to the periplasmic space. (3) **P**umps—some gram-negative bacteria, such as *P. aeruginosa*, have efflux pumps that prevent the accumulation of penicillins within the periplasm. Although these pumps by themselves may only cause a marginal change in susceptibility, they can work together with penicillinases and porins to have a dramatic effect. (4) **P**enicillinases—many bacteria, both gram-positive (staphylococci) and gram-negative (some *Neisseria* and *Haemophilus* strains, many of the enteric

CH_2

FIGURE 5-6. R side chain of penicillin G.

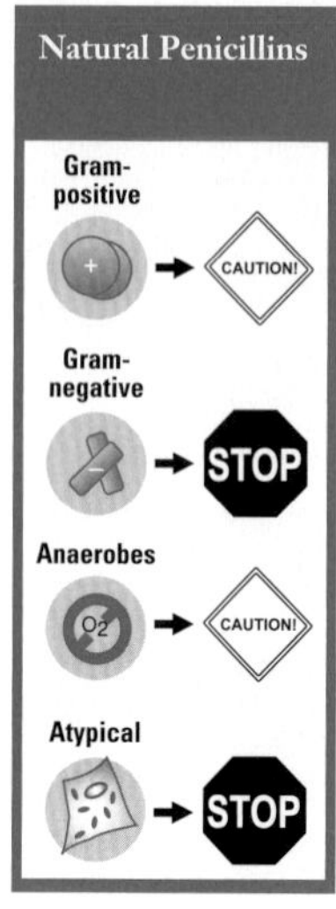

Table 5-3 Antimicrobial Activity of Natural Penicillins

Gram-positive bacteria	*Streptococcus pyogenes* Viridans group streptococci Some *Streptococcus pneumoniae* Some enterococci *Listeria monocytogenes*
Gram-negative bacteria	*Neisseria meningitidis* Some *Haemophilus influenzae*
Anaerobic bacteria	*Clostridia* spp. (except *C. difficile*) *Actinomyces israelii*
Spirochetes	*Treponema pallidum* *Leptospira* spp.

species not listed in (2), and some anaerobes, such as *Bacteroides fragilis*), make penicillinases that degrade the natural penicillins. (5) **P**BPs—some bacteria produce PBPs that do not bind natural penicillins with a high affinity (e.g., some strains of *Streptococcus pneumoniae*). (6) **P**eptidoglycan—some bacteria, such as *Mycoplasma* and *Chlamydia* spp., do not make peptidoglycan and therefore are not affected by the natural penicillins.

Despite these limitations, natural penicillins are still used to treat infections caused by some gram-positive bacteria, especially the streptococci, some anaerobic bacteria, and some spirochetes (Table 5-3). Even a few gram-negative bacteria, such as *Neisseria meningitidis* and some strains of *Haemophilus influenzae* that do not make β-lactamases, remain susceptible to penicillin.

ANTISTAPHYLOCOCCAL PENICILLINS

The antistaphylococcal penicillins (also called the "penicillinase-resistant penicillins") have bulky residues on their R side chains that prevent binding by the staphylococcal β-lactamases (Fig. 5-7). As a result, these penicillins are useful in treating infections caused by *S. aureus* and *Staphylococcus epidermidis*. However, they are unable to bind the PBPs of two special groups of staphylococci called methicillin-resistant *S. aureus* (MRSA) and methicillin-resistant *S. epidermidis* (MRSE).

OC_2H_5

FIGURE 5-7. R side chain of nafcillin.

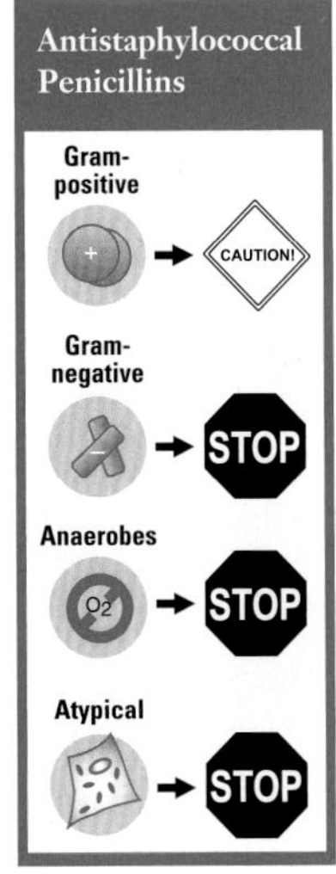

Table 5-4 Antimicrobial Activity of the Antistaphylococcal Penicillins

Gram-positive bacteria	Some *Staphylococcus aureus* Some *Staphylococcus epidermidis*

Because they cannot bind the PBPs of MRSA and MRSE bacteria, antistaphylococcal penicillins are inactive against them. (Note that methicillin is an antistaphylococcal penicillin that is no longer commercially available but is representative of the entire class of antistaphylococcal penicillins in its spectrum of activity.) Antistaphylococcal penicillins are also less effective than natural penicillins against streptococci and are usually not used to treat them. Nor are these penicillins active against enterococci. Likewise, the bulkiness of the side chains limits the ability of these agents to penetrate most other bacteria, and they are generally only used to treat staphylococcal infections (Table 5-4). This group of antibiotics includes **nafcillin**, **oxacillin**, and **dicloxacillin**.

AMINOPENICILLINS

The aminopenicillins, **ampicillin** and **amoxicillin**, have spectra of activity similar to the natural penicillins with one exception: An additional amino group in their side chain increases their hydrophilicity and allows them to pass through the porins in the outer membranes of some enteric gram-negative rods, such *E. coli*, *P. mirabilis*, *S. enterica*, and *Shigella* spp. (Fig. 5-8). This extends the spectra of the aminopenicillins to include these bacteria. Aminopenicillins, however, share the natural penicillins' vulnerability to β-lactamases, and many of the gram-negative bacteria that were initially susceptible to the aminopenicillins are now resistant due to the acquisition of β-lactamase encoding genes (Table 5-5).

$$\text{C}_6\text{H}_5\text{—CH(NH}_2\text{)—}$$

FIGURE 5-8. R side chain of ampicillin.

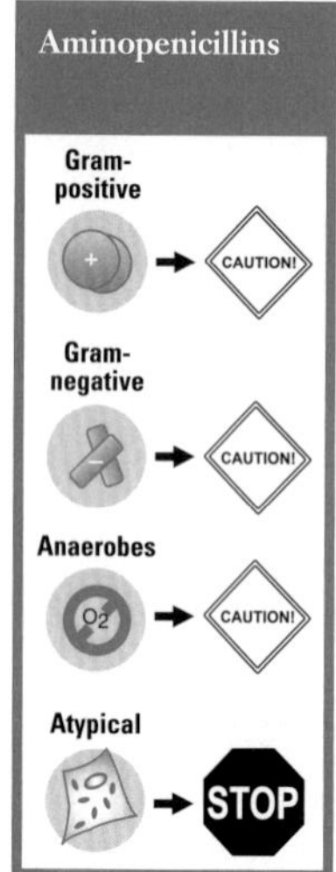

Table 5-5 Antimicrobial Activity of Aminopenicillins

Gram-positive bacteria	*Streptococcus pyogenes* Viridans streptococci Some *Streptococcus pneumoniae* Some enterococci *Listeria monocytogenes*
Gram-negative bacteria	*Neisseria meningitidis* Some *Haemophilus influenzae* Some Enterobacteriaceae
Anaerobic bacteria	*Clostridia* spp. (except *C. difficile*) *Actinomyces israelii*
Spirochetes	*Borrelia burgdorferi*

AMINOPENICILLIN/β-LACTAMASE INHIBITOR COMBINATIONS

Compounds have been developed to inhibit the β-lactamases of many gram-positive and gram-negative bacteria. These inhibitors are structurally similar to penicillin and therefore bind β-lactamases, which results in the inactivation of the β-lactamases. Two of these inhibitors, clavulanate and sulbactam, are used in conjunction with the aminopenicillins to greatly expand their spectra of activity. **Ampicillin-sulbactam** is the parenteral formulation and **amoxicillin-clavulanate** is the oral formulation of these combinations. Sulbactam and clavulanate inactivate the β-lactamases of many gram-positive, gram-negative, and anaerobic bacteria. As a result, they dramatically broaden the antimicrobial spectrum of the aminopenicillins (Table 5-6).

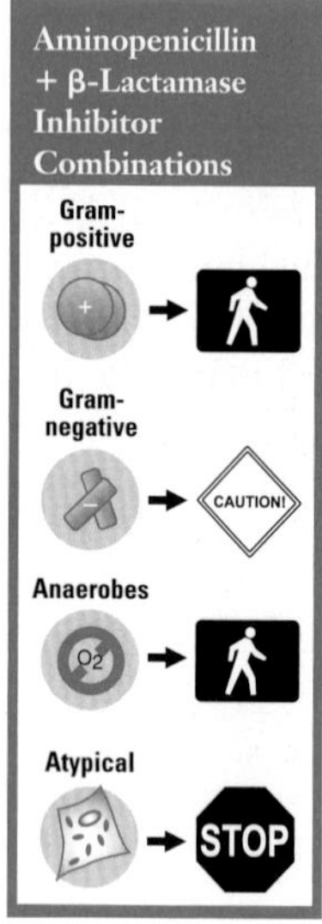

Table 5-6 Antimicrobial Activity of Aminopenicillin + β-Lactamase Inhibitor Combinations

Gram-positive bacteria	Some *Staphylococcus aureus* *Streptococcus pyogenes* Viridans streptococci Some *Streptococcus pneumoniae* Some enterococci *Listeria monocytogenes*
Gram-negative bacteria	*Neisseria* spp. *Haemophilus influenzae* Many Enterobacteriaceae
Anaerobic bacteria	*Clostridia* spp. (except *C. difficile*) *Actinomyces israelii* *Bacteroides* spp.
Spirochetes	*Borrelia burgdorferi*

FIGURE 5-9. R side chain of piperacillin.

EXTENDED-SPECTRUM PENICILLINS

The extended-spectrum penicillins consist of **piperacillin** and **ticarcillin**. The side chains of these agents allow for even greater penetration into gram-negative bacteria than is seen with the aminopenicillins. For example, the side chain of piperacillin is polar, which increases its ability to pass through the outer membrane porins of some gram-negative bacteria (Fig. 5-9). (Incidentally, piperacillin got its name from its side chain, which contains a piperazine derivative.) In addition, the extended-spectrum penicillins are in general more resistant to cleavage by gram-negative β-lactamases than are aminopenicillins, although they remain susceptible to some of these enzymes. Thus, compared to the aminopenicillins, the extended-spectrum penicillins are more active against gram-negative bacilli, including many strains of *P. aeruginosa*. They maintain some of the gram-positive activity of the natural penicillins but, like the natural penicillins, are susceptible to the β-lactamases of staphylococci. They have modest activity against anaerobes (Table 5-7). Piperacillin has broader activity than ticarcillin.

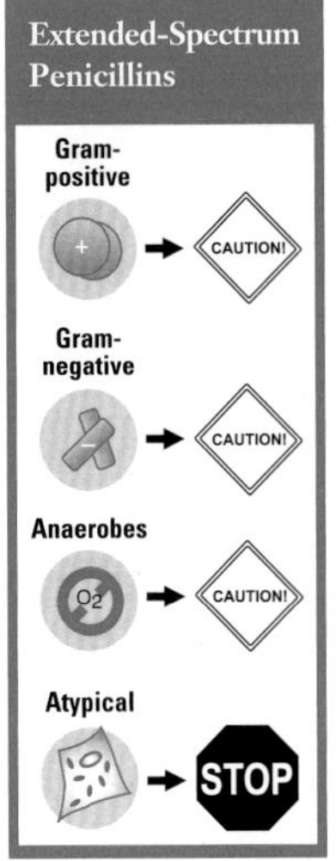

Table 5-7 Antimicrobial Activity of Extended-Spectrum Penicillins

Gram-positive bacteria	*Streptococcus pyogenes* Viridans streptococci Some *Streptococcus pneumoniae* Some enterococci
Gram-negative bacteria	*Neisseria meningitidis* Some *Haemophilus influenzae* Some Enterobacteriaceae *Pseudomonas aeruginosa*
Anaerobic bacteria	*Clostridia* spp. (except *C. difficile*) Some *Bacteroides* spp.

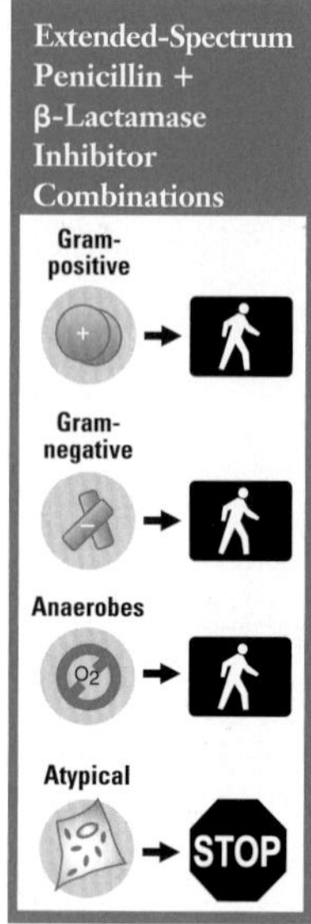

Table 5-8 Antimicrobial Activity of Extended-Spectrum Penicillin + β-Lactamase Inhibitor Combinations

Gram-positive bacteria	Some *Staphylococcus aureus* *Streptococcus pyogenes* Viridans streptococci Some *Streptococcus pneumoniae* Some enterococci *Listeria monocytogenes*
Gram-negative bacteria	*Neisseria* spp. *Haemophilus influenzae* Most Enterobacteriaceae *Pseudomonas aeruginosa*
Anaerobic bacteria	*Clostridia* spp. (except *C. difficile*) *Bacteroides* spp.

EXTENDED-SPECTRUM PENICILLIN/β-LACTAMASE INHIBITOR COMBINATIONS

The fullest antimicrobial potential of the penicillins has been achieved by combining extended-spectrum penicillins with β-lactamase inhibitors. The two available combinations are **piperacillin-tazobactam** and **ticarcillin-clavulanate**. The β-lactamase inhibitors neutralize many of the β-lactamases that otherwise inactivate the extended-spectrum penicillins, resulting in a marked enhancement of their activity. Thus, piperacillin-tazobactam and ticarcillin-clavulanate are the decathletes of the penicillins, with activity against most aerobic gram-positive bacteria, including many β-lactamase–producing staphylococci, most aerobic gram-negative bacteria, and nearly all anaerobic bacteria except *Clostridium difficile* (Table 5-8). As would be expected based on the activity of their penicillin components, piperacillin-tazobactam has a broader spectrum than ticarcillin-clavulanate. Its excellent activity against gram-positive, gram-negative, and anaerobic bacteria makes piperacillin-tazobactam one of the most powerful antibiotics available today.

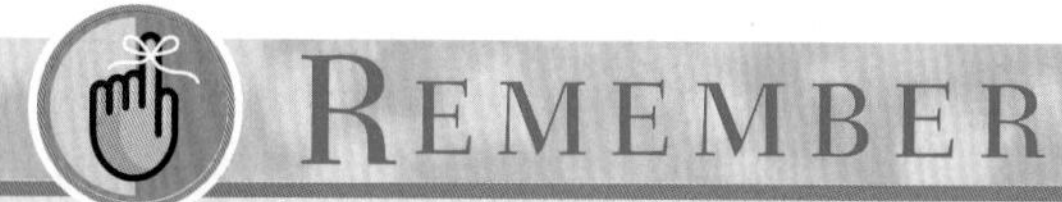

Penicillin G and penicillin V: which is oral and which is parenteral?

The letters in penicillin G and penicillin V can be used to remember how these agents are usually administered. Although not actually true, pretend that the "G" in penicillin G means that this drug is destroyed in the stomach ("gastric") and that the "V" in penicillin V means that this drug is destroyed in "veins." Therefore, penicillin G is given intravenously and penicillin V is given orally.

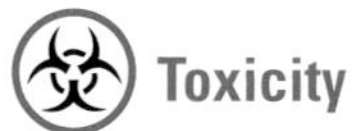

Toxicity

Adverse reactions to the penicillins are relatively common; an estimated 3% to 10% of people are allergic to these agents. Like most antibiotics, penicillins can cause nausea, vomiting, and diarrhea. They also have been associated with drug fever, rash, serum sickness, interstitial nephritis, hepatotoxicity, neurologic toxicity, and hematologic abnormalities. Urticaria, angioedema, and anaphylaxis occur and are referred to as immediate hypersensitivity reactions. Of these, the most feared is anaphylaxis, which is rare but life threatening. Persons allergic to one penicillin should be considered allergic to all penicillins, and cross-allergenicity may extend to other β-lactam antibiotics.

The penicillins vary markedly in their activities, especially against gram-negative bacteria. The activities of these agents against gram-negative bacteria can be summarized as follows: (1) The antistaphylococcal penicillins are inactive against gram-negative bacteria. (2) The natural penicillins have activity against *N. meningitidis* and some strains of *H. influenza*, but few other gram-negative bacteria. (3) The spectrum of the aminopenicillins is expanded to include these organisms plus some enteric gram-negative rods, such as certain strains of *E. coli*, *P. mirabilis*, *S. enterica*, and *Shigella* spp. that do not produce β-lactamases. (4) The extended-spectrum penicillins are active against even more enteric gram-negative rods and, importantly, *P. aeruginosa*. (5) Finally, the addition of a β-lactamase inhibitor to an extended-spectrum penicillin extends this list to include most enteric gram-negative bacilli.

QUESTIONS

5. Penicillins all share the same basic structure, which consists of a thiazolidine ring linked to a ________________ with a modifiable ________________.
6. Penicillins act by binding ________________, which are bacterial enzymes that function to assemble ________________.
7. Natural penicillins have moderate activity against aerobic gram-positive bacteria and anaerobic bacteria but poor activity against aerobic ________________ bacteria and most atypical bacteria.
8. Antistaphylococcal penicillins are useful in treating infections caused by ________________.
9. Compared to natural penicillins, aminopenicillins have improved activity against ________________.
10. Addition of a β-lactamase inhibitor to an aminopenicillin expands the spectra of these agents to include many ________________ as well as additional ________________ and anaerobes.
11. Compared to aminopenicillins, extended-spectrum penicillins have improved activity against aerobic ________________, including ________________.
12. When used in combination with β-lactamase inhibitors, extended-spectrum penicillins are among the most powerful antibacterial agents available today, and are active against most aerobic ________________, aerobic ________________, and ________________.

ADDITIONAL READINGS

Donowitz GR, Mandell GL. Beta-lactam antibiotics (1). *N Engl J Med.* 1988;318:419–426.
Donowitz GR, Mandell GL. Beta-lactam antibiotics (2). *N Engl J Med.* 1988;318:490–500.
Lax E. *The Mold in Dr. Florey's Coat: The Story of the Penicillin Miracle.* New York, NY: Henry Holt and Co.; 2004.
Novak R, Charpentier E, Braun JS, et al. Signal transduction by a death signal peptide: uncovering the mechanism of bacterial killing by penicillin. *Mol Cell.* 2000;5:49–57.
Park MA, Li JT. Diagnosis and management of penicillin allergy. *Mayo Clin Proc.* 2005;80:405–410.
Petri WA Jr. Penicillins, cephalosporins, and other beta-lactam antibiotics. In: Brunton LL, Lazo JS, Parker KL, eds. *Goodman & Gilman's The Pharmacological Basis of Therapeutics.* 10th ed. New York, NY: McGraw-Hill; 2006:1127–1154.
Sanders WE Jr, Sanders CC. Piperacillin/tazobactam: a critical review of the evolving clinical literature. *Clin Infect Dis.* 1996;22:107–123.

Cephalosporins

The cephalosporins received their name from the fungus *Cephalosporium acremonium*, which was the source of the first members of this class. Even more so than penicillins, these agents constitute a large extended family of antibiotics within the β-lactam group. As such, they are appropriately categorized by "generation." Since agents in each generation have somewhat similar spectra of activity, this organizational scheme is helpful in remembering the properties of the many cephalosporins.

Each cephalosporin is composed of a nucleus with two side chains (Fig. 5-10). The nucleus is 7-aminocephalosporanic acid, which is similar to the nucleus of penicillin except that the β-lactam ring is fused to a six-member dihydrothiazine ring instead of a five-member thiazolidine ring (compare Fig. 5-10 to Fig. 5-5). The cephalosporin core has two major advantages over the penicillin core: (1) It is intrinsically more resistant to cleavage by β-lactamases and (2) it has two sites, R1 and R2, at which it can be modified. This in part explains the large number of cephalosporins commercially available today.

Like other β-lactam antibiotics, the cephalosporins exert their effects by attaching to and inhibiting PBPs, thereby preventing the appropriate synthesis of peptidoglycan.

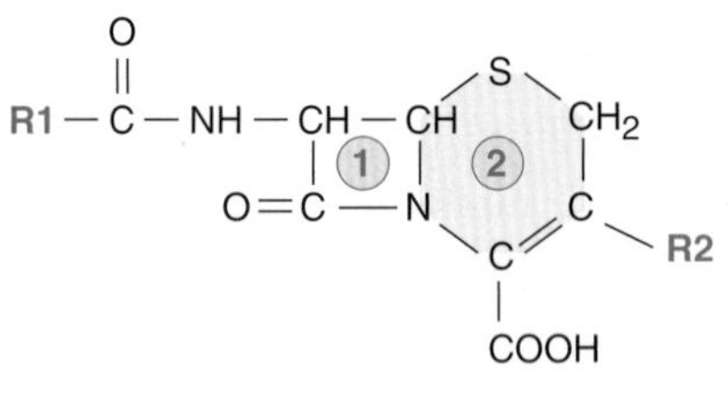

(1) β-lactam ring
(2) Dihydrothiazine ring
R1 Side chain of the β-lactam ring
R2 Side chain of the dihydrothiazine ring

FIGURE 5-10. The structure of cephalosporins.

Although peptidoglycan is a constituent of most bacteria, cephalosporins are not active against certain species and strains of bacteria. As was the case for penicillins, the six **P**s explain resistance to cephalosporins: (1) **P**enetration—cephalosporins, like most β-lactams, penetrate poorly into the intracellular compartment of human cells, so bacteria that for the most part reside in this compartment, such as *Rickettsia* and *Legionella*, are protected from them. (2) **P**orins—some gram-negative bacteria, such as *P. aeruginosa*, have porins in their outer membranes that do not allow passage of many cephalosporins into the periplasmic space. (3) **P**umps—some bacteria, such as *P. aeruginosa*, use efflux pumps to remove antibiotics from the periplasmic space. (4) **P**enicillinases (actually β-lactamases)—many gram-negative bacteria, such as *Enterobacter* and *Citrobacter* spp., make β-lactamases that degrade many cephalosporins. (5) **P**BPs—some bacteria, such as the enterococci and *Listeria monocytogenes*, produce PBPs that do not bind most cephalosporins with a high affinity. (6) **P**eptidoglycan—some bacteria such as *Mycoplasma* and *Chlamydia* do not make peptidoglycan and therefore are not affected by the cephalosporins.

Several generalizations about the spectra of activity of cephalosporins can be made. First, with the exception of the new fifth-generation agents, each successive generation of agents has broader activity against aerobic gram-negative bacteria. Second, also with several important exceptions, cephalosporins have limited activity against anaerobes. Third, the activities of these agents against aerobic gram-positive bacteria are variable, with the fifth-generation agent ceftaroline having the strongest activity against these bacteria.

FIRST-GENERATION CEPHALOSPORINS

Commonly used first-generation cephalosporins include **cefadroxil** and **cefazolin** (Table 5-9). All agents in this group share similar activities against the different types of bacteria.

The strength of the first-generation cephalosporins is their activity against aerobic gram-positive cocci such as staphylococci and streptococci (Table 5-10). The R1 side chains of these agents protect their β-lactam rings from cleavage by the

Table 5-9 The Cephalosporins

Generation	Parenteral Agents	Oral Agents
First generation	Cefazolin	Cefadroxil, cephalexin
Second generation	Cefotetan,* cefoxitin,* cefuroxime	Cefaclor, cefprozil, cefuroxime axetil, loracarbef
Third generation	Cefotaxime, ceftazidime, ceftriaxone	Cefdinir, cefditoren, cefpodoxime proxetil, ceftibuten, cefixime
Fourth generation	Cefepime	
Fifth generation	Ceftaroline	

*Cephamycins

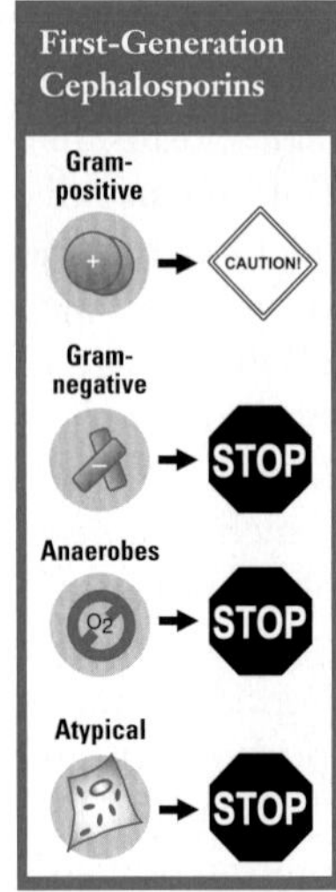

Table 5-10 Antimicrobial Activity of First-Generation Cephalosporins

Gram-positive bacteria	*Streptococcus pyogenes* Some viridans streptococci Some *Staphylococcus aureus* Some *Streptococcus pneumoniae*
Gram-negative bacteria	Some *Escherichia coli* Some *Klebsiella pneumoniae* Some *Proteus mirabilis*

staphylococcal β-lactamase (Fig. 5-11). As a result, they are useful in the treatment of infections caused by many strains of *Staphylococcus aureus*. First-generation cephalosporins cannot bind the PBPs of MRSA and MRSE or many highly penicillin-resistant *Streptococcus pneumoniae*; these agents are ineffective against these bacteria. As mentioned previously, most cephalosporins also lack activity against *L. monocytogenes* and the enterococci.

First-generation cephalosporins have limited activity against aerobic and facultative gram-negative bacteria, primarily because the side chains of these agents, although capable of protecting the β-lactam ring from cleavage by staphylococcal β-lactamases, do not afford protection from the β-lactamases of most gram-negative bacteria. Nonetheless, some strains of *E. coli*, *Klebsiella pneumoniae*, and *P. mirabilis* are susceptible.

First-generation cephalosporins have moderate to poor activity against anaerobes, intracellular bacteria, and spirochetes.

SECOND-GENERATION CEPHALOSPORINS

Second-generation cephalosporins are divided into two groups: the true cephalosporins, such as **cefuroxime**, and the cephamycins, which include **cefotetan** and **cefoxitin** (see Table 5-9). The cephamycins are derivatives of a parent compound originally isolated from the bacterium *Streptomyces lactamdurans* instead of the fungus *C. acremonium*.

N=CH N—CH$_2$ N=N R1 N—N C C CH$_2$S S CH$_3$ R2

FIGURE 5-11. Structure of cefazolin.

FIGURE 5-12. Structure of cefotetan. The methoxy group characteristic of the cephamycins is circled.

They have a methoxy group in place of the hydrogen on the β-lactam ring of the cephalosporin core (Fig. 5-12). Thus, these agents are not actually cephalosporins but are included in this group because they are chemically and pharmacologically similar.

Individual second-generation cephalosporins differ in their activity against aerobic gram-positive bacteria (Table 5-11). The true cephalosporins are in general as active against aerobic gram-positive cocci as the first-generation agents. The cephamycins (cefotetan and cefoxitin) have relatively limited activity against this group of bacteria. The strength of the second-generation agents is their increased activity against aerobic and facultative gram-negative bacteria. Second-generation agents are more potent against *E. coli*, *K. pneumoniae*, and *P. mirabilis* than first-generation agents and are also active against *Neisseria* spp. and, in the case of the true cephalosporins, *H. influenzae* (including β-lactamase-producing strains). Because of the additional methoxy group on the β-lactam ring (Fig. 5-12), the cephamycins also have enhanced stability to the β-lactamases of some anaerobes, such as *B. fragilis*. However, this added anaerobic activity comes at a cost; it is the methoxy group that results in the diminished activity of the cephamycins against staphylococci and streptococci because of decreased affinity for the PBPs of these bacteria.

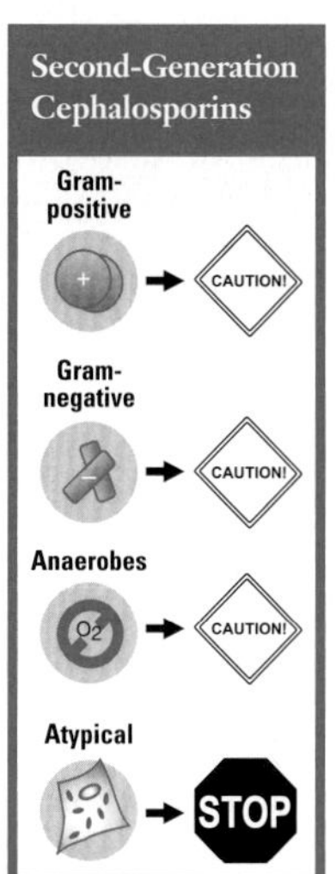

Table 5-11 Antimicrobial Activity of Second-Generation Cephalosporins

Gram-positive bacteria	True cephalosporins have activity equivalent to first-generation agents Cefoxitin and cefotetan have little activity
Gram-negative bacteria	*Escherichia coli* *Klebsiella pneumoniae* *Proteus mirabilis* *Haemophilus influenzae* *Neisseria* spp.
Anaerobic bacteria	Cefoxitin and cefotetan have moderate anaerobic activity

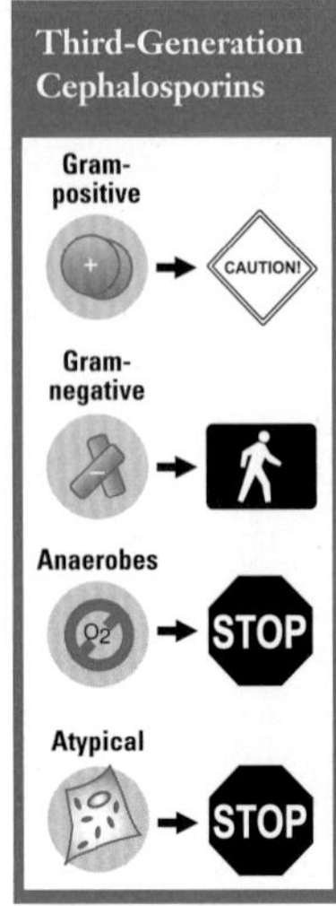

Table 5-12 Antimicrobial Activity of Third-Generation Cephalosporins

Gram-positive bacteria	*Streptococcus pyogenes* Viridans streptococci Many *Streptococcus pneumoniae* Modest activity against *Staphylococcus aureus*
Gram-negative bacteria	*Escherichia coli* *Klebsiella pneumoniae* *Proteus* spp. *Haemophilus influenzae* *Neisseria* spp. Some Enterobacteriaceae
Spirochetes	*Borrelia burgdorferi*

THIRD-GENERATION CEPHALOSPORINS

Commonly used third-generation cephalosporins include **ceftriaxone**, **cefotaxime**, and **ceftazidime** (see Table 5-9). In general, compounds in this group have moderate activity against aerobic gram-positive bacteria (Table 5-12) and inhibit most strains of penicillin-susceptible *S. pneumoniae*. Third-generation cephalosporins are also active against the spirochete *Borrelia burgdorferi* but have little activity against anaerobic bacteria.

A modification common to many of the third-generation cephalosporins is the use of an aminothiazolyl group at R1 (Fig. 5-13). The presence of this structure at R1 results in increased penetration of these agents through the bacterial outer membrane, increased affinity for PBPs, and increased stability in the presence of some of the plasmid-encoded β-lactamases of aerobic and facultative gram-negative bacteria. Thus, these agents have enhanced activity against *E. coli*, *Klebsiella* spp., *Proteus* spp., *Neisseria* spp., and *H. influenzae* relative to the second-generation cephalosporins. In addition, many other strains of the Enterobacteriaceae, including *Enterobacter* spp., *Citrobacter freundii*, *Providencia* spp., *Morganella morganii*, and *Serratia* spp., also initially show susceptibility to third-generation cephalosporins. However, these bacteria

FIGURE 5-13. Structure of cefotaxime. The aminothiazolyl group at R1 is typical of many third-generation cephalosporins.

harbor chromosomally encoded inducible AmpC β-lactamases that may allow the emergence of resistance during treatment. Thus, it is now felt that infections caused by these organisms should either not be treated with third-generation cephalosporins or should be treated with these agents in conjunction with a second active agent, even if they appear to be susceptible by in vitro testing.

One shortcoming of most of the third-generation cephalosporins is their lack of activity against *P. aeruginosa*. To address this, the aminothiazolyl R1 side chain of ceftazidime was modified by the addition of a carboxypropyl group, which dramatically increases antipseudomonal activity. Unfortunately, this modification also results in decreased affinity for the PBPs of staphylococci. As a result, ceftazidime has enhanced activity against *P. aeruginosa* but limited activity against *S. aureus*.

Among the third-generation cephalosporins, ceftriaxone is notable for its long half-life. This agent is widely used because of the convenience of its once per day dosing.

FOURTH-GENERATION CEPHALOSPORINS

As mentioned earlier, the third-generation cephalosporins are powerful antimicrobial agents but suffer from susceptibility to the chromosomally encoded inducible AmpC β-lactamases of many of the Enterobacteriaceae. In addition, activity against *P. aeruginosa* is gained only at the expense of diminished antistaphylococcal activity. Attempts to address these deficiencies led to modifications of the R2 side chain of the third-generation cephalosporins while leaving the highly successful aminothiazolyl group at R1 unchanged (Fig. 5-14). The result of these efforts was the fourth-generation cephalosporin **cefepime**. The side chains of cefepime allow more rapid penetration through the outer membrane of many gram-negative bacteria, including *P. aeruginosa*. It also binds at a high affinity to many of the PBPs of these bacteria but is relatively resistant to hydrolysis by gram-negative β-lactamases, including the chromosomally encoded inducible AmpC β-lactamases of the Enterobacteriaceae (although the clinical relevance of this is controversial). These properties are attained without the loss of activity against aerobic gram-positive cocci. Thus, this incredibly powerful antibiotic has the best features of the various third-generation cephalosporins (antipseudomonal activity without loss of antistaphylococcal activity) and may also have enhanced activity against many of the Enterobacteriaceae. Cefepime has very limited anaerobic activity (Table 5-13).

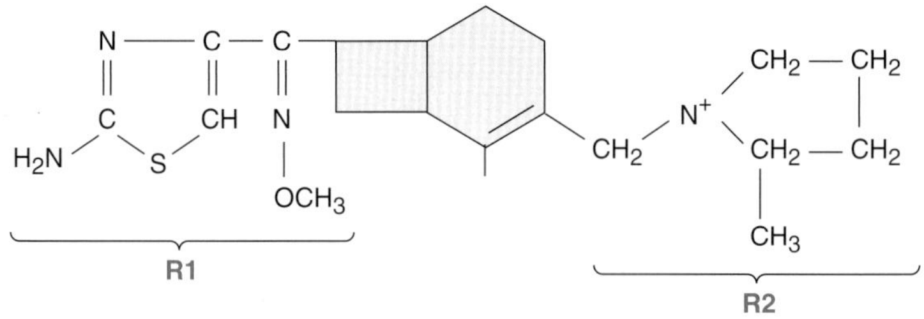

FIGURE 5-14. Structure of cefepime. The aminothiazolyl group typical of many third-generation cephalosporins is at R1, whereas a polar pyrrolidine group is at R2.

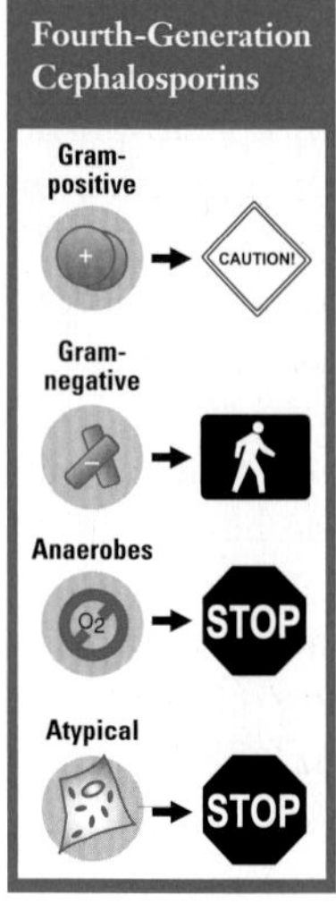

Table 5-13 Antimicrobial Activity of Fourth-Generation Cephalosporins

Gram-positive bacteria	*Streptococcus pyogenes* Viridans streptococci Many *Streptococcus pneumoniae* Modest activity against *Staphylococcus aureus*
Gram-negative bacteria	*Escherichia coli* *Klebsiella pneumoniae* *Proteus* spp. *Haemophilus influenzae* *Neisseria* spp. Many other Enterobacteriaceae *Pseudomonas aeruginosa*

FIFTH-GENERATION CEPHALOSPORINS

Ceftaroline is a new cephalosporin that has expanded activity against aerobic gram-positive cocci, causing some experts to refer to it as a fifth-generation agent. A 1,3-thiazole ring has been added to the R2 side chain of this cephalosporin, which confers upon it the ability to bind to the PBP of methicillin-resistant staphylococci (Fig. 5-15). As a result, ceftaroline has excellent activity against aerobic gram-positive cocci, including methicillin-resistant *Staphylococcus aureus* and *Staphylococcus epidermidis* and penicillin-resistant *Streptococcus pneumoniae* strains (Table 5-14). Its activities against aerobic gram-negative bacteria are similar to that of cefotaxime and ceftriaxone; it lacks antipseudomonal activity. Ceftaroline also has activity against anaerobic gram-positive bacteria but not against anaerobic gram-negative bacteria. This agent is administered as the inactive prodrug ceftaroline fosamil, which is rapidly converted to ceftaroline.

FIGURE 5-15. Structure of ceftaroline. The circled 1,3-thiazole ring in the R-2 side chain confers activity against methicillin-resistant *Staphylococcus aureus* strains.

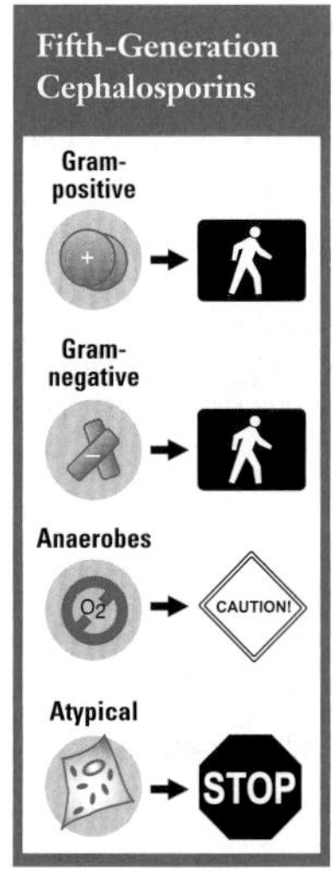

Table 5-14 Antimicrobial Activity of Fifth-Generation Cephalosporins

Gram-positive bacteria	*Streptococcus pyogenes* Viridans streptococci *Streptococcus pneumoniae* Staphylococci
Gram-negative bacteria	*Escherichia coli* *Klebsiella pneumoniae* *Proteus* spp. *Haemophilus influenzae* *Neisseria* spp. Some Enterobacteriaceae
Anaerobic bacteria	Some *Clostridium* spp.

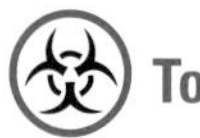

Toxicity

One of the attractions of the cephalosporins is their relatively favorable safety profile. Rarely, these agents cause immediate hypersensitivity reactions consisting of rash, urticaria, or anaphylaxis. In this regard, approximately 5% to 10% of individuals allergic to penicillin will also have a reaction to cephalosporins. Thus, it is usually recommended that individuals with a history of severe immediate hypersensitivity reactions, such as urticaria and anaphylaxis, to penicillin not be treated with cephalosporins. Other rare adverse effects include reversible neutropenia, thrombocytosis, hemolysis, diarrhea, and elevated liver function tests. Cefotetan may cause hypoprothrombinemia and, when used with alcohol, a disulfiram-like reaction. Both of these effects are associated with the methylthiotetrazole moiety at R2 of this agent (see Fig. 5-12). Since ceftriaxone is eliminated by biliary excretion, high doses of this agent may result in biliary sludging.

History

Cephalosporins were discovered by the Italian scientist Giuseppe Brotzu in the 1940s. He noted that the seawater in the vicinity of a sewage outlet in Cagliari, Italy, periodically cleared, a phenomenon he suspected was due to the production of an inhibitory compound by a microbe growing in the water. He eventually identified the microbe as *Cephalosporium acremonium* and showed that it did indeed produce a substance that inhibited bacterial growth. This substance became the backbone from which early cephalosporins were synthesized.

Abraham EP. Cephalosporins 1945–1986. In: Williams JD, ed. *The Cephalosporin Antibiotics.* Auckland, New Zealand: Adis Press; 1987.

In summary, the cephalosporins vary markedly in their activities, but the following generalizations can be made: (1) First-generation agents have good activity against aerobic gram-positive bacteria. (2) Second-generation agents have modest activity against aerobic gram-positive, aerobic gram-negative, and (in some cases) anaerobic bacteria. (3) Third-generation agents have strong activity against aerobic gram-negative bacteria. (4) Fourth-generation agents have especially enhanced activity against aerobic gram-negative bacteria. (5) Fifth-generation agents have strong activity against aerobic gram-negative bacteria and excellent activity against aerobic gram-positive bacteria.

QUESTIONS

13. Cephalosporins are grouped into ________________ and are all part of the larger class of antibiotics known as ________________.

14. Like penicillins, cephalosporins act by binding ________________, which are bacterial enzymes that function to assemble peptidoglycan.

15. First-generation cephalosporins are most useful in the treatment of infections caused by aerobic ________________ bacteria.

16. Compared to first-generation agents, second-generation cephalosporins have enhanced activity against aerobic ________________ bacteria. Some of these agents are also active against ________________ bacteria.

17. Third-generation cephalosporins are most useful in the treatment of infections caused by aerobic ________________ bacteria.

18. Compared to third-generation agents, fourth-generation cephalosporins have a broader spectrum of activity against aerobic gram-negative bacteria, including ________________ and additional members of the ________________.

19. Unlike other cephalosporins, fifth-generation cephalosporins have activity against ________________ *S. aureus* strains.

20. Use of high doses of ________________ has been associated with biliary sludging.

21. Cephalosporins should be used with caution in individuals with severe immediate hypersensitivity reactions to ________________.

ADDITIONAL READINGS

Allan JD Jr, Eliopoulos GM, Moellering RC Jr. Antibiotics: future directions by understanding structure-function relationships. In: Root RK, Trunkey DD, Sande MA, eds. *New Surgical and Medical Approaches in Infectious Diseases*. Vol. 6. New York, NY: Churchill Livingstone; 1987: 262–284.

Endimiani A, Perez F, Bonomo RA. Cefepime: a reappraisal in an era of increasing antimicrobial resistance. *Expert Rev Anti Infect Ther*. 2008;6:805–824.

Petri WA Jr. Penicillins, cephalosporins, and other beta-lactam antibiotics. In: Brunton LL, Lazo JS, Parker KL, eds. *Goodman and Gilman's The Pharmacological Basis of Therapeutics*. 11th ed. New York, NY: McGraw-Hill; 2006:1127–1154.

Prober CG. Cephalosporins: an update. *Pediatr Rev*. 1998;19:118–127.

Zhanel GG, Sniezek G, Schweizer F, et al. Ceftaroline: a novel broad-spectrum cephalosporin with activity against meticillin-resistant Staphylococcus aureus. *Drugs*. 2009;69:809–831.

Carbapenems

If β-lactams are viewed as a large extended family of antibiotics, then carbapenems are the arrogant young sons who drive a high-powered sports car and wear flashy clothes. These antibiotics are among the most broadly active antibiotics in use today. As such, they are often the last line of defense against many organisms that are resistant to other antimicrobial agents. Four members of this class, **imipenem**, **meropenem**, **doripenem**, and **ertapenem**, are commercially available (Table 5-15).

The structure of carbapenems is related to that of penicillins and cephalosporins (Fig. 5-16). A β-lactam ring is fused to a five-membered ring with variable side chains. The five-membered ring differs from the thiazolidine ring of penicillin in two ways (see circles in Fig. 5-16): A methylene group replaces sulfur, and the ring contains a double bond.

The structure of the carbapenems results in three properties that account for their incredibly broad spectra of activity. First, these molecules are quite small and have charge characteristics that allow them to utilize special porins in the outer membrane of gram-negative bacteria to gain access to the PBPs. Second, the structures of the carbapenems make them resistant to cleavage by most β-lactamases. Third, the carbapenems have an affinity for a broad range of PBPs from many different kinds of bacteria. As a result of these three properties, the carbapenems are adept at gaining access to the periplasm, resisting destruction by β-lactamases that reside there, and binding to PBPs to cause bacterial cell death.

Resistance to carbapenems occurs when bacteria overcome the advantageous aspects of these antibiotics. For example, *P. aeruginosa* is prone to develop resistance by acquiring mutations that result in loss of production of the outer membrane porin used by carbapenems to gain access to the periplasm. This often occurs together with overproduction of efflux pumps that limit accumulation of the drugs in the periplasmic space. *Enterococcus faecium* and methicillin-resistant staphylococci are resistant because they produce altered PBPs that do not bind these carbapenems. Finally, some bacteria have acquired the ability to produce extremely powerful β-lactamases that are capable of cleaving carbapenems.

IMIPENEM

Imipenem was the first commercially available carbapenem in the United States. Structurally, this compound differs from the other carbapenems in that it lacks an R1

Table 5-15 The Carbapenems

Parenteral Agents	Oral Agents
Imipenem/cilastatin	None
Meropenem	
Doripenem	
Ertapenem	

FIGURE 5-16. The structure of carbapenems. Circles indicate differences from the penicillin core structure.

side chain (Fig. 5-16). It is rapidly destroyed in the kidney by an enzyme called dehydropeptidase I. As a result, it is administered with cilastatin, an inhibitor of this enzyme.

Imipenem is active against many species of pathogenic bacteria (Table 5-16). Most streptococci, including many penicillin-resistant *S. pneumoniae* strains, are sensitive to this agent, as are many staphylococci (but not the "methicillin-resistant" staphylococci). Imipenem has truly remarkable activity against many different aerobic gram-negative bacteria, including *P. aeruginosa* and many of the highly resistant Enterobacteriaceae, such as *Enterobacter* and *Citrobacter* species. It also has excellent anaerobic coverage and is among the most useful agents in treating infections caused by these organisms. Like most antibiotics, however, it is not active against *C. difficile*.

MEROPENEM

The structure of meropenem differs from that of imipenem at both the R1 and R2 side chains (Fig. 5-16). Importantly, whereas imipenem lacks an R1 side chain, meropenem has a methyl group at this position, which makes the molecule resistant to cleavage by

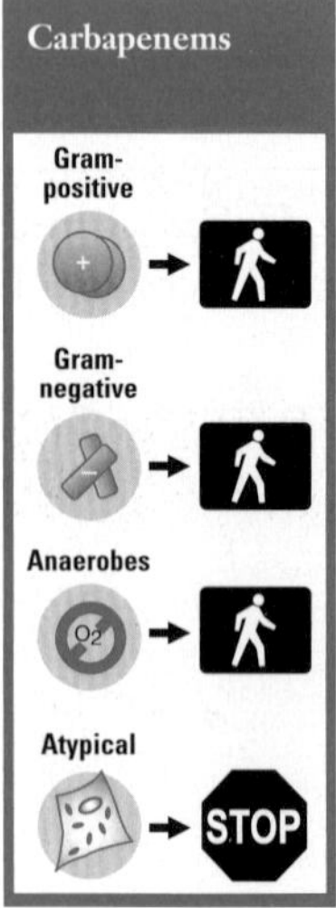

Table 5-16 Antimicrobial Activity of Carbapenems

Gram-positive bacteria	*Streptococcus pyogenes* Viridans group streptococci *Streptococcus pneumoniae* Modest activity against *Staphylococcus aureus* Some enterococci *Listeria monocytogenes*
Gram-negative bacteria	*Haemophilus influenzae* *Neisseria* spp. Enterobacteriaceae *Pseudomonas aeruginosa*
Anaerobic bacteria	*Bacteroides fragilis* Most other anaerobes

the renal dehydropeptidase. As a result, meropenem does not need to be administered in conjunction with cilastatin.

Meropenem's spectrum of activity is essentially the same as imipenem. Thus, this agent also has excellent activity against aerobic gram-positive, aerobic gram-negative, and anaerobic bacteria.

DORIPENEM

Doripenem is a recently approved carbapenem. Like meropenem, it has a methyl group at R1 (see Fig. 5-16) and is not cleaved by renal dehydropeptidase. It differs from the other carbapenems at its R2 side chain, but in general is similar to imipenem and meropenem in its spectrum of activity. In vitro evidence suggests that doripenem is associated with a lower rate of emergence of resistance in *P. aeruginosa* than the other carbapenems, although the clinical significance of this finding remains unclear.

ERTAPENEM

Ertapenem also has a methyl group at R1 (see Fig. 5-16) and therefore is not cleaved by renal dehydropeptidase. It differs from imipenem, meropenem, and doripenem at its R2 side chain, which accounts for its somewhat distinctive antimicrobial and pharmacologic properties; it is less active against aerobic gram-positive bacteria, *P. aeruginosa*, and *Acinetobacter* spp. than the other carbapenems. Ertapenem compensates for this weakness by requiring only once per day dosing.

Toxicity

Carbapenem use is associated with several adverse events, including nausea and vomiting, diarrhea, rash, and drug fever. A more worrisome complication associated with carbapenems is seizures. Patients with preexisting central nervous system disease and with renal insufficiency are most at risk for this complication and should be given these drugs with caution. Initially, meropenem was felt to be less likely to cause seizures than imipenem, but this is now controversial. Results of animal experiments suggest that doripenem is less likely to cause seizures than the other carbapenems.

In summary, carbapenems have excellent activity against a broad spectrum of bacteria, including many aerobic gram-positive bacteria, most aerobic gram-negative bacteria, and most anaerobes. As a result, these compounds are among the most powerful antibacterial agents in use today.

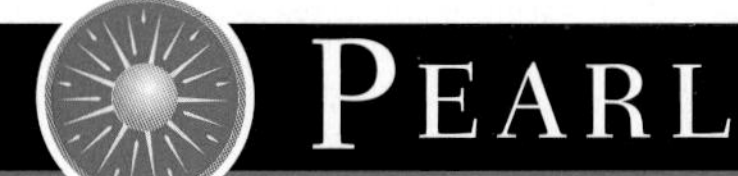

Strains of *Enterococcus faecalis* that are susceptible to penicillin are also susceptible to carbapenems (except ertapenem). *Enterococcus faecium*, however, is resistant to all carbapenems.

Edwards JR. Meropenem: a microbiological overview. *J Antimicrob Chemother.* 1995;36(suppl A):1–17.

QUESTIONS

22. Imipenem is hydrolyzed by dehydropeptidase I in the kidney and therefore must be given with ________________.

23. Carbapenems have excellent aerobic ________________, aerobic ________________, and ________________ activity.

24. Compared to other carbapenems, ertapenem is less active against aerobic gram-positive bacteria, ________________, and ________________.

ADDITIONAL READINGS

Birnbaum J, Kahan FM, Kropp H, et al. Carbapenems, a new class of beta-lactam antibiotics. Discovery and development of imipenem/cilastatin. *Am J Med.* 1985;78:3–21.

Giske CG, Buarø L, Sundsfjord A, et al. Alterations of porin, pumps, and penicillin-binding proteins in carbapenem resistant clinical isolates of Pseudomonas aeruginosa. *Microb Drug Resist.* 2008;14:23–30.

Nicolau DP. Carbapenems: a potent class of antibiotics. *Expert Opin Pharmacother.* 2008;9:23–37.

Paterson DL, Depestel DD. Doripenem. *Clin Infect Dis.* 2009;49:291–298.

Zhanel GG, Johanson C, Embil JM, et al. Ertapenem: review of a new carbapenem. *Expert Rev Anti Infect Ther.* 2005;3:23–39.

Monobactams

Many of the newer β-lactam antibiotics have extremely broad spectra of activity, but the monobactams go against this trend. **Aztreonam**, the only commercially available monobactam, does only one thing but does it quite well: It kills aerobic gram-negative bacteria. It is available for parenteral use only.

The term *monobactam* has been used to describe several bacterially derived antibiotics that consist of a lone β-lactam ring as opposed to the linked two-ring structures of the penicillins, cephalosporins, and carbapenems (Fig. 5-17). Aztreonam is a totally synthetic monobactam that combines some of the useful features of other β-lactam antibiotics.

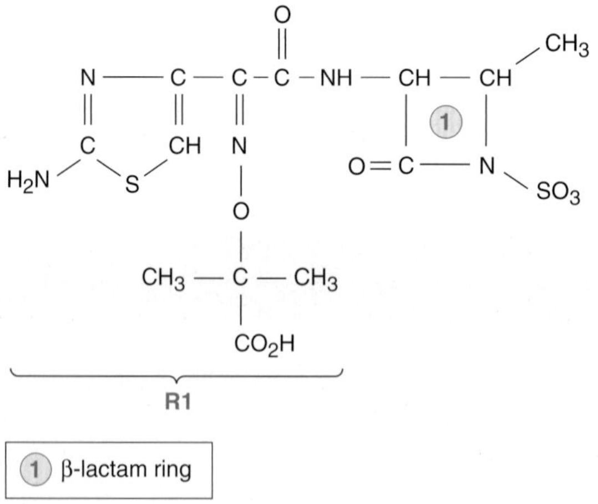

FIGURE 5-17. The structure of aztreonam. The R1 side chain is similar to that of ceftazidime.

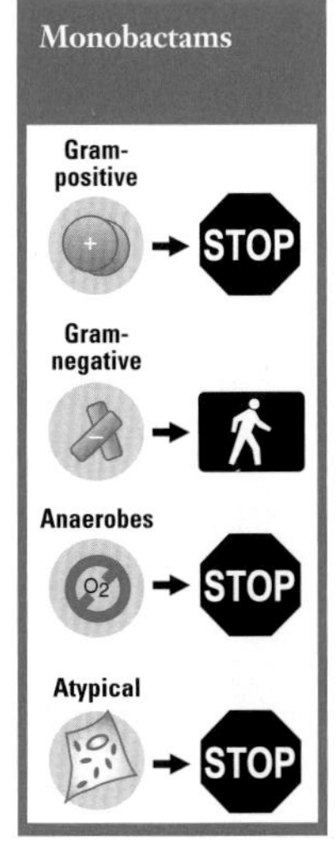

Table 5-17	Antimicrobial Activity of Monobactams
Gram-negative bacteria	*Haemophilus influenzae* *Neisseria* spp. Most Enterobacteriaceae Many *Pseudomonas aeruginosa*

For example, one of the side chains of aztreonam incorporates the aminothiazolyl group that dramatically improves the aerobic gram-negative coverage of third-generation cephalosporins (compare Fig. 5-17 with Fig. 5-13 in the "Cephalosporins" discussion).

As a result of its designer structural properties, aztreonam gains access to and binds quite well to the PBPs of aerobic gram-negative bacteria and is stable against many of the β-lactamases produced by these organisms (Table 5-17). It has excellent activity against *Neisseria* and *Haemophilus* spp. and intermediate activity against *P. aeruginosa*. Unfortunately, it does not bind the PBPs of gram-positive or anaerobic bacteria and therefore is not useful for infections caused by these organisms.

Resistance to aztreonam does occur in some members of the Enterobacteriaceae and *P. aeruginosa*, usually as the result of changes in the permeability of the outer membrane of these bacteria or of destruction by β-lactamases.

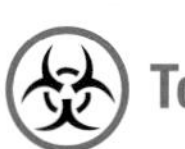

Toxicity

One of the major advantages of aztreonam is its safety profile. It is not associated with nephrotoxicity and can be viewed as a renal-sparing alternative to the aminoglycosides, since both agents have activity against aerobic gram-negative bacteria. Importantly, there are no allergic cross-reactions between aztreonam and other β-lactams, so aztreonam is safe to use in patients with penicillin allergies.

In summary, aztreonam, the only commercially available monobactam, has excellent activity against aerobic gram-negative bacteria but is not useful against gram-positive or anaerobic bacteria. It is a relatively safe drug and can be used in individuals with allergies to other β-lactam agents.

Questions

25. ________________ is the only commercially available monobactam.

26. Aztreonam has excellent activity against aerobic ________________ bacteria but lacks activity against aerobic ________________ bacteria and ________________ bacteria.

27. A particularly useful feature of aztreonam is that it can be used in patients with allergies to other ________________ antibiotics.

ADDITIONAL READINGS

Asbel LE, Levison ME. Cephalosporins, carbapenems, and monobactams. *Infect Dis Clin North Am*. 2000;14:435–447.

Sykes RB, Bonner DP. Aztreonam: the first monobactam. *Am J Med*. 1985;78:2–10.

Sykes RB, Bonner DP. Discovery and development of the monobactams. *Rev Infect Dis*. 1985; 7(suppl 4):S579–S593.

Glycopeptides

Glycopeptide antibiotics are peptides with sugar moieties attached to them. **Vancomycin and telavancin** are two members of this group. Intact glycopeptides are poorly absorbed in the gastrointestinal tract, so these agents must be given intravenously to treat systemic infections. Relative to other antibiotics, they are extremely large (Fig. 5-18), which prevents them from passing through porins in the outer membranes of gram-negative bacteria. Thus, their activity is restricted to gram-positive organisms (Table 5-18). Within this group, though, their coverage is impressive. Vancomycin and telavancin are active against nearly all staphylococci and streptococci, including methicillin-resistant staphylococci and strains of penicillin-resistant *S. pneumoniae*. Susceptibility among enterococci is now variable. Although *L. monocytogenes* usually appears susceptible in vitro, clinical failures have been reported with vancomycin, and these agents should not be used to

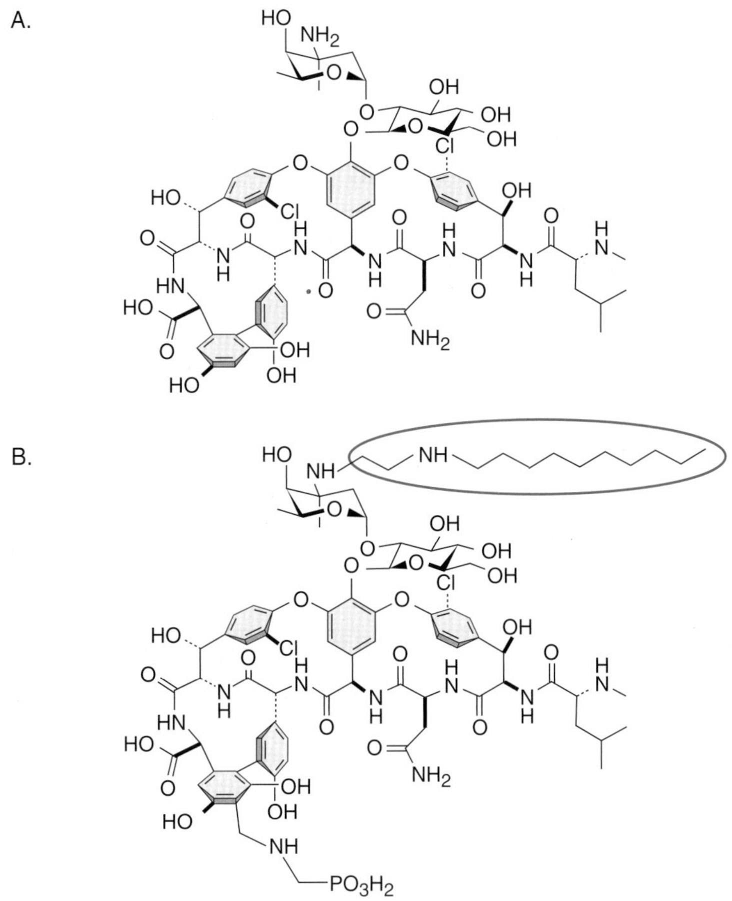

FIGURE 5-18. The structure of glycopeptides. **A.** Vancomycin. **B.** Telavancin. The lipophilic decylaminoethyl side chain of telavancin is circled.

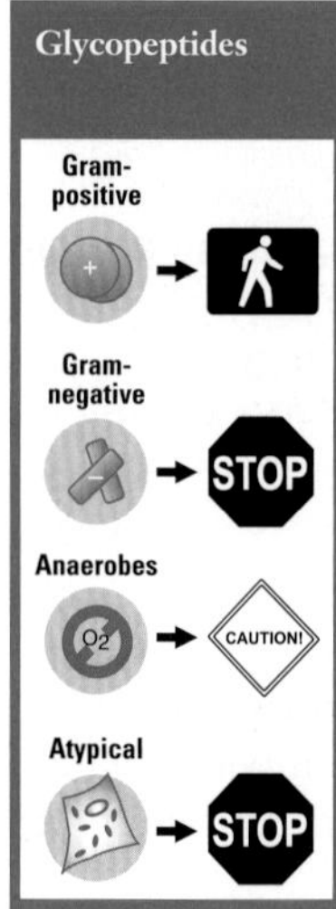

Table 5-18 Antimicrobial Activity of Glycopeptides

Gram-positive bacteria	*Staphylococcus aureus* *Staphylococcus epidermidis* *Streptococcus pyogenes* Viridans group streptococci *Streptococcus pneumoniae* Some enterococci
Anaerobic bacteria	*Clostridium* spp. Other gram-positive anaerobes

treat infections caused by this organism. Glycopeptides also have good activity against anaerobic gram-positive bacteria, including *C. difficile*.

Like the β-lactams, glycopeptides kill bacteria by preventing synthesis of the cell wall. They bind to the D-alanyl–D-alanine portion of the peptide side chain of precursor peptidoglycan subunits. Because of the bulk of the large glycopeptide molecule, this binding prevents these subunits from being accessed by the PBPs that would normally incorporate them into the growing peptidoglycan polymer (Fig. 5-19A).

Some enterococci have developed an ingenious way of resisting glycopeptides. These bacteria encode genes that modify the structure of the peptidoglycan precursor such that the D-alanyl–D-alanine dipeptide is changed, most often to D-alanyl–D-lactate (Fig. 5-19B). Glycopeptides are no longer able to recognize and bind to these altered precursors. Unfortunately, the gene clusters that encode this activity in enterococci are transferable and have already been found in *S. aureus*. Thus, it is anticipated that glycopeptide resistance will occur with increasing frequency in staphylococci as well.

HISTORY

Vancomycin was discovered when a missionary from Borneo sent a soil sample to his friend who was an organic chemist at Eli Lilly and Company. The soil sample turned out to harbor a bacterium that made a compound with potent activity against gram-positive bacteria. Eventually the compound was purified and named vancomycin, which is derived from the word "vanquish."

Griffith RS. Vancomycin use—an historical review. *J Antimicrob Chemother.* 1984;14(suppl D):1–5.

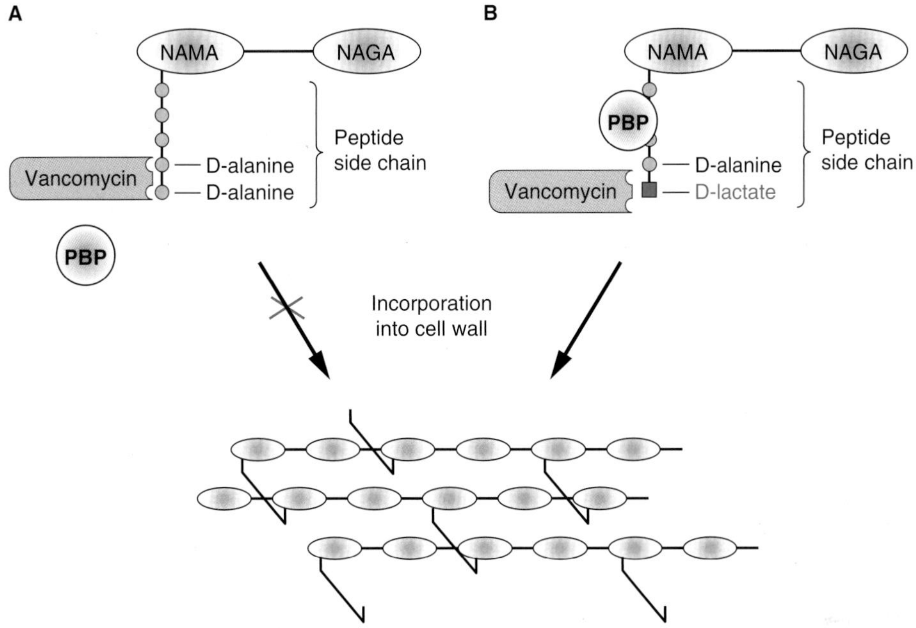

FIGURE 5-19. **A.** Vancomycin binds to the D-alanyl–D-alanine dipeptide on the peptide side chain of newly synthesized peptidoglycan subunits, preventing them from being incorporated into the cell wall by penicillin-binding proteins (PBPs). **B.** In many vancomycin-resistant strains of enterococci, the D-alanyl–D-alanine dipeptide is replaced with D-alanyl–D-lactate, which is not recognized by vancomycin. Thus, the peptidoglycan subunit is appropriately incorporated into the cell wall.

VANCOMYCIN

Vancomycin is the most commonly used member of this class (see Fig. 5-18A). It is an old drug initially associated with substantial toxicity. This toxicity, however, is now known to be due to contaminants that resulted from the crude purification process. Newer production techniques have greatly enhanced the safety profile of vancomycin, while other agents, such as the penicillins, have been progressively limited in their use by increasing resistance. As a result, vancomycin has become a workhorse among antibacterial agents. With increasing use, however, its preeminent position, too, has been threatened by emerging resistance, especially among the enterococci. Although usually given intravenously, it can be given orally to treat bowel infections, such as diarrhea caused by *C. difficile*, but it is not absorbed when administered in this way.

TELAVANCIN

Telavancin is a recently developed derivative of vancomycin with a lipophilic decylaminoethyl side chain added to the peptide core, which classifies it as a lipoglycopeptide (see Fig. 5-18B). This modification enhances binding to D-alanine–D-alanine-containing peptidoglycan intermediates relative to vancomycin and confers upon telavancin a greater ability to inhibit peptidoglycan synthesis. The lipophilic side chain also promotes binding to bacterial cell membranes, which may lead to loss of membrane potential, pore formation, and leakage of cytosolic contents. Thus, telavancin has two modes of antibacterial activity and, theoretically, may be more potent than vancomycin, although more studies are necessary to confirm this. Telavancin is approved for the treatment of complicated skin and skin structure infections.

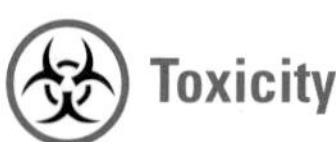

Toxicity

Vancomycin may cause hearing loss, especially when administered along with an aminoglycoside. Rapid infusion has been associated with "red man" syndrome, in which patients develop pruritus and an erythematous rash on the face, neck, and upper torso. Red man syndrome is not a true allergy and can often be avoided by infusing vancomycin at a slower rate. Rarely, neutropenia may occur with use of this agent. Telavancin has been associated with effects involving the central nervous system (insomnia, psychiatric disorders, and headache), gastrointestinal system (metallic/soapy taste, nausea, vomiting), and the urinary tract (foamy urine).

In summary, glycopeptides antibiotics have excellent activity against most aerobic and anaerobic gram-positive bacteria. Despite increasing resistance, they should continue to be workhorses in the treatment of infections caused by gram-positive bacteria for years to come.

QUESTIONS

28. Glycopeptides have excellent activity against both aerobic and anaerobic ________________ bacteria.

29. Recently, resistance to vancomycin has become more common among the ________________.

30. Like the β-lactam antibiotics, glycopeptides kill bacteria by preventing proper synthesis of ________________.

31. Unlike vancomycin, telavancin possesses a lipophilic side chain, which classifies it as a ________________.

ADDITIONAL READINGS

Charneski L, Patel PN, Sym D. Telavancin: a novel lipoglycopeptide antibiotic. *Ann Pharmacother*. 2009;43:928–938.

Courvalin P. Vancomycin resistance in gram-positive cocci. *Clin Infect Dis*. 2006;42(suppl 1):S25–S34.

Kirst HA, Thompson DG, Nicas TI. Historical yearly usage of vancomycin. *Antimicrob Agents Chemother*. 1998;42:1303–1304.

Saravolatz LD, Stein GE, Johnson LB. Telavancin: a novel lipoglycopeptide. *Clin Infect Dis*. 2009;49:1908–1914.

Stevens, DL. The role of vancomycin in the treatment paradigm. *Clin Infect Dis*. 2006;42(suppl 1): S51–S57.

Walsh C. Deconstructing vancomycin. *Science*. 1999;284:442–443.

Weigel LM, Clewell DB, Gill SR, et al. Genetic analysis of a high-level vancomycin-resistant isolate of Staphylococcus aureus. *Science*. 2003;302:1569–1571.

Daptomycin

Daptomycin is a novel cyclic lipopeptide antibiotic that was approved for use in the United States in 2003 (Fig. 5-20). The lipid portion of this drug inserts into the bacterial cytoplasmic membrane, where it forms an ion-conducting channel. This channel allows ions to escape from the bacterium, resulting in bacterial death. Daptomycin is active against many aerobic gram-positive bacteria, including highly resistant strains such as MRSA, penicillin-resistant *S. pneumoniae*, and some vancomycin-resistant enterococci (Table 5-19). Daptomycin is not active against gram-negative organisms because it cannot penetrate the gram-negative outer membrane to reach the cytoplasmic membrane. Unfortunately, daptomycin has poor activity in the lungs and should not be used to treat pneumonia. It has been primarily studied in the treatment of skin and soft tissue infections. An oral formulation is not available.

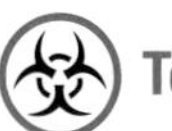

Toxicity

Daptomycin is relatively well tolerated, but reversible myopathy has been observed at higher doses. Phlebitis, rash, and gastrointestinal adverse effects also occur.

In summary, daptomycin has promise as a potent agent against aerobic gram-positive bacteria, but additional clinical trials are necessary to determine whether it is effective for the treatment of infections other than those involving the skin and soft tissues.

Questions

32. The structure of daptomycin is a ________________.

33. Daptomycin has excellent activity against aerobic ________________ bacteria.

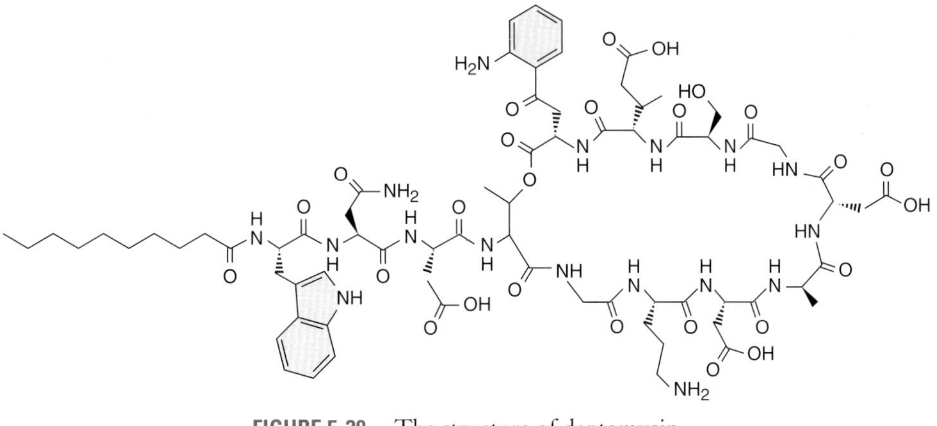

FIGURE 5-20. The structure of daptomycin.

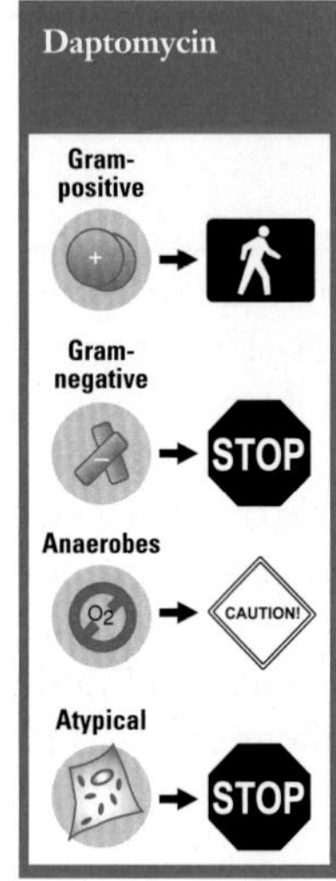

Table 5-19 Antimicrobial Activity of Daptomycin

Gram-positive bacteria	*Streptococcus pyogenes* Viridans group streptococci *Streptococcus pneumoniae* Staphylococci Enterococci
Anaerobic bacteria	Some *Clostridium* spp.

ADDITIONAL READINGS

Carpenter CF, Chambers HF. Daptomycin: another novel agent for treating infections due to drug-resistant gram-positive pathogens. *Clin Infect Dis*. 2004;38:994–1000.

Rybak MJ. The efficacy and safety of daptomycin: first in a new class of antibiotics for Gram-positive bacteria. *Clin Microbiol Infect*. 2006;12(suppl 1):24–32.

Colistin

Colistin is the prodigal son of antibiotics. After first being used in the 1950s, it fell into disfavor in the early 1980s because of its perceived toxicities and the availability of safer alternatives. In recent years, however, colistin has again become a popular choice of clinicians faced with few options in the treatment of multidrug-resistant gram-negative bacteria.

Colistin belongs to the polymyxin group of antibiotics. It is a cationic (positively charged) cyclic decapeptide with a fatty acid side chain (Fig. 5-21). The positive charge allows colistin to bind to the negatively charged lipopolysaccharide molecules in the bacterial outer membrane, displacing Ca^{++} and Mg^{++} ions that normally stabilize these lipids. The fatty acid tail facilitates further insertion of colistin into the outer membrane. The bulkiness of colistin disrupts the normally tightly packed

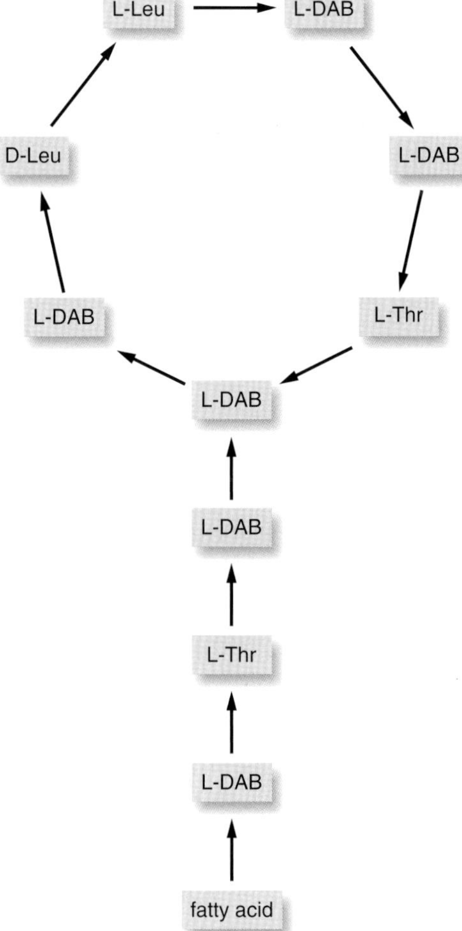

FIGURE 5-21. The structure of colistin. *Leu*, leucine; *Thr*, threonine; *DAB*, diaminobutyric acid.

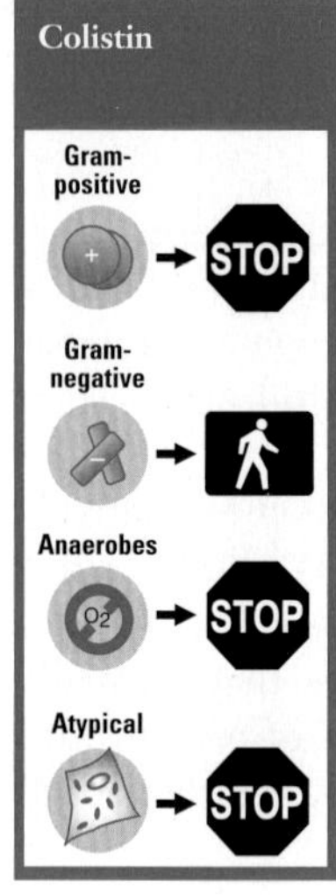

Table 5-20 Antimicrobial Activity of Colistin	
Gram-negative bacteria	*Pseudomonas aeruginosa* many Enterobacteriaceae *Haemophilus influenzae*

lipopolysaccharide molecules, leading to increased permeability and, eventually, lysis of the bacterium. Resistance occurs by several mechanisms, such as alteration of the negative charge associated with lipopolysaccharide, which in turn decreases the interaction between colistin and lipopolysaccharide. As would be expected, colistin has activity against many aerobic gram-negative bacteria, including *P. aeruginosa*, *E. coli*, and *Klebsiella* spp. (Table 5-20). Because colistin has been infrequently used over the last several decades, many multidrug-resistant strains of these bacteria remain susceptible to it. Colistin lacks activity against other gram-negative bacteria (e.g., *Proteus* and *Serratia* spp.), gram-positive bacteria, and anaerobic bacteria.

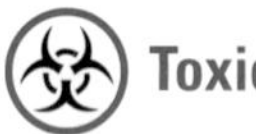

Toxicity

The toxicity of colistin, which earlier led to its disuse, has now been found to be less than previously believed. Nonetheless, it is associated with nephrotoxicity (decreased creatinine clearance) and neurotoxicity (e.g., dizziness, weakness, ataxia, paresthesias, vertigo).

In summary, colistin has activity against many aerobic gram-negative bacilli and is useful in the treatment of infections caused by these bacteria when resistance precludes use of other agents.

QUESTIONS

34. Colistin binds to and disrupts ________________ in the bacterial outer membrane.

35. Colistin has activity against aerobic ________________ bacteria.

ADDITIONAL READINGS

Falagas ME, Kasiakou SK. Colistin: the revival of polymyxins for the management of multidrug-resistant Gram-negative bacterial infections. *Clin Infect Dis*. 2005;40:1333–1341.

Falagas ME, Rafailidis PI, Matthaiou DK. Resistance to polymyxins: mechanisms, frequency and treatment options. *Drug Resist Updat*. 2010;13:132–138.

Nation RL, Li J. Colistin in the 21st century. *Curr Opin Infect Dis*. 2009;22:535–543.

CHAPTER 6

Antibiotics that Block Protein Production

"Vercingetorix had now suffered a series of setbacks, at Vellaunodunum, Cenabum, and Noviodunum. He therefore called his supporters to a council of war, and pointed out to them that the war must be waged in quite a different way from hitherto. They must direct all their efforts towards cutting the Romans off from forage and supplies. . . . All villages and isolated buildings must be set on fire in every direction from the Romans' line of march as far as foragers seemed likely to be able to reach."

—The Battle of Gaul, Julius Caesar

Bacteria must constantly use the resources available in their environment to produce new biomolecules that replace old worn-out ones and to build new bacteria. For example, new proteins are continuously being manufactured in a process that involves the synthesis of mRNA from DNA genes (transcription) and the subsequent generation of proteins from the mRNA templates (translation). Because these processes are crucial for the growth and multiplication of bacteria, they can be targeted by antibiotics. In the following sections, we discuss the antimicrobial agents that inhibit bacterial transcription and translation.

Rifamycins

The **rifamycins** are "accessory" antibiotics. Just as a stylish purse or sparkling necklace is used to adorn a dress, these antimicrobial agents are added to traditional treatment wardrobes that require a little accentuation for the optimal effect. The rifamycins consist of **rifampin** (also called rifampicin), **rifabutin**, **rifapentine**, and **rifaximin** (Table 6-1). Each has a similar structure that includes an aromatic nucleus linked on both ends by an aliphatic "handle" (Fig. 6-1).

Rifamycins act by inhibiting bacterial RNA polymerase. They nestle deep into the DNA/RNA tunnel of this enzyme and, once lodged in this position, sterically block elongation of the nascent mRNA molecule. Resistance develops relatively easily and can result from one of several single mutations in the bacterial gene that encodes RNA polymerase. These mutations each change only a single amino acid at the site where the rifamycins bind to RNA polymerase but are sufficient to prevent this binding. Because single mutations are sufficient to lead to resistance, rifamycins are usually used in combination with other agents to prevent the emergence of resistant strains.

Many of the rifamycins are frequently used in combination regimens for the treatment of mycobacterial infections (Table 6-2). Of the rifamycins, rifampin has been used along with other antibiotics to treat staphylococcal infections. Rifampin is also effective as monotherapy for prophylaxis against *Neisseria meningitidis* and *Haemophilus influenzae*. The use of rifampin alone in prophylaxis is justified by the fact that, usually, very few bacteria are present in the absence of overt disease, thus minimizing the chance that a rifampin-resistance mutation will spontaneously occur.

RIFAMPIN

Rifampin is the oldest and most widely used of the rifamycins. It is also the most potent inducer of the cytochrome P-450 system.

RIFABUTIN

Rifabutin is favored over rifampin in individuals who are simultaneously being treated for tuberculosis and HIV infection because it inhibits the cytochrome P-450 system to a lesser degree than rifampin or rifapentine and thus can be more easily administered along with the many antiretroviral agents that also interact with this system.

Table 6-1 The Rifamycins

Parenteral Agents	Oral Agents
Rifampin	Rifampin
	Rifabutin
	Rifapentine
	Rifaximin

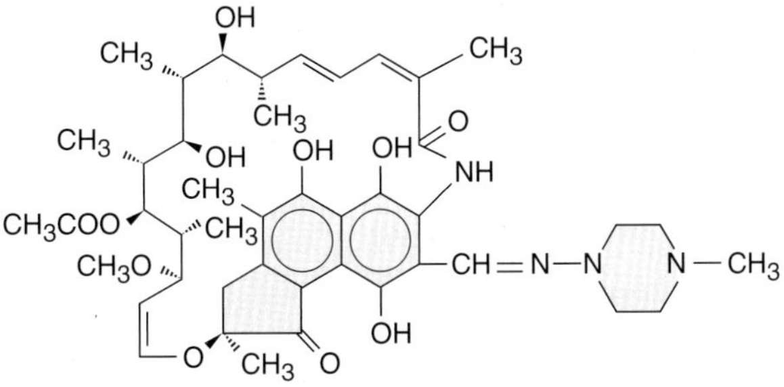

FIGURE 6-1. The structure of rifampin.

RIFAPENTINE

Rifapentine has a long serum half-life, which has led to its use in once-weekly regimens for immunocompetent patients with tuberculosis.

RIFAXIMIN

Rifaximin is a poorly absorbed rifamycin that is used for the treatment of travelers' diarrhea. Because it is not systemically absorbed, it has limited activity against invasive bacteria, such as *Salmonella* and *Campylobacter* spp.

Toxicity

The rifamycins are potent inducers of the cytochrome P-450 system. Thus, they may dramatically affect the levels of other drugs metabolized by this system. Rifamycins also commonly cause gastrointestinal complaints such as nausea, vomiting, and diarrhea and have been associated with hepatitis. Skin rashes and hematologic abnormalities may also occur. Of note, rifampin causes an orange-red discoloration of tears,

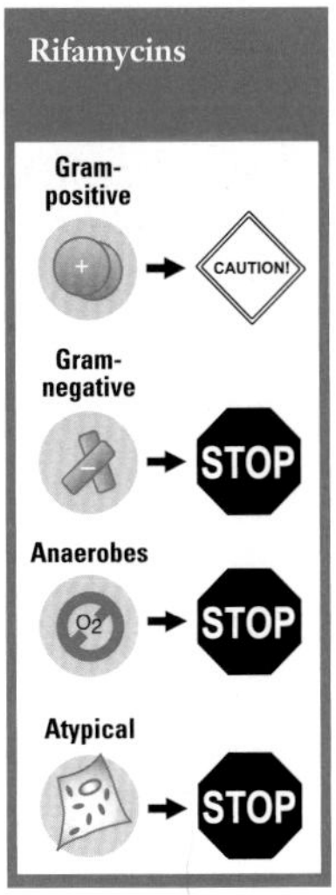

Rifamycins

Gram-positive → CAUTION!

Gram-negative → STOP

Anaerobes → STOP

Atypical → STOP

Table 6-2 Antimicrobial Activity of Rifamycins

Gram-positive bacteria	Staphylococci
Gram-negative bacteria	*Haemophilus influenzae* *Neisseria meningitidis*
Mycobacteria	*Mycobacterium tuberculosis* *Mycobacterium avium* complex *Mycobacterium leprae*

HISTORY

The name *rifamycin* was derived from the French movie Rififi, which was popular at the time these agents were discovered.

Sensi P. History of the development of rifampin. *Rev Infect Dis.* 1983;5(suppl 3):S402–S406.

urine, and other body fluids, which can lead to patient anxiety and the staining of contact lenses. Rifabutin has been associated with uveitis.

The rifamycins are used primarily as components of multidrug regimens for mycobacterial infections and some staphylococcal infections. The ease with which bacteria develop resistance to these agents precludes their use as monotherapy in active disease.

QUESTIONS

1. Rifampin binds bacterial ________________ and inhibits synthesis of ________________.
2. Rifampin is used primarily in the treatment of diseases caused by ________________ and ________________.
3. The rifamycins are usually used in conjunction with other antimicrobial agents because ________________ to rifamycins develops during monotherapy.

ADDITIONAL READINGS

Burman WJ, Gallicano K, Peloquin C. Comparative pharmacokinetics and pharmacodynamics of the rifamycin antibacterials. *Clin Pharmacokinet.* 2001;40:327–341.

Campbell EA, Korzheva N, Mustaev A, et al. Structural mechanism for rifampicin inhibition of bacterial RNA polymerase. *Cell.* 2001;104:901–912.

Huang DB, DuPont HL. Rifaximin—a novel antimicrobial for enteric infections. *J Infect.* 2005;50:97–106.

Munsiff SS, Kambili C, Ahuja SD. Rifapentine for the treatment of pulmonary tuberculosis. *Clin Infect Dis.* 2006;43:1468–1475.

Aminoglycosides

The **aminoglycosides** are among the oldest antibiotics, dating back to the purification of **streptomycin** from the bacterium *Streptomyces griseus* in 1944. **Neomycin** became available in 1949, followed by **gentamicin** in 1963, **tobramycin** in 1967, and **amikacin** in 1972 (Table 6-3). Like penicillin, these agents initially were active against both gram-negative and gram-positive bacteria. Unlike penicillin, though, the aminoglycosides have maintained their effectiveness against many of these bacteria despite over 30 years of use and today are commonly administered antibiotics.

The aminoglycosides are positively charged molecules that are quite large (Fig. 6-2), although still only one-third the size of vancomycin. Each aminoglycoside molecule consists of two or more sugars bound by a glycosidic linkage to a central six-membered ring that contains amino group substituents. The name *aminoglycoside* is derived from the *amino* groups and the *glycosidic* linkage. Unlike vancomycin, the aminoglycosides have excellent activity against aerobic gram-negative bacteria because their size does not prevent their passage through the bacterial outer membrane. Rather, the positively charged nature of aminoglycosides allows them to bind to the negatively charged outer membrane and results in the formation of transient holes through which the antibiotic molecules move. Access to the bacterial ribosomes, which are the targets of aminoglycosides, still requires penetration of the bacterial cytoplasmic membrane. This is accomplished by an energy-dependent active bacterial transport mechanism that requires oxygen and an active proton motive force. For these reasons, aminoglycosides work poorly in anaerobic and acidic environments such as abscesses and have no activity against anaerobic bacteria. Each aminoglycoside acts by binding to the 30S subunit of the bacterial ribosome, which causes mismatching between the mRNA codon and the charged aminoacyl-tRNA. This in turn promotes protein mistranslation.

For reasons that are unclear, resistance to aminoglycoside antibiotics remains relatively rare. When it does occur, it is usually the result of one of three mechanisms (Fig. 6-3): (1) decreased accumulation within the bacterium, which most likely reflects the presence of efflux pumps; (2) bacterial enzymes such as acetyltransferases, nucleotidyltransferases, and phosphotransferases, which modify the drug and prevent it from binding ribosomes; and (3) mutation of the bacterial ribosome in such a way that the aminoglycoside can no longer bind to it. (This last mechanism appears to be

Table 6-3 The Aminoglycosides

Parenteral Agents	Oral Agents
Streptomycin	Neomycin*
Gentamicin	
Tobramycin	
Amikacin	

*Not absorbed when given orally. Used for bowel decontamination.

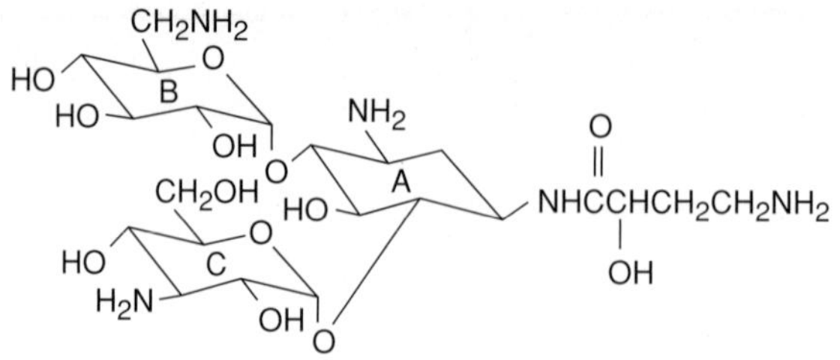

FIGURE 6-2. The structure of the aminoglycoside amikacin. Features of aminoglycosides include amino sugars **(B, C)** bound by glycosidic linkages to a relatively conserved six-membered ring **(A)** that itself contains amino group substituents.

relatively rare.) Resistance is not always classwide. For example, because of its unique side chains, amikacin is resistant to modification by some bacterial enzymes that are active against gentamicin and tobramycin.

Aminoglycosides have excellent activity against aerobic gram-negative bacteria (Table 6-4). These agents are commonly used to treat infections caused by members of the Enterobacteriaceae and *Pseudomonas aeruginosa*. Because of disappointing results in animal studies, aminoglycosides are usually used in combination with another active agent, even against bacterial strains that are highly sensitive. These agents are active to a lesser degree against aerobic gram-positive bacteria. Uptake of aminoglycosides is enhanced by antibiotics that inhibit bacterial cell wall synthesis, such as β-lactams and vancomycin. Thus, in some aerobic gram-positive bacteria such as enterococci, aminoglycosides have synergistic efficacy when used with these agents even when the bacterium is moderately resistant to aminoglycosides. Lower amounts of aminoglycosides, referred to as *synergistic dosing*, are given when they are used with cell wall–active agents to treat aerobic gram-positive bacteria. Some of the aminoglycosides are also

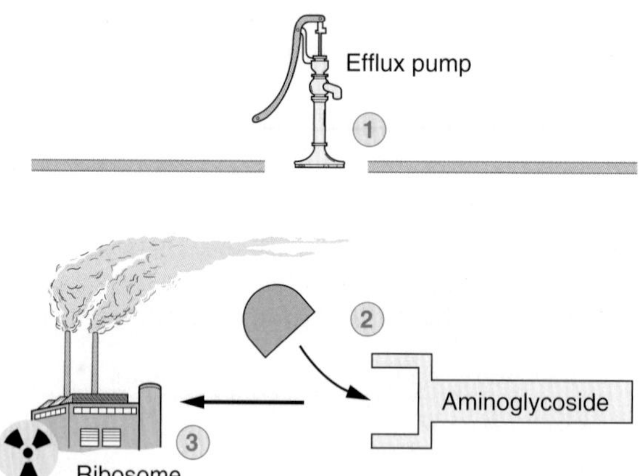

FIGURE 6-3. Bacterial resistance to aminoglycosides occurs via one of three mechanisms that prevent the normal binding of the antibiotic to its ribosomal target: (1) Efflux pumps prevent accumulation of the aminoglycoside in the cytosol of the bacterium. (2) Modification of the aminoglycoside prevents binding to the ribosome. (3) Mutations within the ribosome prevent aminoglycoside binding.

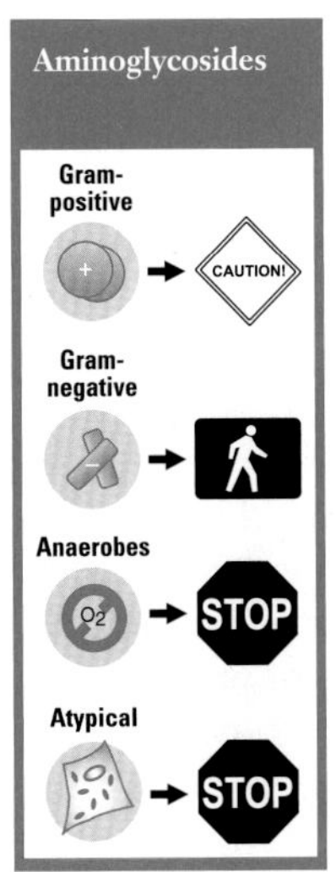

Table 6-4 Antimicrobial Activity of Aminoglycosides

Gram-positive bacteria	Used synergistically against some: Staphylococci Streptococci Enterococci *Listeria monocytogenes*
Gram-negative bacteria	*Haemophilus influenzae* Enterobacteriaceae *Pseudomonas aeruginosa*
Mycobacteria	*Mycobacterium tuberculosis* *Mycobacterium avium* complex

active against certain mycobacteria species such as *Mycobacterium tuberculosis* and *Mycobacterium avium* complex.

STREPTOMYCIN

Streptomycin is the oldest aminoglycoside and is rarely used today. It is still a second-line agent in the treatment of tuberculosis. Also, because of differences in resistance mechanisms, streptomycin remains effective against some strains of enterococci that are resistant to the synergistic effects of gentamicin and other aminoglycosides.

GENTAMICIN

Gentamicin is the most commonly used of the aminoglycosides. It is active against both aerobic gram-negative and aerobic gram-positive bacteria.

TOBRAMYCIN

For practical purposes, tobramycin has the same spectrum of activity as gentamicin and is used similarly. In general, most gentamicin-resistant strains also lack susceptibility to tobramycin. Unlike gentamicin, however, tobramycin lacks activity against enterococci and should not be used for infections caused by this bacterium.

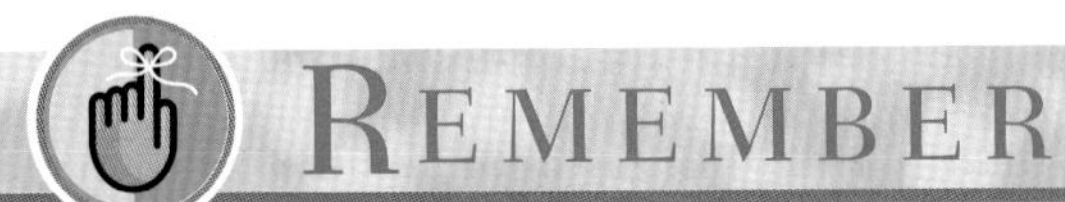

Unlike tobramycin, neomycin, and streptomycin, the aminoglycoside gentamicin is spelled without a "y." This has led to it being one of the most commonly misspelled medical words. Other contenders include "pruritic" and "guaiac."

AMIKACIN

Strains of aerobic gram-negative bacteria that are resistant to gentamicin and tobramycin may remain susceptible to amikacin. Thus, this agent has better overall activity against these bacteria. Like tobramycin, however, amikacin lacks clinically significant activity against enterococci.

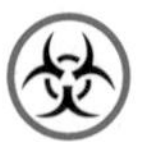

Toxicity

The major factor limiting the use of aminoglycosides is their toxicity. These agents are associated with relatively high frequencies of nephrotoxicity and ototoxicity. Aminoglycosides penetrate human cells poorly except for proximal renal tubule cells, where they are concentrated. As a result, approximately 5% to 10% of patients who receive aminoglycosides will develop nephrotoxicity or decreased renal function. This incidence can be as high as 50% in patients who have specific risk factors for toxicity, such as increased age and concomitant exposure to other renal toxins. Fortunately, the damage to the kidneys is usually reversible, and renal function often returns to normal after discontinuation of the drug. Note that renal toxicity is usually only observed after 4 to 5 days of therapy, so aminoglycosides can be safely given for a short period without placing the patient at significant risk for this adverse effect. Ototoxicity consists of two types: auditory impairment, which may lead to irreversible hearing loss, and vestibular toxicity, which results in disturbances in balance. Streptomycin has been associated with especially high rates of vestibular toxicity.

The aminoglycosides remain potent agents for the treatment of many infections caused by aerobic gram-negative bacteria. They also possess synergistic activity with cell wall–active agents and are useful as adjunctive therapy against some aerobic gram-positive bacteria. Toxicity continues to be a concern with their use.

QUESTIONS

4. The aminoglycosides have excellent activity against aerobic ________________ bacteria.
5. The aminoglycosides are used at synergistic doses along with cell wall–active agents to treat some aerobic ________________ bacteria.
6. The two major toxicities associated with the aminoglycosides are ________________ and ________________.

ADDITIONAL READINGS

Chambers HF. Aminoglycosides. In: Burunton LL, Lazo JS, Parker KL, eds. *Goodman and Gilman's the Pharmacological Basis of Therapeutics*. 11th ed. New York, NY: McGraw-Hill; 2006:1155–1172.

Gonzalez LS III, Spencer JP. Aminoglycosides: a practical review. *Am Fam Physician*. 1998;58: 1811–1820.

Mingeot-Leclercq MP, Glupczynski Y, Tulkens PM. Aminoglycosides: activity and resistance. *Antimicrob Agents Chemother*. 1999;43:727–737.

Vakulenko SB, Mobashery S. Versatility of aminoglycosides and prospects for the future. *Clin Microbiol Rev*. 2003;16:430–450.

Macrolides and Ketolides

Macrolide antibiotics follow the old adage "jack of all trades, master of none." These agents are active against some gram-positive bacteria, some gram-negative bacteria, some atypical bacteria, some mycobacteria, and even some spirochetes. But they are not reliably effective against most bacteria in any one group. Nonetheless, they remain very useful agents for the treatment of specific types of infections, such as respiratory infections, and for treatment directed toward specific organisms. The macrolide group of antibiotics consists of **erythromycin**, **clarithromycin**, and **azithromycin** (Table 6-5). **Telithromycin** is a recently approved member of a structurally related class of antibiotics called the ketolides and also will be discussed here.

All macrolides consist of a large cyclic core called a macrocyclic lactone ring (Fig. 6-4) (hence the name *macrolide*). This ring is decorated with sugar residues. Macrolides bind tightly to the 50S subunit of the bacterial ribosome at a location that blocks the exit of the newly synthesized peptide. Thus, macrolides function in a manner similar to the aminoglycosides in that they target ribosomes and prevent protein production. Resistance is becoming increasingly common and occurs by one of several mechanisms: (1) inhibition of drug entry and accumulation—macrolides have difficulty penetrating the outer membrane of most aerobic gram-negative bacilli and are actively pumped out of some resistant bacteria. For example, some gram-positive bacteria, such as *Streptococcus pneumoniae*, contain a *mef* gene that encodes an efflux pump that impairs accumulation of macrolides within the bacterium. (2) Enzyme-mediated ribosome binding site alteration—some bacteria acquire resistance to macrolides by methylating the portion of the 50S ribosome normally bound by these drugs, preventing this interaction. For example, this type of resistance is encoded by the *erm* gene in *S. pneumoniae*. Methylation of the ribosome in this way also results in resistance to clindamycin and streptogramins, which act by binding the bacterial ribosome and inhibiting protein translation as well. (3) Mutation of the ribosome binding site—rarely, mutations occur that affect the portion of the bacterial ribosome bound by macrolides. Regardless of the mechanism, resistance to one member of the macrolide group usually implies resistance to all members.

As a group, the macrolides are active against various bacteria (Table 6-6). They are effective against some staphylococci and streptococci, although not usually

Table 6-5 The Macrolides and Ketolides

Parenteral Agents	Oral Agents
Erythromycin	Erythromycin
	Clarithromycin
Azithromycin	Azithromycin
	Telithromycin

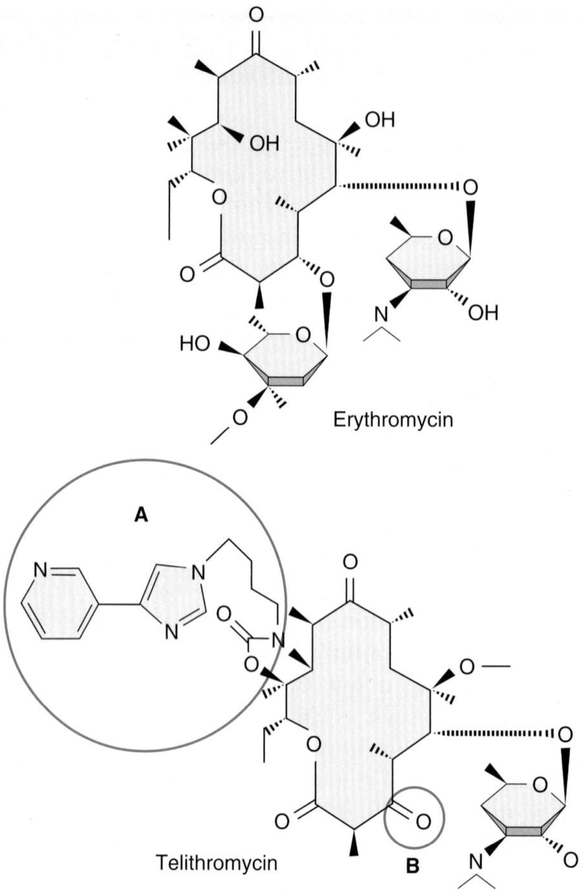

FIGURE 6-4. The structures of erythromycin **(top)** and telithromycin **(bottom)**. Circled substituents **A** and **B** distinguish telithromycin from the macrolides. Substituent **A** allows telithromycin to bind to a second site on the bacterial ribosome.

methicillin-resistant staphylococci and penicillin-resistant streptococci. A large hole in the spectrum of macrolides is that most aerobic gram-negative bacilli are resistant, but some *Neisseria*, *Bordetella*, and *Haemophilus* strains are susceptible. Macrolides are not useful in the treatment of most anaerobic infections. On the other hand, they are active against many atypical bacteria and some mycobacteria and spirochetes.

ERYTHROMYCIN

Erythromycin, the oldest of the macrolides, was discovered in 1952 and contains a 14-member macrocyclic lactone ring (Fig. 6-4). It is less useful than the other macrolides in the treatment of respiratory infections because it lacks significant activity against *H. influenzae*. Because it has a spectrum of activity similar to clarithromycin and azithromycin but is less well tolerated, it is being replaced by these newer agents.

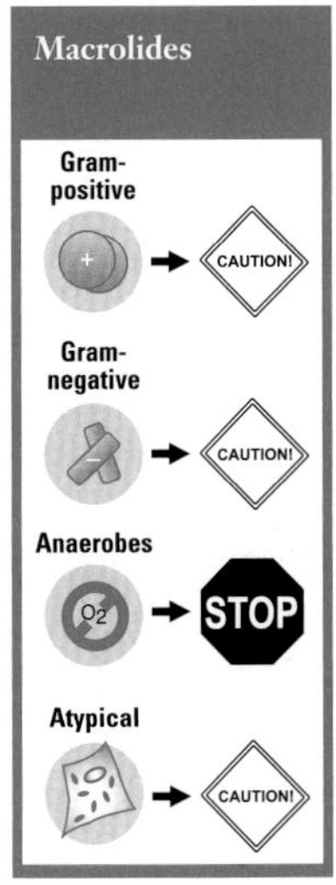

Table 6-6 Antimicrobial Activity of Macrolides

Gram-positive bacteria	Some *Streptococcus pyogenes* Some viridans streptococci Some *Streptococcus pneumoniae* Some *Staphylococcus aureus*
Gram-negative bacteria	*Neisseria* spp. Some *Haemophilus influenzae* *Bordetella pertussis*
Atypical bacteria	*Chlamydia* spp. *Mycoplasma* spp. *Legionella pneumophila* Some *Rickettsia* spp.
Mycobacteria	*Mycobacterium avium* complex *Mycobacterium leprae*
Spirochetes	*Treponema pallidum* *Borrelia burgdorferi*

CLARITHROMYCIN

Clarithromycin is a semisynthetic derivative of erythromycin and also consists of a 14-member macrocyclic lactone ring. It has somewhat greater activity against aerobic gram-positive bacteria and *H. influenzae* than erythromycin.

AZITHROMYCIN

Azithromycin has a modified 15-member macrocyclic lactone ring that allows it to better penetrate the outer membrane of some aerobic gram-negative bacteria. Hence, it has somewhat better activity against these bacteria and is useful in the treatment of *H. influenzae*. One of its main advantages is that it is taken up in high amounts by tissues and then slowly released over subsequent days. Thus, a 5-day course of oral therapy results in therapeutic drug levels in the blood for 10 days.

TELITHROMYCIN

Telithromycin is the first commercially available member of a new class of antibiotics called *ketolides*. Ketolides are structurally related to the macrolides (Fig. 6-4) but have an expanded spectrum of activity. Telithromycin binds to the same site of the 50S subunit of the bacterial ribosome as the macrolides but has an additional alkyl-aryl extension (labeled "A" in Fig. 6-4), which binds to a second distinct site on the ribosome. Two sites of contact instead of one result in tighter binding and continued interaction even in the presence of some enzymes that methylate the ribosome and result in resistance to macrolides. This tighter binding also limits export of telithromycin by macrolide efflux pumps. Thus, telithromycin is active against many strains of *Streptococcus pneumoniae*, *Staphylococcus aureus*, and *Streptococcus pyogenes* that are resistant to macrolides.

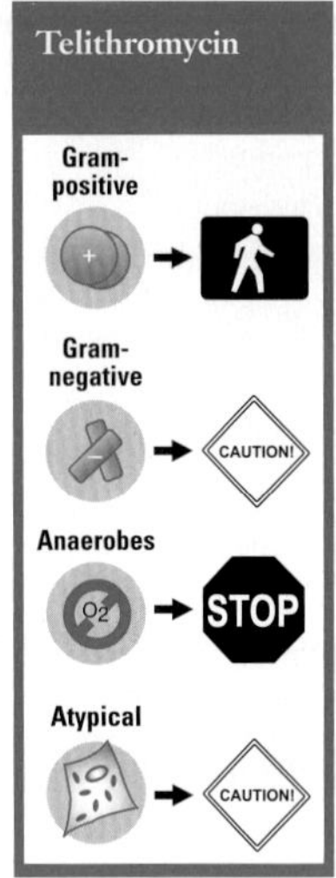

Table 6-7 Antimicrobial Activity of Telithromycin

Gram-positive bacteria	*Streptococcus pyogenes* *Streptococcus pneumoniae* Some *Staphylococcus aureus*
Gram-negative bacteria	Some *Haemophilus influenzae* *Bordetella pertussis*
Atypical bacteria	*Chlamydia* spp. *Mycoplasma* spp. *Legionella pneumophila*

Telithromycin is approved for use in patients with bacterial respiratory infections and has been most carefully studied with organisms that cause these infections (Table 6-7). In this context, it is active against most strains of *S. pneumoniae*, including penicillin-resistant and macrolide-resistant strains. Telithromycin is also active against more strains of staphylococci and other streptococci than are the macrolides, although some strains are resistant because they are capable of modifying their ribosomes in such a way that even telithromycin can no longer bind them. Enterobacteriaceae are resistant to telithromycin, but *H. influenzae* and *Bordetella pertussis* are susceptible. The activity of this agent against *Neisseria* spp. has not been well studied. Many atypical bacteria such as *Chlamydia pneumoniae*, *Mycoplasma pneumoniae*, and *Legionella pneumophila* are susceptible to telithromycin, but its activity against mycobacteria and spirochetes has not yet been defined. Telithromycin is currently only available in an oral formulation.

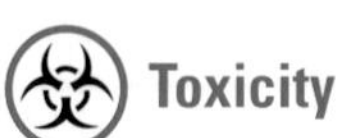

Toxicity

The macrolides are safe drugs, causing several relatively mild adverse reactions. Erythromycin is associated with gastrointestinal symptoms such as nausea, vomiting, and diarrhea and with thrombophlebitis following intravenous administration, but clarithromycin and azithromycin are usually tolerated quite well. QT prolongation leading to polymorphic ventricular tachycardia has been reported with use of these agents. Erythromycin and clarithromycin but not azithromycin are also capable of inhibiting the cytochrome P-450 system and thereby affecting levels of other drugs. Telithromycin is a strong inhibitor of the P-450 system and therefore affects levels of other drugs that are metabolized by this system. Its use has been associated with gastrointestinal complaints, headache, dizziness, and QT prolongation. In addition, this agent may cause visual disturbances such as reversible blurred vision, diplopia, or difficultly focusing. Of concern are recent reports that it may also cause severe liver damage.

The macrolides have some activity against aerobic gram-positive bacteria, aerobic gram-negative bacteria, atypical bacteria, mycobacteria, and spirochetes. Within each of these groups, however, several bacteria are resistant to these agents, and macrolides, therefore, must be used with caution as empiric agents. Telithromycin is an agent belonging to a new class of antibiotics called ketolides that are related to the macrolides. It is notable for its superior activity against *S. pneumoniae*. It has been primarily studied for the treatment of patients with mild to moderate community-acquired pneumonia.

QUESTIONS

7. Among the macrolides, ________________ has the best aerobic gram-negative coverage and is therefore useful against ________________.

8. ________________ and ________________ are macrolides that are better tolerated than erythromycin.

9. Macrolides have relatively poor activity against aerobic gram-negative bacilli and ________________ bacteria.

10. Telithromycin is a member of the ________________ class of antimicrobial agents.

11. Because of its spectrum of activity, telithromycin is most useful in treating ________________ infections.

ADDITIONAL READINGS

Clark JP, Langston E. Ketolides: a new class of antibacterial agents for treatment of community-acquired respiratory tract infections in a primary care setting. *Mayo Clinic Proc.* 2003;78:1113–1124.

Leclercq R. Mechanisms of resistance to macrolides and lincosamides: nature of the resistance elements and their clinical implications. *Clin Infect Dis.* 2002;34:482–492.

Lonks JR, Goldmann DA. Telithromycin: a ketolide antibiotic for treatment of respiratory tract infections. *Clin Infect Dis.* 2005;40:1657–1664.

Neu HC. New macrolide antibiotics: azithromycin and clarithromycin. *Ann Intern Med.* 1992;116:517–519.

Zuckerman JM. The newer macrolides: azithromycin and clarithromycin. *Infect Dis Clin North Am.* 2000;14:449–462.

Tetracyclines and Glycylcyclines

The **tetracyclines** are another class of antibiotics that date back to the 1950s. Today, three members of this group are commonly used: **tetracycline**, **doxycycline**, and **minocycline** (Table 6-8). **Tigecycline**, a member of a related class of antibiotics called the **glycylcyclines**, has recently been approved for use.

The core structure of the tetracyclines consists of four fused six-membered rings (Fig. 6-5). This structure allows the tetracyclines to interact with the 30S subunit of the bacterial ribosome and prevent binding by tRNA molecules loaded with amino acids. In this way, protein synthesis is blocked. Resistance to tetracyclines most commonly occurs by one of two mechanisms. Exogenous genes are acquired that encode efflux pumps, which prevent intracellular accumulation of these drugs. Alternatively, genes may be acquired that encode ribosomal protection proteins. These factors alter the conformation of the bacterial ribosome such that tetracyclines no longer bind them but protein translation remains unaffected.

Tetracyclines are active against some aerobic gram-positive bacteria, such as *S. pneumoniae*, and some aerobic gram-negative bacteria, such as *H. influenzae* and *N. meningitidis* (Table 6-9). These agents also have some anaerobic activity and can be used to treat infections caused by some spirochetes, such as *Borrelia burgdorferi* and *Treponema pallidum*. The strength of this class of drugs, however, is its activity against atypical bacteria, including rickettsiae, chlamydiae, and mycoplasmas.

TETRACYCLINE

Tetracycline was discovered in 1953 but is still used today. It is available in an oral formulation.

DOXYCYCLINE

The spectrum of activity of doxycycline is essentially the same as tetracycline. It is more commonly used because of its longer half-life, which allows for twice per day dosing.

Table 6-8 The Tetracyclines and Glycylcyclines

Parenteral Agents	Oral Agents
Doxycycline	Tetracycline
Tigecycline	Doxycycline
	Minocycline

FIGURE 6-5. The structure of tetracycline.

MINOCYCLINE

The spectrum of activity of minocycline is similar to that of the other tetracyclines except that this agent is preferable for the treatment of methicillin-resistant staphylococcal infections. Minocycline is also occasionally used for leprosy caused by *Mycobacterium leprae*.

TIGECYCLINE

Tigecycline is not actually a tetracycline but a member of a structurally related class of antibiotics called the glycylcyclines, of which tigecycline is the only commercially available member. The key modification present in glycylcyclines is the addition of a glycyl amide group to the terminal six-membered ring of the core tetracycline structure (Fig. 6-6). This addition prevents recognition of tigecycline by many bacterial efflux pumps and makes it insensitive to modifications of the 30S ribosomal subunit that confer resistance to tetracyclines. Because these mechanisms account for the bulk of the resistance to tetracyclines, tigecycline has an impressively broad antimicrobial spectrum. It is active against most aerobic gram-negative bacteria, including multidrug-resistant *Acinetobacter* spp. However, *P. aeruginosa* and *Proteus* spp., which produce efflux pumps that do recognize this agent, are usually resistant (Table 6-10).

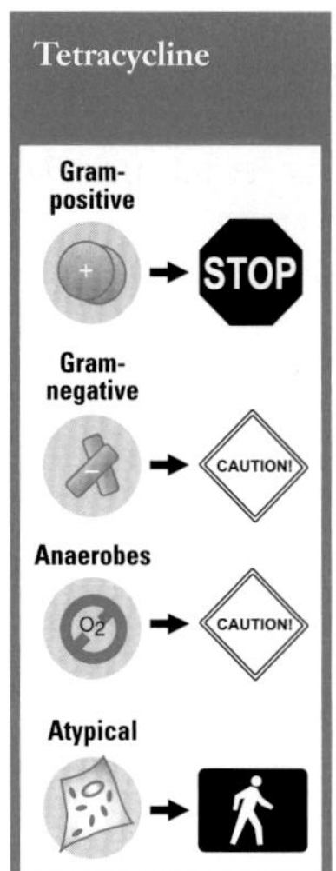

Table 6-9 Antimicrobial Activity of Tetracycline

Gram-positive bacteria	Some *Streptococcus pneumoniae*
Gram-negative bacteria	*Haemophilus influenzae* *Neisseria meningitidis*
Anaerobic bacteria	Some *Clostridia* spp.
Spirochetes	*Borrelia burgdorferi* *Treponema pallidum*
Atypical bacteria	*Rickettsia* spp. *Chlamydia* spp. *Mycoplasma* spp.

FIGURE 6-6. The structure of tigecycline.

Most aerobic gram-positive bacteria, including methicillin-resistant staphylococci, vancomycin-resistant enterococci, and penicillin-resistant *S. pneumoniae*, are susceptible to tigecycline. It also has good activity against anaerobic bacteria, although it is inferior to carbapenems and piperacillin-tazobactam in this regard. As would be expected of a tetracycline-related agent, tigecycline appears to have excellent activity against atypical bacteria.

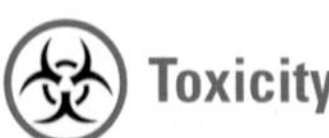

Toxicity

The tetracyclines are relatively safe drugs, but several contraindications must be kept in mind. One of the core rings of these agents is a potent chelator of metal ions such as calcium. This may result in the gray to yellow discoloration of actively forming teeth and deposition in growing bone. For these reasons, the tetracyclines should not be given to pregnant women and given cautiously to children younger than the age of 8 years. Hypersensitivity reactions such as rashes and anaphylaxis occur but are not common. An exception is the blue-black hyperpigmentation of skin and mucous membranes observed relatively frequently with minocycline use. The tetracyclines are also associated with phototoxicity. Gastrointestinal side effects such as nausea, vomiting, and esophageal ulceration are also seen, as is hepatotoxicity.

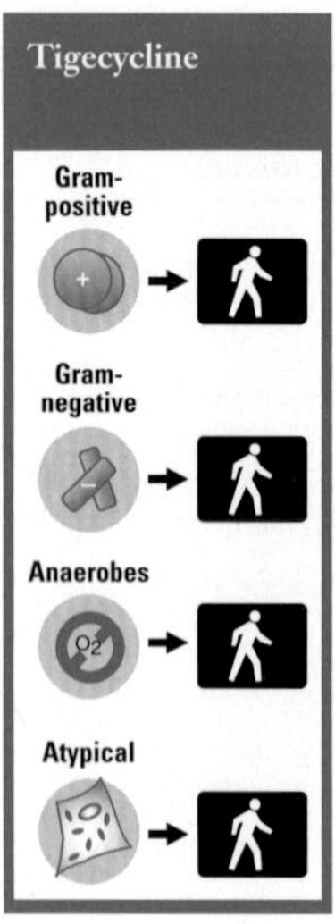

Table 6-10 Antimicrobial Activity of Tigecycline

Gram-positive bacteria	*Streptococcus pyogenes* Viridans group streptococci *Streptococcus pneumoniae* Staphylococci Enterococci *Listeria monocytogenes*
Gram-negative bacteria	*Haemophilus influenzae* *Neisseria* spp. Enterobacteriaceae
Anaerobic bacteria	*Bacteroides fragilis* Many other anaerobes
Atypical bacteria	*Mycoplasma* spp.

The tetracyclines are an old class of antibiotics that are still used for treating infections caused by certain organisms, particularly atypical pathogens. The glycylcycline tigecycline is a newer variant of these agents with broad activity against aerobic and anaerobic bacteria, including some species resistant to many other antibiotics. Toxicity precludes their use in pregnant women and requires that they be used cautiously in young children.

QUESTIONS

12. Tetracyclines inhibit bacterial growth by binding to bacterial ________________.

13. Tetracyclines have excellent activity against ________________ bacteria.

14. Because of problems with discoloration of teeth and deposition in bones, tetracyclines should not be used in ________________ and should be used with caution in ________________.

15. Tigecycline is a member of the class of antibiotics called ________________.

16. Tigecycline has activity against many highly resistant aerobic ________________ and ________________ bacteria.

ADDITIONAL READINGS

Chopra I, Roberts M. Tetracycline antibiotics: mode of action, applications, molecular biology, and epidemiology of bacterial resistance. *Microbiol Mol Biol Rev*. 2001;65:232–260.

Joshi N, Miller DQ. Doxycycline revisited. *Arch Intern Med*. 1997;157:1421–1428.

Livermore DM. Tigecycline: what is it, and where should it be used? *J Antimicrob Chemother*. 2005;56:611–614.

Roberts MC. Tetracycline therapy: update. *Clin Infect Dis*. 2003;36:462–467.

Slover CM, Rodvold KA, Danziger LH. Tigecycline: a novel broad-spectrum antimicrobial. *Ann Pharmacother*. 2007;41:965–972.

Chloramphenicol

Chloramphenicol is a very old antibiotic that was first available for clinical use in 1947. Although it remains effective against various bacteria, toxicity has limited its use to situations in which cost or resistance precludes alternatives. The structure of chloramphenicol (Fig. 6-7) allows for binding to the 50S subunit of the ribosome, where it blocks binding of tRNA loaded with an amino acid. Resistance occurs when bacteria acquire genes that encode for an enzyme that acetylates chloramphenicol, which prevents it from effectively binding to its target. Efflux pumps that recognize this agent have also been described. Chloramphenicol is only available in a parenteral formulation in the United States, but capsules for oral ingestion are available in other parts of the world.

Chloramphenicol has a broad spectrum of activity against many different categories of bacteria (Table 6-11). It is effective against many aerobic gram-positive streptococci, including a high proportion of *S. pneumoniae* and *S. pyogenes* strains. Many aerobic gram-negative bacteria are also susceptible, including strains of *H. influenzae*, *Neisseria* spp., *Salmonella* spp., and *Shigella* spp. Chloramphenicol is one of the most effective antibiotics against anaerobic bacteria and can be used to treat infections caused by *Bacteroides fragilis* and some *Clostridium* spp. Finally, this agent has excellent activity against atypical bacteria, including *Chlamydia trachomatis*, *M. pneumoniae*, and *Rickettsia* spp.

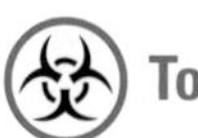

Toxicity

It is not possible to summarize chloramphenicol without discussing its toxicity profile, which has had a major impact on the usefulness of this agent. The most serious of these effects involves the bone marrow. Chloramphenicol commonly causes reversible dose-dependent bone marrow suppression during the course of therapy. This toxicity is thought to result from binding of chloramphenicol to the mitochondrial ribosome, which resembles the bacterial ribosome. More feared but much more rare is the development of irreversible aplastic anemia, which typically occurs after completion of a course of therapy. As might be expected, both these toxicities have dramatically limited the use of chloramphenicol. This agent can also lead to a fatal condition in neonates called *gray baby syndrome* and to neurologic abnormalities such as optic neuritis.

In summary, chloramphenicol has a broad spectrum of activity that includes many aerobic gram-positive, aerobic gram-negative, anaerobic, and atypical bacteria. Its use, however, has been severely limited by its toxicity profile.

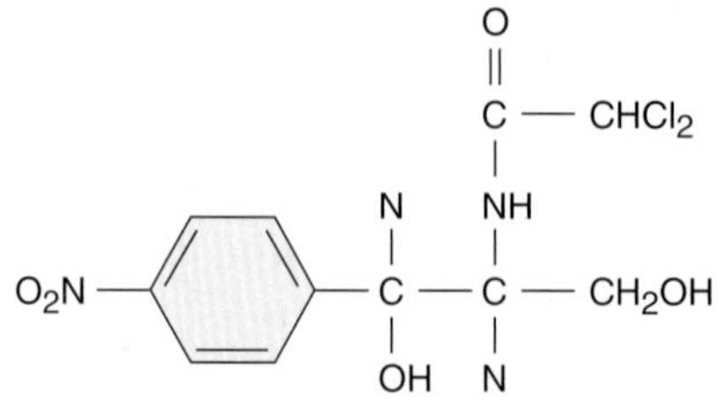

FIGURE 6-7. The structure of chloramphenicol.

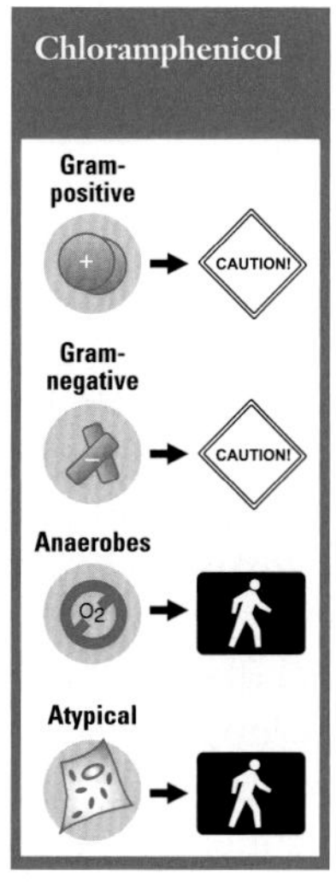

Table 6-11 Antimicrobial Activity of Chloramphenicol

Gram-positive bacteria	*Streptococcus pyogenes* Viridans group streptococci Some *Streptococcus pneumoniae*
Gram-negative bacteria	*Haemophilus influenzae* *Neisseria* spp. *Salmonella* spp. *Shigella* spp.
Anaerobic bacteria	*Bacteroides fragilis* Some *Clostridia* spp. Other anaerobic gram-positive and gram-negative bacteria
Atypical bacteria	*Rickettsia* spp. *Chlamydia trachomatis* *Mycoplasma* spp.

QUESTIONS

17. Chloramphenicol inhibits bacterial growth by binding to bacterial ________________.

18. Chloramphenicol has excellent activity against ________________ and ________________ bacteria. It is also active against many aerobic gram-positive and aerobic gram-negative bacteria.

19. Resistance to chloramphenicol may occur when bacteria acquire the ability to inactivate the drug by ________________ or produce ________________ ________________ that prevent its accumulation.

20. The major factor limiting the use of chloramphenicol is its ________________, which primarily consists of reversible ________________ ________________ suppression and irreversible ________________ ________________.

ADDITIONAL READINGS

Feder HM Jr, Osier C, Maderazo EG. Chloramphenicol: a review of its use in clinical practice. *Rev Infect Dis*. 1981;3:479–491.

Trevett AJ, Naraqi S. Saint or sinner? A look at chloramphenicol. *PNG Med J*. 1992;35:210–216.

Wallerstein RO, Condit PK, Kasper CK, et al. Statewide study of chloramphenicol therapy and fatal aplastic anemia. *JAMA*. 1969;208:2045–2050.

Clindamycin

Clindamycin, which was introduced in 1966, is a synthetic derivative of the antibiotic lincomycin. Together, these agents comprise the lincosamide antibiotic group and are characterized by the common structure of an amino acid linked to an amino sugar (Fig. 6-8). Only clindamycin, which is available in both oral and intravenous forms, is commonly used today. Recently, there has been a resurgence of interest in clindamycin because of its activity against many strains of community-acquired methicillin-resistant *S. aureus* and because of its potential efficacy in the treatment of toxin-mediated diseases caused by staphylococci and streptococci.

The lincosamide antibiotics bind to the 50S subunit of the bacterial ribosome and inhibit protein synthesis. Theoretically, then, these agents should prevent production of bacterial toxins, and they are often used for this reason as adjunctive therapy in toxic shock syndrome caused by streptococci or staphylococci. Clindamycin's mechanism of action is very similar to that of the macrolides. In fact, their binding sites overlap. Thus, some strains of bacteria that are resistant to erythromycin because of ribosomal modification are also resistant to clindamycin. Most gram-negative bacteria are intrinsically resistant to clindamycin because their outer membranes resist penetration by this drug.

Clindamycin's utility lies in its activity against two groups of bacteria: aerobic gram-positive bacteria and anaerobic bacteria (Table 6-12). In particular, it is active against many staphylococci and streptococci, including some strains of community-acquired methicillin-resistant *S. aureus*. Likewise, it has relatively broad activity against anaerobic bacteria, although some *B. fragilis* and clostridial strains are resistant. As mentioned previously, it is not useful against aerobic gram-negative bacteria.

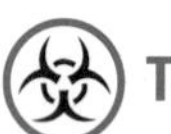

Toxicity

The major toxicity of clindamycin, which has limited its use, is the occurrence of *Clostridium difficile* colitis in 0.01% to 10% of individuals who receive it. Clindamycin kills many components of the normal bacterial flora in the bowel, allowing for overgrowth by *C. difficile*, which is resistant to this drug. In the most serious form of *C. difficile* colitis, plaques of necrotic debris are seen lining the colon, which is referred to as *pseudomembranous colitis*. Clindamycin has also been associated with diarrhea not caused by *C. difficile* and with rash.

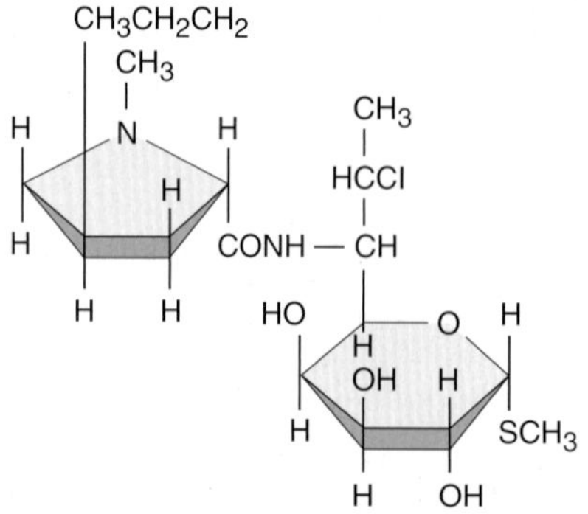

FIGURE 6-8. The structure of clindamycin.

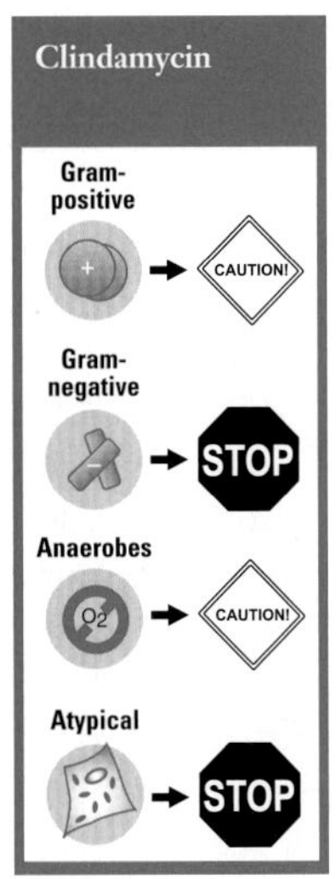

Table 6-12 Antimicrobial Activity of Clindamycin

Gram-positive bacteria	Some *Streptococcus pyogenes* Some viridans group streptococci Some *Streptococcus pneumoniae* Some *Staphylococcus aureus*
Anaerobic bacteria	Some *Bacteroides fragilis* Some *Clostridium* spp. Most other anaerobes

Clindamycin remains a useful drug for the treatment of some infections caused by aerobic gram-positive and anaerobic bacteria. It is not active against aerobic gram-negative bacteria. Caution must be exercised regarding the relatively frequent occurrence of *C. difficile* colitis associated with its use.

QUESTIONS

21. Clindamycin is active against many aerobic ________________ bacteria and ________________ bacteria.

22. Resistance to ________________ may also lead to resistance to clindamycin in some bacteria.

23. Use of clindamycin may lead to life-threatening ________________.

ADDITIONAL READINGS

Falagas ME, Gorbach SL. Clindamycin and metronidazole. *Med Clin North Am.* 1995;79:845–867.

Fass RJ, Scholand JF, Hodges GR, et al. Clindamycin in the treatment of serious anaerobic infections. *Ann Intern Med.* 1973;78:853–859.

Russell NE, Pachorek RE. Clindamycin in the treatment of streptococcal and staphylococcal toxic shock syndromes. *Ann Pharmacother.* 2000;34:936–939.

Sutter VL. In vitro susceptibility of anaerobes: comparison of clindamycin and other antimicrobial agents. *J Infect Dis.* 1977;135(suppl):S7–S12.

HISTORY

The class of lincosamide antibiotics received its name from the site where the bacterium that produced lincomycin was isolated: Lincoln, Nebraska.

Mason KJ, Dietz A, Deboer C. Lincomycin, a new antibiotic, I: discovery and biologic properties. *Antimicrob Agents Chemother.* 1962;2:554–559.

Streptogramins

Over the last few decades, we have found that certain combinations of antibiotics work synergistically to kill bacteria. Not surprisingly, bacteria themselves discovered this ages before we did. *Streptomyces* spp. naturally secrete pairs of antibiotics from the streptogramin family that work together to kill other bacteria. It is difficult to label the streptogramins as either old or new. They were isolated in 1953, but it was not until 1968 that the first agent of this class, pristinamycin, was marketed in Europe and not until 1999 that a pair of members of this group, quinupristin/dalfopristin, became available in the United States. Currently, quinupristin/dalfopristin in an intravenous formulation is the only streptogramin available in the United States.

Streptogramins consist of two different macrocyclic compounds (Fig. 6-9), each of which binds to the 50S subunit of the bacterial ribosome to inhibit protein synthesis. Whereas each component alone has moderate antibacterial activity, the two together are quite potent. This synergy is explained by the fact that each compound alone inhibits a different step in the process of protein elongation and that dalfopristin induces a conformational change in the ribosome that enhances binding of quinupristin.

Resistance to streptogramins occurs by three mechanisms: modification of the 50S ribosomal subunit such that a conformational change in the subunit prevents streptogramin binding, enzymatic inactivation of the streptogramins, and production of efflux pumps. Because quinupristin and dalfopristin bind to the same region of the

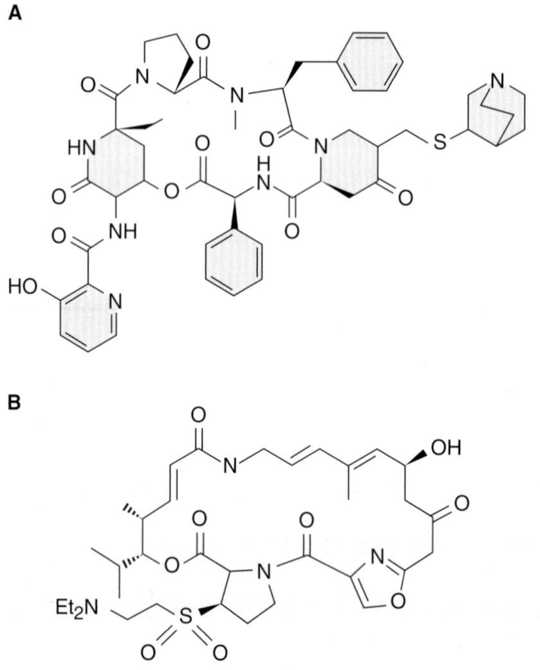

A. Quinupristin
B. Dalfopristin

FIGURE 6-9. The structure of quinupristin/dalfopristin.

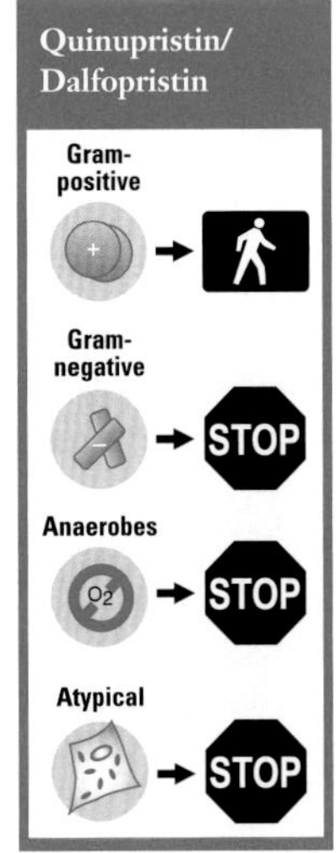

Table 6-13 Antimicrobial Activity of Quinupristin/Dalfopristin

Gram-positive bacteria	*Streptococcus pyogenes* Viridans group streptococci *Streptococcus pneumoniae* *Staphylococcus aureus* Some enterococci

ribosome as macrolides and clindamycin, the first of these mechanisms sometimes leads to cross-resistance between these three agents.

Quinupristin/dalfopristin has activity against a who's who list of troublesome aerobic gram-positive bacteria, including methicillin-resistant staphylococci, penicillin-resistant *S. pneumoniae*, and some vancomycin-resistant enterococci (Table 6-13). Most other aerobic gram-positive bacteria are also susceptible. Although quinupristin/dalfopristin has in vitro activity against some aerobic gram-negative bacteria and some anaerobic bacteria, its clinical efficacy in treating these infections is currently unclear, and it should not be used for these purposes.

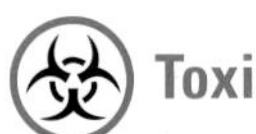

Toxicity

Adverse effects related to the site of infusion are very common when quinupristin/dalfopristin is given through a peripheral intravenous catheter. These include pain, inflammation, and thrombophlebitis. For this reason, it is recommended that this drug be given through a central venous catheter. Arthralgias, myalgias, and hyperbilirubinemia are also common. Quinupristin/dalfopristin inhibits the cytochrome P-450 system and can therefore affect the levels of other drugs.

Quinupristin/dalfopristin is active against highly resistant staphylococci, streptococci, and some enterococci. It is, however, associated with several adverse effects.

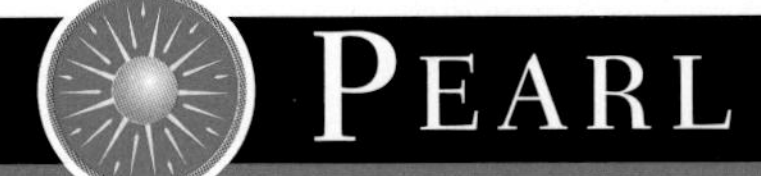

PEARL

Quinupristin/dalfopristin is active against *Enterococcus faecium* but not *Enterococcus faecalis. E. faecalis* actively pumps this antibiotic out of the bacterial cell.

Jones RN, Ballow CH, Biedenbach DJ, et al. Antimicrobial activity of quinupristin-dalfopristin (RP 59500, Synercid) tested against over 28,000 recent clinical isolates from 200 medical centers in the United States and Canada. *Diagn Microbiol Infect Dis.* 1998;31:437–451.

QUESTIONS

24. Streptogramins consist of ________________ antibiotics that work synergistically together.

25. Quinupristin/dalfopristin has excellent activity against aerobic ________________ bacteria.

26. The strength of quinupristin/dalfopristin is its activity against ________________-resistant staphylococci, ________________-resistant *Streptococcus pneumoniae*, and some ________________-resistant enterococci.

ADDITIONAL READING

Allington DR, Rivey MP. Quinupristin/dalfopristin: a therapeutic review. *Clin Ther*. 2001;23:24–44.

Bouanchaud DH. In-vitro and in-vivo antibacterial activity of quinupristin/dalfopristin. *J Antimicrob Chemother*. 1997;39(suppl A):15–21.

Cocito C, Di Giambattista M, Nyssen E, et al. Inhibition of protein synthesis by streptogramins and related antibiotics. *J Antimicrob Chemother*. 1997;39(suppl A):7–13.

Linezolid

Linezolid is a recently approved member of a novel class of antibacterial agents called *oxazolidinones*. Unlike many of the drugs discussed up to this point, which were isolated from bacteria or fungi, oxazolidinones are completely synthetic compounds. Linezolid's structure consists of an oxazolidinone core that has been modified at several sites (Fig. 6-10). By binding the 50S subunit of the bacterial ribosome, it prevents association of this subunit with the 30S subunit, thus precluding ribosome assembly. It also inhibits protein synthesis by preventing formation of the first peptide bond of the nascent peptide. Although linezolid is a new agent not found in nature and its structure unique among antimicrobial agents, resistance has already been detected. It is the consequence of a single amino acid mutation within the gene encoding a portion of the ribosome. Interestingly, some aerobic gram-negative bacilli such as *Escherichia coli* are intrinsically resistant to linezolid because they produce efflux pumps active against this compound.

Linezolid has excellent activity against most aerobic gram-positive bacteria, including methicillin-resistant staphylococci, penicillin-resistant *S. pneumoniae*, and vancomycin-resistant enterococci (Table 6-14). It also has in vitro activity against some aerobic gram-negative, anaerobic, and atypical bacteria, but it currently is not used to treat infections caused by these organisms. Linezolid is available in both oral and intravenous formulations and achieves similarly high serum levels when given by either route.

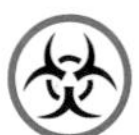

Toxicity

Linezolid is in general well tolerated. Like most antibiotics, it causes gastrointestinal symptoms such as nausea, vomiting, and diarrhea. Thrombocytopenia, anemia, and leukopenia occur relatively frequently but are reversible. Linezolid should not be given with monoamine oxidase (MAO) inhibitors. It should be used with caution with serotonin receptor inhibitors because this combination can lead to the serotonin syndrome, which consists of fever, agitation, mental status changes, and tremors.

Linezolid is an important addition to our antimicrobial armamentarium. This drug has excellent activity against aerobic gram-positive bacteria, including many of those resistant to other antibiotics.

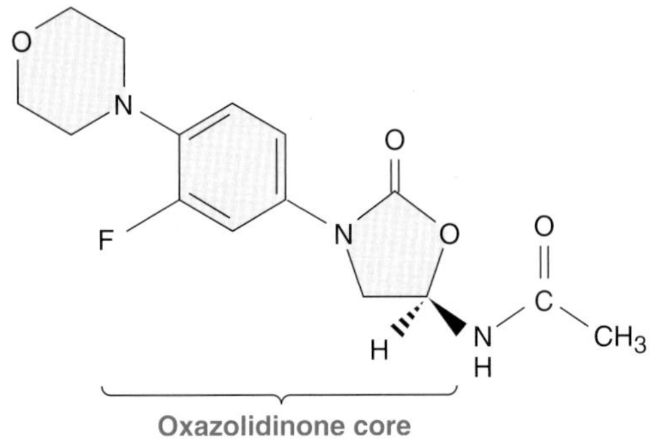

Oxazolidinone core

FIGURE 6-10. The structure of linezolid.

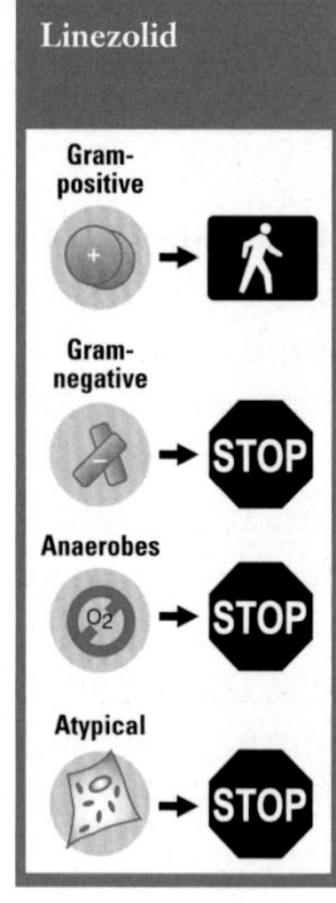

Table 6-14 Antimicrobial Activity of Linezolid

Gram-positive bacteria	*Streptococcus pyogenes* Viridans group streptococci *Streptococcus pneumoniae* Staphylococci Enterococci

QUESTIONS

27. Linezolid has excellent activity against resistant gram-positive bacteria such as ________________-resistant staphylococci and ________________-resistant enterococci.

28. This agent binds to bacterial ________________ and inhibits protein synthesis.

29. One advantage of linezolid is that it achieves similarly high serum levels whether given ________________ or ________________.

ADDITIONAL READINGS

Hamel JC, Stapert D, Moerman JK, et al. Linezolid, critical characteristics. *Infection*. 2000;28:60–64.

Moellering RC. Linezolid: the first oxazolidinone antimicrobial. *Ann Intern Med*. 2003;138:135–142.

Swaney SM, Aoki H, Ganoza MC, et al. The oxazolidinone linezolid inhibits initiation of protein synthesis in bacteria. *Antimicrob Agents Chemother*. 1998;42:3251–3255.

Nitrofurantoin

Nitrofurantoin is an old drug, having been first marketed in 1953. It belongs to a group of compounds called the *nitrofurans* (Fig. 6-11). Because nitrofurantoin achieves only low levels in the blood but is concentrated in urine, it has been used almost exclusively for the treatment of acute cystitis. It is not recommended for pyelonephritis because these infections are often associated with bacteremia. The mechanism of action of nitrofurantoin remains poorly characterized but it may bind ribosomes and inhibit translation. This, in turn, may adversely affect carbohydrate metabolism within bacteria. Nitrofurantoin has activity against many of the organisms that commonly cause urinary tract infections, including aerobic gram-negative bacteria (except *Proteus* spp. and *P. aeruginosa*) and aerobic gram-positive bacteria, such as enterococci and *Staphylococcus saprophyticus* (Table 6-15). Contributing to its longevity is that emergence of resistance has been rare. Nitrofurantoin is only available in an oral formulation.

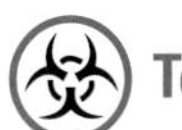

Toxicity

Nitrofurantoin use has been associated with several adverse reactions, including nausea, vomiting, rash, pulmonary hypersensitivity reactions and interstitial pneumonitis, hepatitis, hemolytic anemia, and peripheral neuropathy.

Nitrofurantoin is a "niche" antibiotic with excellent activity against many of the bacteria that commonly cause acute cystitis. It does not achieve therapeutically active levels in body tissues outside the urinary tract and should not be used to treat other types of infections.

QUESTIONS

30. Nitrofurantoin has excellent activity against many of the aerobic ______________ and ______________ bacteria that commonly cause acute cystitis.

31. Nitrofurantoin does not achieve high ______________ levels and therefore should not be used to treat systemic infections or pyelonephritis.

32. Despite decades of use, very little ______________ to nitrofurantoin has emerged.

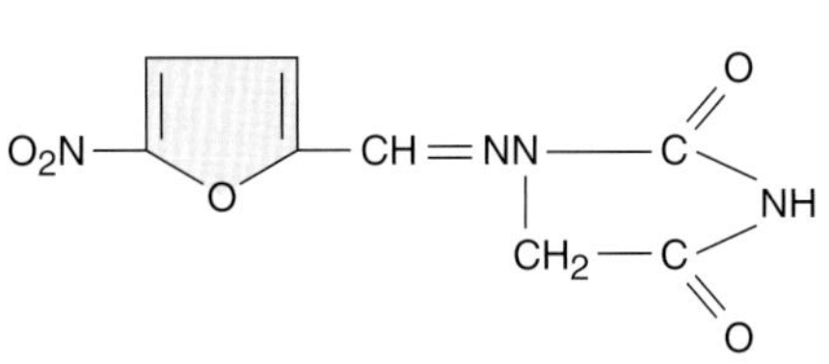

FIGURE 6-11. The structure of nitrofurantoin.

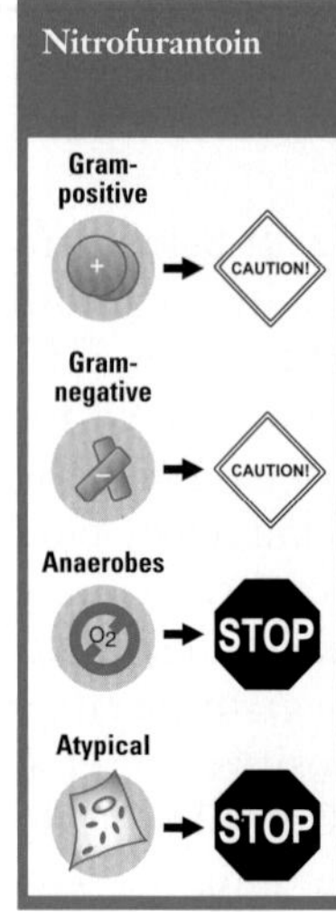

Table 6-15	Antimicrobial Activity of Nitrofurantoin*
Gram-positive bacteria	*Staphylococcus saprophyticus* Enterococci
Gram-negative bacteria	Most Enterobacteriaceae

*Only in context of acute cystitis.

ADDITIONAL READINGS

Cunha BA. Nitrofurantoin: an update. *Obstet Gynecol Surv*. 1989;44:399–406.

Cunha BA. New uses for older antibiotics: nitrofurantoin, amikacin, colistin, polymyxin B, doxycyline, and minocycline revisited. *Med Clin North Am*. 2006;90:1089–1107.

Mandell GL, Bennett JE, Dolin R. *Mandell, Douglas, and Bennett's Principles and Practice of Infectious Disease*. 7th ed. Philadelphia, PA: Churchill Livingstone/Elsevier; 2010:515–520.

CHAPTER 7

Antibiotics that Target DNA and Replication

"What made the French naval effort so formidable was their excellent Admiral, Jean de Vienne, whose aim was to control the Channel and prevent English reinforcements reaching Guyenne and Brittany."

—THE HUNDRED YEARS WAR, DESMOND SEWARD

In the battle between bacterial invaders and the human immune response, superiority in numbers is often crucial. Bacteria have an advantage in this regard because they are capable of rapidly dividing; in a sense, they continuously reinforce themselves through rapid replication. Several antibiotics block the arrival of these reinforcements by inhibiting bacterial DNA replication and thus bacterial multiplication. In the following sections, we will discuss these antimicrobial agents in detail.

Sulfa Drugs

Sulfa drugs are very old and date back to the early part of the 20th century. Thus, this class of antibiotics predates even the penicillins. In this section, we will discuss two members of this group that are still widely used: **trimethoprim-sulfamethoxazole** and **dapsone** (Table 7-1). A third member, sulfisoxazole, is used in conjunction with erythromycin to treat otitis media in children.

As its name suggests, trimethoprim-sulfamethoxazole is actually a combination of two antimicrobial agents: trimethoprim and sulfamethoxazole. Trimethoprim is not a sulfa drug but acts on the same general pathway as these drugs. It is not as old as the sulfa drugs but nonetheless traces its roots back to the 1950s and 1960s. The breakthrough in the development of trimethoprim-sulfamethoxazole, however, came when it was discovered in 1968 that these two agents had potent activity when used in combination. Over the past 30 years, trimethoprim-sulfamethoxazole has been used to treat various bacterial infections.

Trimethoprim-sulfamethoxazole inhibits bacterial growth by preventing the synthesis of *tetrahydrofolate* (THF), the active form of folic acid. THF is an essential cofactor for metabolic pathways that generate deoxynucleotides, which are the building blocks of DNA (Fig. 7-1). Sulfamethoxazole does this by mimicking *para*-aminobenzoate (PABA) and thereby competitively inhibiting the enzyme dihydropteroate synthase that normally incorporates PABA into the synthesis pathway of THF (Figs. 7-1 and 7-2). Trimethoprim, on the other hand, is a structural analog of dihydrofolate and therefore inhibits dihydrofolate reductase, which is required for conversion of dihydrofolate to THF (Figs. 7-1 and 7-3). Thus, these two antibiotics inhibit distinct steps in the same pathway, and in that way block the production of compounds essential for bacterial growth while decreasing the probability that bacterial resistance will develop. Nonetheless, the emergence of resistant strains has limited the use of trimethoprim-sulfamethoxazole. Bacteria become resistant to both of these agents by producing altered forms of their target enzymes that are not inhibited by the antibiotics or by changes in permeability that prevent the accumulation of the antibiotics within bacteria. Some strains overproduce PABA, which at high concentrations is capable of successfully competing with sulfamethoxazole for dihydropteroate synthase, resulting in sulfamethoxazole resistance.

Trimethoprim-sulfamethoxazole has activity against a broad range of aerobic gram-positive and aerobic gram-negative bacteria (Table 7-2). However, as might be expected with an agent that has been widely used for such an extended period,

Table 7-1 Sulfa Drugs

Parenteral Agents	Oral Agents
Trimethoprim-sulfamethoxazole	Trimethoprim-sulfamethoxazole
	Dapsone
	Sulfisoxazole (with erythromycin)

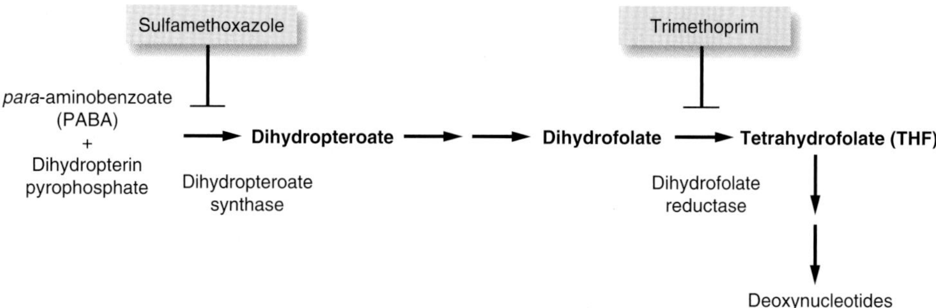

FIGURE 7-1. Inhibition of tetrahydrofolate synthesis by trimethoprim-sulfamethoxazole.

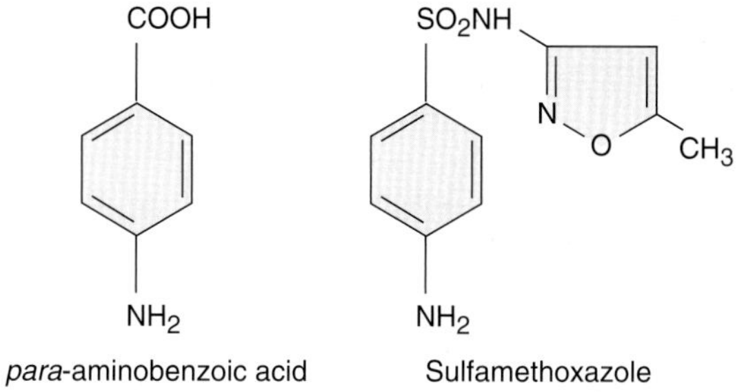

COOH

NH_2

para-aminobenzoic acid

SO_2NH

N O CH_3

NH_2

Sulfamethoxazole

FIGURE 7-2. The structure of sulfamethoxazole is similar to that of *para*-aminobenzoic acid.

NH_2 N N NH_2 CH_2 OCH_3 OCH_3 OCH_3

Trimethoprim

H_2N N H N N N OH CH_2 — N H O H CO_2H C — N — CH CH_2 CH_2 CO_2H

Dihydrofolic acid

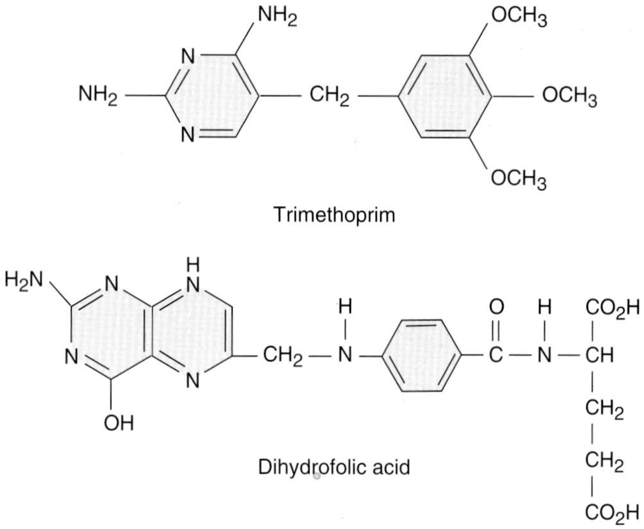

FIGURE 7-3. The structure of trimethoprim is similar to that of dihydrofolic acid.

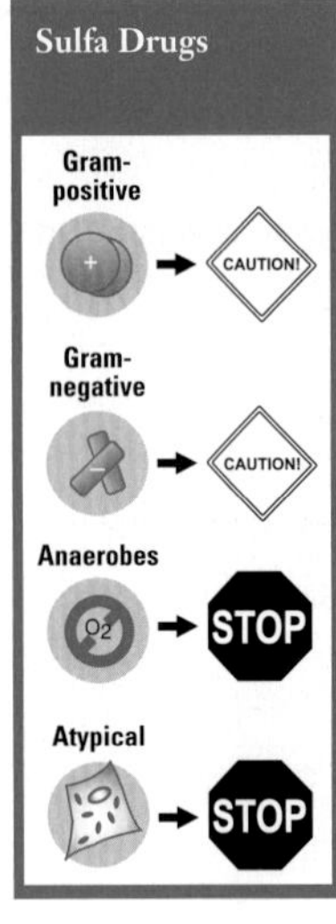

Table 7-2 Antimicrobial Activity of Sulfa Drugs

Trimethoprim-sulfamethoxazole	
Gram-positive bacteria	Some *Streptococcus pneumoniae* Some staphylococci *Listeria monocytogenes*
Gram-negative bacteria	Some *Haemophilus influenzae* Some Enterobacteriaceae
Dapsone	*Mycobacterium leprae*

many strains that were intrinsically susceptible have now acquired resistance. Still, many streptococci and staphylococci remain susceptible to this drug combination, as does *Listeria monocytogenes*. Some strains of Enterobacteriaceae such as *Escherichia coli*, *Salmonella* spp., and *Shigella* spp. are also susceptible, as are some strains of *Haemophilus influenzae*. Anaerobes and atypical bacteria tend to be resistant to trimethoprim-sulfamethoxazole. This agent is available in both oral and parenteral formulations. When given orally, both drugs are well absorbed, and serum levels approach those achieved with IV administration.

Dapsone is a second sulfa drug that is frequently used today. Its structure is related to that of sulfamethoxazole (Fig. 7-4) and it acts by the same mechanism. Its spectrum of activity, however, is quite distinct. Dapsone's use as an antibacterial agent is limited to the treatment of leprosy, which is caused by *Mycobacterium leprae* (Table 7-2).

FIGURE 7-4. Comparison of the structures of sulfamethoxazole and dapsone.

History

Sulfa drugs were the first antibacterial agents used in the United States. In 1935, sulfachrysoidine was used to treat a 10-year-old girl with meningitis caused by *Haemophilus influenzae*. The patient's father, who was a physician, had heard about the use of this sulfa drug in Germany to successfully treat bacterial infections. He therefore asked whether some sulfachrysoidine could be obtained for treatment of his daughter. This was done, but the therapy unfortunately failed and the girl died.

Carithers HA. The first use of an antibiotic in America. *Am J Dis Child.* 1974;128:207–211.

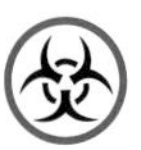

Toxicity

Because human cells do not synthesize folic acid, they lack dihydropteroate synthase, the target of sulfamethoxazole. Human cells do contain dihydrofolate reductase, which they use to recycle THF to dihydrofolate, but trimethoprim is 50,000 to 100,000 times more active against the bacterial enzyme than the human enzyme. Thus, one might expect that trimethoprim-sulfamethoxazole would be associated with relatively little toxicity, but this turns out not to be the case. It is associated with gastrointestinal effects as well as fever, rash (including Stevens-Johnson syndrome), leukopenia, thrombocytopenia, hepatitis, and hyperkalemia. For reasons that are unclear, HIV-infected individuals are particularly prone to trimethoprim-sulfamethoxazole toxicity. Dapsone causes similar adverse effects and, in addition, has been associated with hemolysis and methemoglobinemia.

Sulfa drugs are very old antibiotics that are still frequently used today. Trimethoprim-sulfamethoxazole is used for treatment of some infections caused by aerobic gram-positive and aerobic gram-negative bacteria. Dapsone is an agent of choice for leprosy.

Pearl

Some bacteria, like human cells, are capable of taking up folic acid from their environment and thus do not need to synthesize this factor. For example, enterococci are inhibited by trimethoprim-sulfamethoxazole when grown on laboratory medium, which does not contain folic acid. Trimethoprim-sulfamethoxazole, however, is not useful in treating enterococcal infections because these bacteria are capable of using folic acid present in the human body.

Wisell KT, Kahlmeter G, Giske CG. Trimethoprim and enterococci in urinary tract infections: new perspectives on an old issue. *J Antimicrob Chemother.* 2008;62:35–40.

QUESTIONS

1. Trimethoprim and sulfamethoxazole are structurally unrelated antibiotics that both inhibit the synthesis of ________________.
2. This combination of antibiotics has activity against some aerobic ________________ and aerobic ________________ bacteria.
3. Individuals infected with ________________ are particularly prone to the toxicity of trimethoprim-sulfamethoxazole.
4. Dapsone's primary antibacterial use is for the treatment of ________________.

ADDITIONAL READINGS

Burchall JJ. Mechanism of action of trimethoprim-sulfamethoxazole. II. *J Infect Dis.* 1973;128 (suppl):437–441.

Huovinen P. Increases in rates of resistance to trimethoprim. *Clin Infect Dis.* 1997;24(suppl 1): S63–S66.

Masters PA, O'Bryan TA, Zurlo J, et al. Trimethoprim-sulfamethoxazole revisited. *Arch Intern Med.* 2003;163:402–410.

Meyers WM. Leprosy. *Dermatol Clin.* 1992;10:73–96.

Quinolones

The **quinolones**, like the penicillins, are a group of antibiotics that resulted from serendipity flavored with a healthy dose of rational drug design. The discovery of this class of antimicrobial agents can be traced to the observation that a byproduct generated during the synthesis of chloroquine, an antimalarial compound, possessed modest activity against gram-negative bacteria. The subsequent modification of this compound has led to agents with potent activity against aerobic gram-negative, aerobic gram-positive, and even some anaerobic bacteria. Broad spectra of activity, high absorbance when given orally, and favorable toxicity profiles have caused the quinolones to become some of the most commonly used antibiotics today. Of the quinolones, **ciprofloxacin**, **levofloxacin**, **ofloxacin**, **moxifloxacin**, and **gemifloxacin** are the most frequently prescribed (Table 7-3).

All commercially available quinolones possess a core dual ring structure (Fig. 7-5). During modification of this core, it was discovered that addition of a fluorine enhanced potency, and, as a result, this alteration has been incorporated into all the quinolones commonly used today. For this reason, these drugs are called *fluoroquinolones* to distinguish them from older agents such as nalidixic acid that lacked this fluorine.

Quinolones work by inhibiting two topoisomerases, bacterial enzymes that regulate DNA supercoiling. These topoisomerases are named DNA gyrase and topoisomerase IV. Quinolones stabilize the complex that forms between topoisomerases and DNA at the stage of DNA strand breakage but before religation, resulting in the accumulation of double-stranded breaks in the chromosome. These breaks cause arrest of the DNA replication machinery, leading to inhibition of DNA synthesis and eventually bacterial death.

Resistance to quinolones results from spontaneous mutations that occur in specific regions of the genes encoding DNA gyrase and topoisomerase IV. Unfortunately, a single mutation in one of these genes is often sufficient to significantly reduce sensitivity to the quinolones. Bacteria with such a mutation are better able to survive in the presence of quinolones, thus allowing for the occurrence of secondary mutations over time that further increase the resistance to the quinolones. Eventually, bacteria with specific mutations in both the DNA gyrase and topoisomerase genes emerge; such bacteria are highly resistant to quinolones. Because a single mutation is capable of starting this process, it is not surprising that quinolone resistance is the

Table 7-3 The Quinolones

Parenteral Agents	Oral Agents
Ciprofloxacin	Ciprofloxacin
Levofloxacin	Levofloxacin
Moxifloxacin	Moxifloxacin
	Gemifloxacin
	Ofloxacin

FIGURE 7-5. The core structure of the quinolones.

major factor limiting the use of these agents. A second mechanism of resistance is the overexpression of efflux pumps in some bacteria. Because these efflux pumps tend to export several different antibiotics in addition to the quinolones, this can lead to cross-resistance between quinolones and other classes of antibiotics.

The quinolones have broad activity against various bacteria (Table 7-4). Their strength is their activity against aerobic gram-negative bacteria. In general, they are highly active against most members of the Enterobacteriaceae, *Haemophilus* spp., and *Neisseria* spp. They are also effective against some staphylococci and streptococci, many atypical bacteria, and even some mycobacteria.

CIPROFLOXACIN

Ciprofloxacin is one of the oldest fluoroquinolones still in common use. Like many of the fluoroquinolones, it contains a piperazine derivative at the R1 side chain, which greatly enhances its activity against aerobic gram-negative bacteria (Fig. 7-6). (Note that addition of a piperazine derivative to the penicillin core structure results in piperacillin, which also has enhanced activity against gram-negative bacteria.) It is the most potent of the quinolones against aerobic gram-negative bacteria and is effective against *Pseudomonas aeruginosa*. This is balanced by rather weak aerobic gram-positive

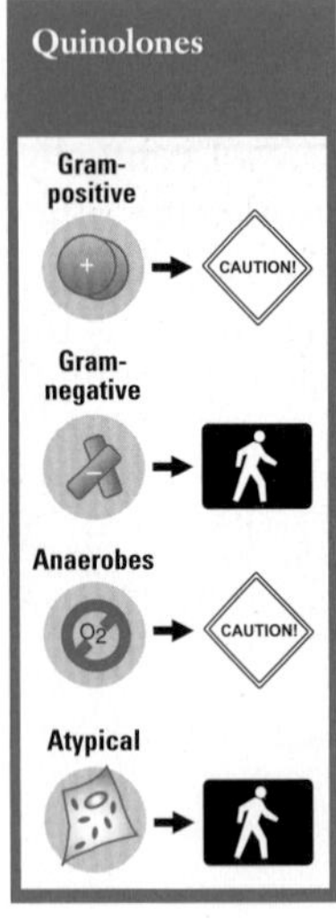

Table 7-4 Antimicrobial Activity of the Quinolones

Gram-positive bacteria	Some *Staphylococcus aureus* *Streptococcus pyogenes* Viridans group streptococci *Streptococcus pneumoniae*
Gram-negative bacteria	*Neisseria* spp. *Haemophilus influenzae* Many Enterobacteriaceae Some *Pseudomonas aeruginosa*
Anaerobic bacteria	Some *Clostridia* spp. Some *Bacteroides* spp.
Atypical bacteria	*Chlamydia* and *Chlamydophila* *Mycoplasma pneumoniae* *Legionella* spp.
Mycobacteria	*Mycobacterium tuberculosis* *Mycobacterium avium* complex *Mycobacterium leprae*

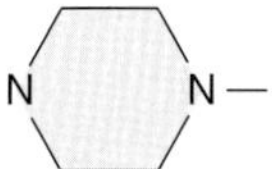

FIGURE 7-6. The R1 side chain of ciprofloxacin is a piperazine derivative, which enhances activity against aerobic gram-negative bacteria.

activity. For example, ciprofloxacin should not be used to treat severe infections caused by *Streptococcus pneumoniae*. Ciprofloxacin is also active against many atypical bacteria and some mycobacteria.

LEVOFLOXACIN AND OFLOXACIN

Structurally, levofloxacin and ofloxacin are very closely related. *Ofloxacin* is a racemic mixture of an active and an inactive stereoisomer, whereas *levofloxacin* is composed solely of the active stereoisomer. Thus, these two agents have the same spectra of activity, but levofloxacin is generally twofold more potent and, as a result, more commonly used. Levofloxacin is not quite as active as ciprofloxacin against aerobic gram-negative bacteria but is still effective against infections caused by most of these bacteria, including *P. aeruginosa*. Relative to ciprofloxacin, levofloxacin has enhanced activity against aerobic gram-positive bacteria and is effective in the treatment of severe infections caused by *S. pneumoniae*, including those strains that are penicillin resistant.

MOXIFLOXACIN AND GEMIFLOXACIN

These newer agents, especially gemifloxacin, have enhanced activity against *S. pneumoniae* (including penicillin-resistant strains) and atypical bacteria. This comes at the expense of aerobic gram-negative activity, especially against *P. aeruginosa*. Moxifloxacin contains a methoxy group at R2, which increases potency against anaerobic bacteria (Fig. 7-7).

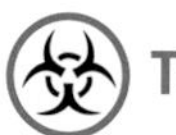

Toxicity

Because human gyrases and topoisomerases are quite dissimilar to the corresponding bacterial enzymes, quinolones are in general well tolerated. Gastrointestinal symptoms are the most common side effect, seen in 5% to 10% of individuals taking these agents. Adverse effects involving the central nervous system such as headache and dizziness occur in approximately 5% of patients, whereas rashes occur in approximately 1% to 2%. Quinolones cause cartilage abnormalities in juvenile animals, so they should be avoided when possible in children younger than 18 years of age and not used at all in pregnant women. Achilles tendon rupture has been reported in the elderly. Quinolone use has been associated with prolongation of the QT interval on electrocardiograms. Thus, these agents may predispose to ventricular arrhythmias

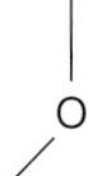

FIGURE 7-7. The R2 side chain of moxifloxacin is a methoxy group, which enhances activity against anaerobic bacteria.

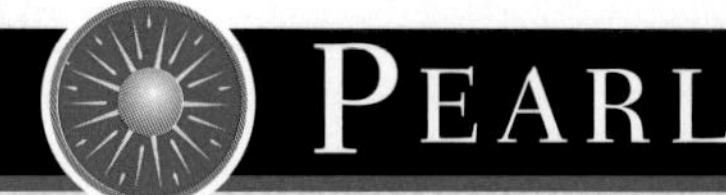

In general, the quinolones have good activity against *Streptococcus pneumoniae* and are especially useful for infections caused by penicillin-resistant strains of this bacterium. However, ciprofloxacin should be used with caution in the treatment of serious infections caused by *S. pneumoniae* because treatment failures have been reported.

Mandell LA, Wunderink RG, Anzueto A, et al. Infectious Diseases Society of America/American Thoracic Society consensus guidelines on the management of community-acquired pneumonia in adults. *Clin Infect Dis.* 2007;44(suppl 2):S27–S72.

such as torsades de pointes, especially when they are used in conjunction with other agents that also prolong the QT interval. Some reports suggest that quinolone use results in the development of *Clostridium difficile*–associated diarrhea more frequently than most antibiotics.

Quinolones are relatively well-tolerated antibiotics that are useful in treating infections caused by aerobic gram-negative bacteria, atypical bacteria, and some aerobic gram-positive bacteria and mycobacteria. Some members also have activity against *P. aeruginosa* or anaerobic bacteria.

Questions

5. The fluoroquinolones are most useful in the treatment of aerobic ______________ infections, although they also have activity against aerobic ______________ bacteria, atypical bacteria, and mycobacteria.
6. Of the fluoroquinolones, ______________ is most active against *Pseudomonas aeruginosa.*
7. ______________ is the most active quinolone against anaerobic bacteria.
8. The quinolones target bacterial ______________ and ______________, which leads to breaks in the bacterial chromosome.
9. Fluoroquinolones should be given to children with caution because of concerns about possible damage to ______________.

Additional Readings

Andriole VT. The quinolones: past, present, and future. *Clin Infect Dis.* 2005;41(suppl 2):S113–S119.
Domagala JM. Structure-activity and structure-side-effect relationships for the quinolone antibacterials. *J Antimicrob Chemother.* 1994;33:685–706.
Jacoby GA. Mechanisms of resistance to quinolones. *Clin Infect Dis.* 2005;41(suppl 2):S120–S126.
O'Donnell JA, Gelone SP. Fluoroquinolones. *Infect Dis Clin North Am.* 2000;14:489–513.
Saravolatz LD, Leggett J. Gatifloxacin, gemifloxacin, and moxifloxacin: the role of 3 newer fluoroquinolones. *Clin Infect Dis.* 2003;37:1210–1215.
Stein GE, Goldstein EJ. Fluoroquinolones and anaerobes. *Clin Infect Dis.* 2006;42:1598–1607.

Metronidazole

Metronidazole, a 5-nitroimidazole, was discovered in the 1950s. It continues to be an important and frequently used antibiotic for the treatment of infections caused by anaerobic bacteria.

Metronidazole is a small molecule that can passively diffuse into bacteria. An important component of its structure is a nitro group that extends from the core five-membered ring (Fig. 7-8). This group must be reduced (i.e., accept electrons) for metronidazole to be active. As part of their metabolic machinery, anaerobic bacteria possess low redox potential electron transport proteins, which are capable of donating electrons to this nitro group. Aerobic bacteria, however, lack these proteins, perhaps because they are incompatible with the presence of oxygen, which itself is an extremely potent electron acceptor. For this reason, metronidazole's spectrum of activity is limited to obligate anaerobic bacteria and some microaerophilic bacteria that normally thrive in the presence of low concentrations of oxygen. Once reduced, the nitro group is thought to form free radicals that lead to breaks in DNA molecules and subsequent bacterial death.

Resistance to metronidazole is rare among obligate anaerobic bacteria. When it does occur, it is thought to result from a decrease in the capacity of the electron transport proteins to reduce the nitro group of metronidazole. The development of resistance in the microaerophilic bacterium *Helicobacter pylori* is more common, although the mechanism remains unclear.

Metronidazole is effective against nearly all anaerobic gram-negative bacteria, including *Bacteroides fragilis*, and most anaerobic gram-positive bacteria, including *Clostridium* spp. (Table 7-5). It is one of the few antibiotics that has activity against *C. difficile* and is the treatment of choice for infections caused by this organism. The microaerophilic (i.e., optimal growth in low levels of oxygen) bacterium *H. pylori* is also frequently susceptible.

Both oral and IV formulations of metronidazole are available. Oral metronidazole is extremely well absorbed and results in serum levels comparable to those following IV administration.

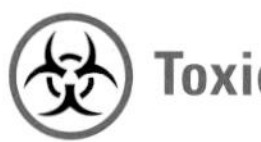

Toxicity

Metronidazole is relatively well tolerated but is associated with some minor toxicities, such as nausea and epigastric discomfort. It can also cause an unpleasant metallic taste and furring of the tongue. Occasionally, metronidazole is associated with neurologic complaints, including headache, dizziness, and peripheral neuropathy. Metronidazole

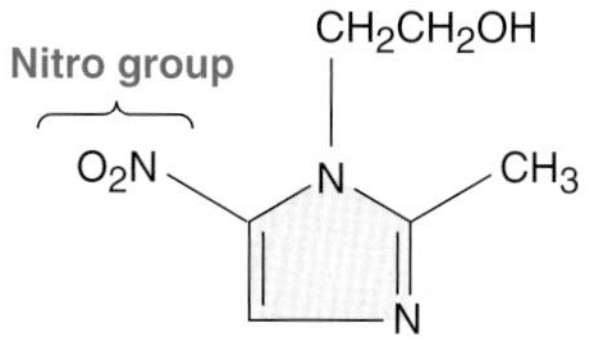

Nitro group
CH_2CH_2OH
O_2N N CH_3
N

FIGURE 7-8. The structure of metronidazole.

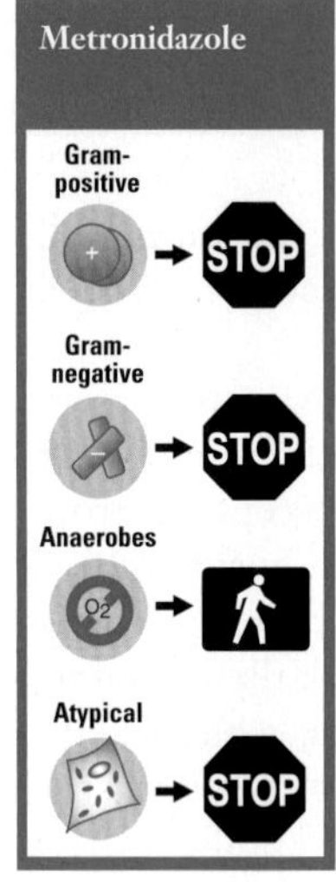

Table 7-5 Antimicrobial Activity of Metronidazole

Anaerobic bacteria	*Bacteroides fragilis* *Clostridium* spp. Most other anaerobes

can lead to a disulfiram-like reaction; ingestion of alcohol should be avoided while taking this drug.

Metronidazole retains excellent activity against obligate anaerobic bacteria and is useful in the treatment of some microaerophilic bacteria, such as *H. pylori*.

Questions

10. Metronidazole has excellent activity against most ________________ bacteria.

11. Metronidazole also has activity against some ________________ bacteria, such as *Helicobacter pylori*.

12. Aerobic bacteria are not killed by metronidazole because they do not ________________ its nitro group.

Additional Readings

Bartlett JG. Metronidazole. *Johns Hopkins Med J*. 1981;149:89–92.
Edwards DI. Nitroimidazole drugs—action and resistance mechanisms. I. Mechanisms of action. *J Antimicrob Chemother*. 1993;31:9–20.
Finegold SM. Metronidazole. *Ann Intern Med*. 1980;93:585–587.

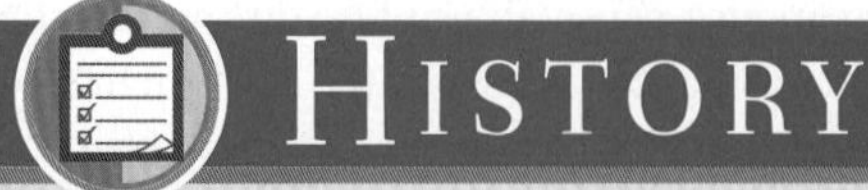

History

Metronidazole was discovered because of its activity against protozoans. However, a patient being treated with metronidazole for *Trichomonas vaginalis* vaginitis, a protozoan infection, was noted to have marked improvement in her gingivitis, which was caused by anaerobic bacteria. This led to investigations of metronidazole's activity against anaerobic bacteria.

Mascaretti OA. *Bacteria versus Antibacterial Agents: An Integrated Approach*. Washington, DC: ASM Press; 2003.

CHAPTER 8

Antimycobacterial Agents

"I do not know nor can I tell all the horrors nor all the tortures that they did to wretched men in this land. And it lasted the 19 years while Stephen was king, and it always grew worse and worse. . . . They robbed and burned all the villages, so that you could well go a whole day's journey and never find anyone occupying a village or land tilled. Then corn was dear, and flesh and cheese and butter, because there was none in the land. Wretched men starved with hunger. . . . Wherever men tilled, the earth bore no corn because the land was all done for by such doings; and they said openly that Christ and His saints slept. Such things, and more than we know how to tell, we suffered 19 years for our sins."

—THE ANGLO-SAXON CHRONICLES, TRANSLATED AND EDITED BY MICHAEL SWANTON

Like residents of regions devastated by prolonged wars, patients afflicted with mycobacterial infections tend to become weakened and emaciated, and may even die due to the chronicity of the disease process. These slowly progressing infections are caused by bacteria that are themselves slow growing. Because many antimicrobial agents have poor activity against slowly dividing bacteria, mycobacteria are prone to develop resistance to antibiotics. As a result, treatment of infections caused by mycobacteria requires multiple antimicrobial agents for extended periods. Different species of mycobacteria cause different diseases, each of which requires its own unique therapeutic regimen. In this chapter, we will focus on several agents used for the treatment of common mycobacterial infections.

Tuberculosis is caused by *Mycobacterium tuberculosis*. *Mycobacterium avium* complex is a group of mycobacteria that frequently cause disease in immunocompromised hosts, particularly those infected with HIV. The disfiguring disease leprosy is caused by *Mycobacterium leprae*. A long list of other mycobacteria, often referred to as atypical mycobacteria, also cause various diseases in humans. Agents commonly used to treat mycobacterial infections include **isoniazid**, **rifampin**, **rifabutin**, **pyrazinamide**, **ethambutol**, **clarithromycin**, and **azithromycin**. Other agents occasionally used in the treatment of mycobacterial infections include amikacin, streptomycin, cycloserine, ethionamide, capreomycin *p*-aminosalicylic acid, clofazimine, dapsone, and the quinolones.

ISONIAZID

Isoniazid has little activity against most bacteria but is capable of killing both intracellular and extracellular *M. tuberculosis*. It is thought to inhibit an enzyme essential for the synthesis of mycolic acid, an important constituent of the *M. tuberculosis* cell envelope. This may explain the specificity of isoniazid for mycobacteria because other bacteria do not make mycolic acid. Resistance occurs with mutations in the gene that encodes catalase-peroxidase, which is required to convert isoniazid to its active form. Likewise, mutations in the gene encoding the target enzyme essential for mycolic acid synthesis also result in resistance. Isoniazid is associated with rash, fever, hepatotoxicity, and peripheral neuropathy. The prophylactic administration of pyridoxine prevents neuropathy.

RIFAMPIN, RIFABUTIN, AND RIFAPENTINE

Unlike isoniazid, the rifamycins are active against a broad spectrum of bacteria. These agents, which inhibit bacterial RNA polymerase, are discussed in more detail in the "Rifamycins" section. Mycobacteria readily become resistant to rifamycins when they are used as monotherapy. Resistance is the result of mutations in the gene that encodes RNA polymerase.

PYRAZINAMIDE

Like isoniazid, pyrazinamide targets an enzyme essential for the synthesis of mycolic acid. This agent only kills mycobacteria at acidic pH. Fortunately, intracellular *M. tuberculosis* resides within an acidic phagosome. Consequently, this drug is active against intracellular organisms. Resistance results from mutations in the gene encoding pyrazinamidase, an enzyme essential for converting pyrazinamide into its active form. Adverse effects include hepatotoxicity and elevated serum levels of uric acid, which may lead to gout.

ETHAMBUTOL

Ethambutol targets an enzyme involved in the synthesis of the mycobacterial cell wall. Mutations in the gene encoding this enzyme result in resistance. The major toxicity is optic neuritis, which may lead to decreased visual acuity and red–green discrimination.

CLARITHROMYCIN AND AZITHROMYCIN

Clarithromycin and azithromycin prevent protein translation by targeting the ribosomes of many different bacteria, including some mycobacteria. These agents are discussed in more detail in the "Macrolides" section.

Several antibiotics are active against mycobacteria. Some of these agents, such as isoniazid, are used specifically to treat mycobacterial infections, whereas other agents, such as rifampin, show activity against a broad range of bacterial genera. Because mycobacteria are prone to develop resistance to antimicrobial compounds and are difficult to eradicate, treatment regimens usually contain multiple agents and continue for months. Toxicity is problematic and must be carefully monitored over the extended periods that these agents are given.

QUESTIONS

1. Mycobacterial infections are usually treated with ______________ drugs for extended periods.
2. ______________, ______________, ______________, and ______________ are first-line agents for the treatment of *Mycobacterium tuberculosis*.
3. Isoniazid, rifampin, and pyrazinamide all may cause ______________.

ADDITIONAL READINGS

Blumberg HM, Burman WJ, Chaisson RE, et al. American Thoracic Society/Centers for Disease Control and Prevention/Infectious Diseases Society of America: treatment of tuberculosis. *Am J Respir Crit Care Med.* 2003;167:603–662.

Di Perri G, Bonora S. Which agents should we use for the treatment of multidrug-resistant Mycobacterium tuberculosis? *J Antimicrob Chemother.* 2004;54:593–602.

Petri WA Jr. Drugs used in the chemotherapy of tuberculosis, Mycobacterium avium complex disease, and leprosy. In: Brunton LL, Lazo JS, Parker KL, eds. *Goodman and Gilman's The Pharmacological Basis of Therapeutics.* 11th ed. New York, NY: The McGraw-Hill Companies; 2006:1203–1224.

Vilchèze C, Wang F, Arai M, et al. Transfer of a point mutation in Mycobacterium tuberculosis inhA resolves the target of isoniazid. *Nature Med.* 2006;12:1027–1029.

CHAPTER 9

Summary of Antibacterial Agents

Now let us take a deep breath and review what we have learned. Probably, the most apparent fact is that there are a lot of antibiotics used to treat bacterial infections! Certainly, it has gotten progressively more difficult to master this topic over the years as more and more antimicrobial agents have been developed. Yet, by grouping these agents based on their spectra of activity, the subject becomes manageable.

Let's start with aerobic gram-positive bacteria. A quick review of the antibiotics in the preceding sections indicates that certain agents have robust activity against gram-positive organisms, whereas other agents have modest activity and still others have very limited or no activity (Fig. 9-1). Those agents with activity against most gram-positive bacteria are β-lactam/β-lactamase inhibitor combinations, carbapenems, glycopeptides, streptogramins, linezolid, and daptomycin. When empirically treating probable gram-positive infections, use of one of these agents will likely be effective. Remember this group of high-power agents! However, even these antibiotics are not perfect—each has its weaknesses. For example, carbapenems and β-lactam/β-lactamase inhibitor combinations are not active against methicillin-resistant *Staphylococcus aureus*. Obviously, vancomycin will not kill vancomycin-resistant enterococci. The streptogramins quinupristin/dalfopristin are not active against *Enterococcus faecalis*. Resistance to linezolid and daptomycin has already been reported among gram-positive bacteria. So do not forget to check susceptibilities and modify treatment accordingly. Many agents have modest activity against gram-positive bacteria (Fig. 9-1). These antibiotics are active against some gram-positive bacteria but not others. Some, such as aminoglycosides and the rifampins, should only be used in combination with other agents active against this class of bacteria.

Aerobic gram-negative bacteria are particularly troublesome causes of infection, and a large number of antimicrobial agents have been developed to target these bacteria (Fig. 9-2). Those with the broadest activity include extended-spectrum penicillin/β-lactamase inhibitor combinations, third-, fourth-, and fifth-generation cephalosporins, carbapenems, monobactams, aminoglycosides, colistin, and quinolones. These agents share the ability to penetrate the outer membrane barrier of most gram-negative pathogens and avoid inactivation by common resistance mechanisms. Nonetheless, a significant number of gram-negative bacteria will be resistant to agents in one or more of these classes, and susceptibilities of individual bacterial strains must still be checked to ensure optimal therapy. A second group of antibiotics has modest activity against gram-negative bacteria; these agents are useful in the treatment of infections caused by some gram-negative bacteria (Fig. 9-2).

Anaerobic bacteria have a propensity to cause mixed infections and are difficult to culture. As a result, these infections are often treated empirically, which requires a thorough understanding of the spectra of activity of individual antibiotics. Five groups of agents are active against an especially broad range of anaerobic bacteria: the aminopenicillin/β-lactamase inhibitor combinations, the extended-spectrum

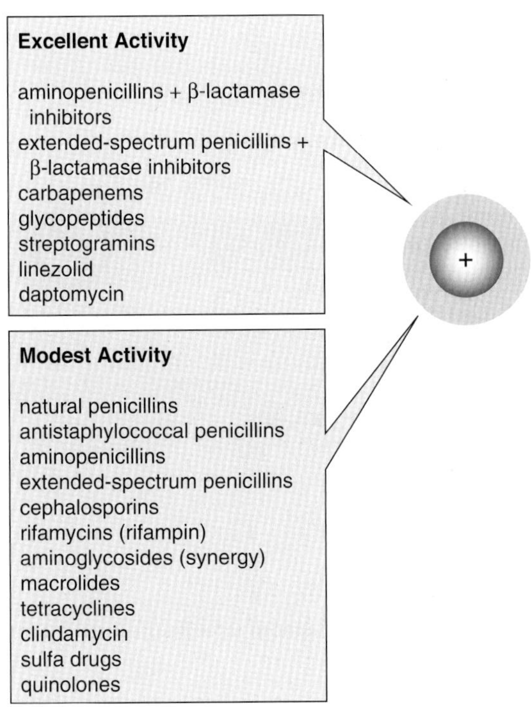

FIGURE 9-1. Antibiotics for the treatment of infections caused by aerobic gram-positive bacteria.

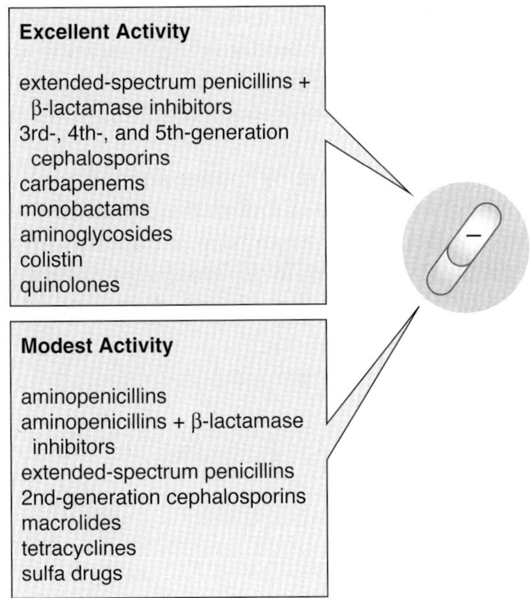

FIGURE 9-2. Antibiotics for the treatment of infections caused by aerobic gram-negative bacteria.

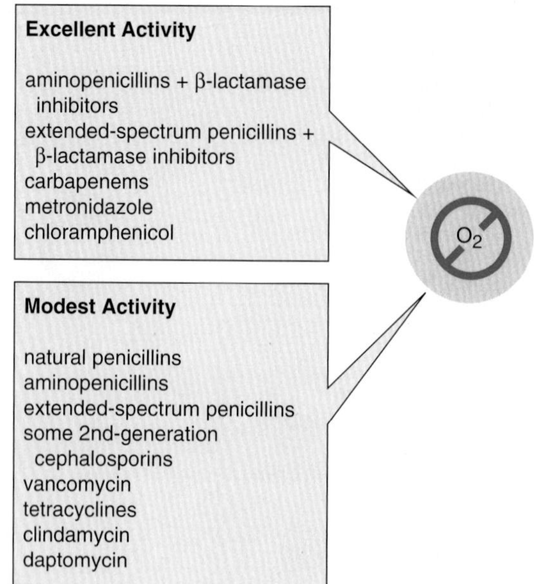

FIGURE 9-3. Antibiotics for the treatment of infections caused by anaerobic bacteria.

penicillin/β-lactamase inhibitor combinations, the carbapenems, metronidazole, and chloramphenicol (Fig. 9-3). These agents will effectively treat most anaerobic bacteria encountered in clinical practice. One important exception is *Clostridium difficile*, a cause of antibiotic-associated diarrhea, which is reliably susceptible to only metronidazole and vancomycin. Although lacking the near-universal spectra of activity of the first group of agents, a large number of antibiotics are still useful in the treatment of anaerobic infections and make up a second tier of anaerobic drugs (Fig. 9-3). These agents are used to treat infections caused by one or a subset of anaerobic bacteria with known susceptibilities.

Atypical bacteria are hard to visualize by routine methods such as Gram staining or are difficult to grow on laboratory media. Although this classification is not perfect, it does allow for a way of thinking about this diverse group of bacteria with regard to antimicrobial therapy. Some of the bacteria included in this group are *Chlamydia/Chlamydophila* spp., *Mycoplasma* spp., *Legionella pneumophila*, *Brucella* spp., *Francisella tularensis*, and *Rickettsia*

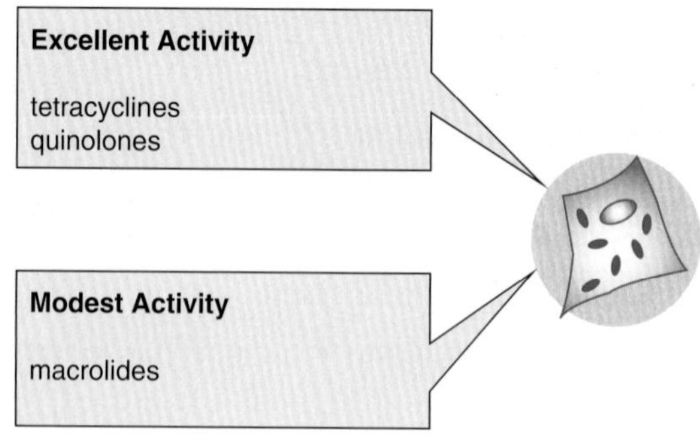

FIGURE 9-4. Antibiotics for the treatment of infections caused by atypical bacteria.

spp. Many of these bacteria reside within macrophages or other host cell types. As a result, antibiotics that penetrate well into host cells have the best activity against these organisms. These include the tetracyclines and the quinolones (Fig. 9-4). The macrolides are also effective against infections caused by many of these bacteria.

Knowing which antibiotic classes have activity against the different groups of bacteria is a useful way to learn how to choose appropriate antimicrobial agents. However, one must remember that the antimicrobial activity of agents within some classes differs significantly. For example, the quinolones are not listed as having anaerobic activity, yet moxifloxacin is effective against infections caused by some of these bacteria. Likewise, tigecycline and telithromycin have much broader activity than the other members of the tetracycline- and macrolide-like antibiotics, respectively. Thus, the activities summarized in this chapter should be thought of as general guidelines with many exceptions.

PART III

Definitive Therapy

"You can attain proficiency in this path by seeing through the opponent's strategy, and by knowing the strengths and weaknesses of the opponent's tactics."

—THE BOOK OF FIVE RINGS, MIYAMOTO MUSASHI

The choice of which antibiotic to prescribe for the treatment of a bacterial infection usually must be made in one of three types of situations. First, a patient may be suspected or known to have a bacterial infection, but the bacterial species responsible for the illness has not yet been identified. Treatment in such cases is referred to as **empiric therapy** and consists of an antimicrobial agent or agents that are active against the bacteria most associated with the disease syndrome (e.g., community-acquired pneumonia) afflicting the patient. Often in such cases, clinical samples will be obtained prior to starting antimicrobial therapy, and these samples will be cultured or otherwise tested in an attempt to identify the causative bacterium. If the bacterial species responsible for the illness is identified, therapy is narrowed to specifically target this particular organism. For example, a sputum sample obtained from a patient with community-acquired pneumonia may grow *Streptococcus pneumoniae*, and it is then the clinician's job to choose the best antibiotic regimen to treat the pneumonia. The prescribed regimen would be referred to as **definitive therapy** because the causative organism is known. A final decision regarding antimicrobial therapy must often be made several days later, when the antibiotic susceptibilities of the cultured bacterium are reported. At that time, activity, cost, convenience of dosing, penetration, and other factors are used to choose the most appropriate antibiotic from the list of agents to which the bacterium is susceptible.

In this section, we will focus on definitive therapy. Essential to choosing the best antimicrobial regimens for definitive therapy is knowing which antibiotics have activity against the individual bacterial pathogens, so we will discuss the preferred antimicrobial agents for the bacteria most commonly encountered in clinical practice. The emphasis will be on parenteral agents used to treat severe infections. As in the preceding sections, we will somewhat arbitrarily divide the common bacterial pathogens into the following groups: gram-positive bacteria, gram-negative bacteria, anaerobic bacteria, and atypical bacteria. In this way, the information presented in this section will review and solidify the knowledge you have gained in the preceding section. Two additional groups of bacteria will also be discussed: spirochetes and mycobacteria.

Note that in clinical practice, a large variety of factors enter into the decision of which antimicrobial agent is prescribed for a particular patient. Consideration is given to the allergy profile of the patient, the penetration of different agents to the site of infection, cost, ease of administration, and the recent antibiotic exposure history, which may suggest a risk of resistance to certain agents. To prevent the emergence of resistance, it is often preferred to use an agent with a narrow spectrum of activity over one with a broad spectrum of activity. Here, however, we will focus only on the susceptibility of specific kinds of bacteria to antibiotics, because this is the point from which most prescribing decisions begin.

CHAPTER 10

Gram-Positive Bacteria

"'A terrible worm in an iron cocoon,' as he was called in an anonymous poem, the knight rode on a saddle rising in a higher ridge above the horse's backbone with his feet resting in very long stirrups so that he was virtually standing up and able to deliver tremendous swinging blows from side to side with any one of his armory of weapons. He began battle with the lance used for unhorsing the enemy, while from his belt hung a two-handed sword at one side and an eighteen-inch dagger on the other. He also had available, either attached to his saddle or carried by his squire, a longer sword for thrusting like a lance, a battle-ax fitted with a spike behind the curved blade, and a club-headed mace with sharpened, ridged edges, a weapon favored by martial bishops and abbots on the theory that it did not come under the rule forbidding clerics 'to smite with the edge of the sword.'"

—A Distant Mirror, Barbara W. Tuchman

Like the medieval knight, gram-positive bacteria harbor an impressive array of offensive and defensive weapons. For protection, they utilize a thick and rigid cell wall. From behind this armor, they brandish an imposing number of toxins designed to subdue the host. These attributes make them formidable foes in their battles against the defenses of the human body.

After a period of relative calm, gram-positive bacteria have burst upon the scene in recent years to once again garner notoriety as causes of serious and difficult-to-treat infections. Much of this is due to marked increases in antibiotic resistance among these bacteria, most notably methicillin resistance in *Staphylococcus aureus*, decreased susceptibility to penicillin in *Streptococcus pneumoniae*, and vancomycin resistance in the enterococci. In this section, we will review some of the major gram-positive pathogens: staphylococci, pneumococci, other streptococci, enterococci, *Listeria monocytogenes*, and *Bacillus anthracis*. We will focus on the appropriate antimicrobial treatment for infections caused by each of these organisms.

Staphylococci

Three species of staphylococci are of major medical importance: *S. aureus*, *Staphylococcus epidermidis*, and *Staphylococcus saprophyticus*. *S. aureus* is the "workaholic" of bacterial pathogens. Not only is this organism a frequent cause of human infections, but it also brings about a remarkable variety of disease manifestations, including bacteremia, endocarditis, skin and soft tissue infections, osteomyelitis, pneumonia, and toxic shock syndrome (Fig. 10-1). It does so by producing a plethora of toxins that damage the host or manipulate its immune response. *S. aureus* is a gram-positive coccus that grows in grape-like clusters and often forms yellow-golden–colored colonies on agar plates (hence the name *aureus*, which means gold). *S. epidermidis* is the most important member of a larger group of bacteria referred to as *coagulase-negative staphylococci*. These bacteria are morphologically similar to *S. aureus* but are less virulent and less versatile. They are mainly associated with infections involving foreign objects, such as intravenous catheters, prosthetic heart valves, and prosthetic joints. *S. saprophyticus* is a member of the coagulase-negative staphylococci that causes community-acquired urinary tract infections.

A historical overview of the attempts to treat *S. aureus* infections is illustrative of the ability of bacteria to counter our best efforts at antimicrobial containment (Fig. 10-2). In the 1940s and 1950s, infections caused by *S. aureus* were treated with **penicillin**, which was active against the thick cell wall of this bacterium. Resistance, however, soon developed in the form of bacteria producing β-lactamases that efficiently cleaved penicillin

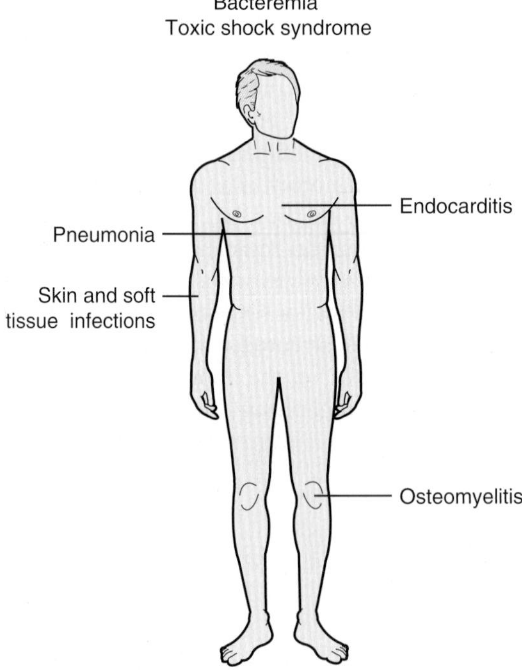

FIGURE 10-1. Sites of *Staphylococcus aureus* infections.

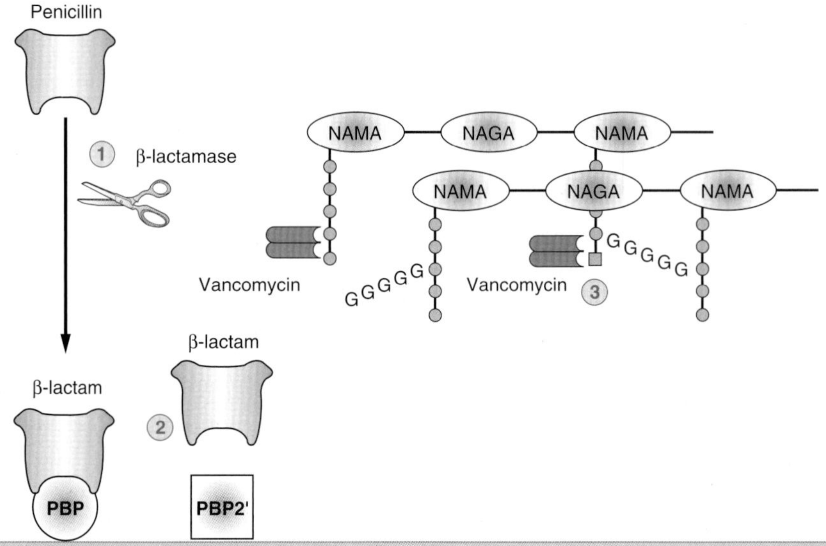

FIGURE 10-2. Mechanisms by which *Staphylococcus aureus* resists the action of antibiotics. **(1)** Although penicillin was initially effective against this bacterium, most strains now produce β-lactamases that cleave penicillin. For this reason, antistaphylococcal penicillins that are resistant to cleavage by staphylococcal β-lactamases were developed. **(2)** Methicillin-resistant *S. aureus* (MRSA) strains, however, produce an altered penicillin-binding protein (PBP) (referred to as PBP2′) that is not recognized by these compounds or other β-lactam agents. Vancomycin, a glycopeptide, overcomes this difficulty by binding to the terminal alanine–alanine group of the peptide side chain of peptidoglycan and thus inhibits peptidoglycan cross-linking without binding to PBPs. **(3)** Vancomycin-resistant strains of *S. aureus* are now being identified. Some of these strains have become resistant to vancomycin by altering the structure of the peptide side chain of newly formed peptidoglycan subunits so that they are not recognized by vancomycin.

(step 1 in Fig. 10-2). Fortunately, antistaphylococcal penicillins, which are modified to resist cleavage by staphylococcal β-lactamases, became available and were highly active against *S. aureus*. This group of agents includes **nafcillin**, **oxacillin**, and methicillin (the last of which is no longer available in the United States) (Table 10-1). Because of their narrow spectra and potency, these antibiotics remain the drugs of choice for many infections caused by *S. aureus*. In addition, cephalosporins resistant to cleavage by the staphylococcal β-lactamases were also developed. First-generation cephalosporins (e.g., **cefazolin**) and some second-generation cephalosporins (e.g., **cefuroxime**) are quite potent in this regard, while third-generation cephalosporins (e.g., **ceftriaxone**, **cefotaxime**) are less potent. Later, the β-lactamase inhibitors clavulanate, sulbactam, and tazobactam, which inactivate the staphylococcal β-lactamases, were developed. Thus, β-lactam/β-lactamase inhibitor combinations, such as **ampicillin-sulbactam**, **piperacillin-tazobactam**, and **ticarcillin-clavulanate**, are now available for the treatment of infections caused by *S. aureus*. Likewise, some carbapenems (**imipenem**, **meropenem**, **doripenem**) are not hydrolyzed by these β-lactamases and are also useful in the treatment of infections caused by this bacterium.

The ever-resourceful *S. aureus* again countered, however, by altering one of its PBPs (step 2 in Fig. 10-2). The variant PBP is called PBP2′, and it does not bind any of the β-lactam compounds. Thus, PBP2′-producing strains of *S. aureus*, referred to as

Table 10-1 Antimicrobial Agents for Treatment of Infections Caused by *Staphylococcus Aureus*

Antibiotic Class	Antibiotic
Antistaphylococcal penicillins	Nafcillin, oxacillin
First-generation cephalosporins	Cefazolin
Second-generation cephalosporins	Cefuroxime
Third-generation cephalosporins	Ceftriaxone, cefotaxime
Fourth-generation cephalosporins	Cefepime
β-Lactam/β-lactamase inhibitor combinations	Ampicillin-sulbactam, piperacillin-tazobactam, ticarcillin-clavulanate
Carbapenems	Imipenem, meropenem, doripenem
Also sometimes active	
Clindamycin	
Sulfa drugs	Trimethoprim-sulfamethoxazole
Quinolones	Ciprofloxacin, levofloxacin, moxifloxacin
Tetracyclines	Minocycline, doxycycline
Macrolides	Erythromycin, azithromycin
Rifamycins	Rifampin
Aminoglycosides	Gentamicin (synergistic doses)
If methicillin-resistant *Staphylococcus aureus*	
Glycopeptides	Vancomycin, telavancin
Linezolid	
Streptogramins	Quinupristin-dalfopristin
Daptomycin	
Tetracycline-like	Tigecycline
Fifth-generation cephalosporins	Ceftaroline

methicillin-resistant *S. aureus* (MRSA) for historical reasons, are actually resistant to all penicillins (including all antistaphylococcal penicillins), cephalosporins, and carbapenems. These strains are a serious and common problem in most intensive care units and are becoming a more frequent cause of community-acquired infections. They are usually treated with **vancomycin**, one of the few antibiotics that reliably retain activity against these strains. Unfortunately, vancomycin-resistant *S. aureus* (VRSA) strains have already been reported. These strains have acquired the ability to alter the part of peptidoglycan normally bound by vancomycin, thus preventing this antibiotic from exerting its effect (step 3 in Fig. 10-2). Only a few relatively new antibiotics, such as **linezolid**, **tigecycline**, **quinupristin-dalfopristin**, **daptomycin**, and **ceftaroline**, are reliably active against these staphylococci.

Other antibiotics, such as **clindamycin**, the quinolones (**ciprofloxacin**, **levofloxacin**, **moxifloxacin**), **trimethoprim-sulfamethoxazole**, some tetracyclines (**minocycline**, **doxycycline**), and the macrolides (**erythromycin**, **azithromycin**), are sometimes active

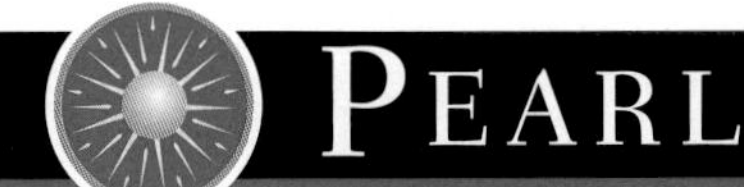

Each year, an increasing number of *Staphylococcus aureus* isolates are resistant to β-lactam antibiotics. In some countries, more than half of isolates from intensive care units are methicillin-resistant *S. aureus* (MRSA) strains. Of great concern is that infections caused by MRSA strains are no longer limited to hospitalized patients. A recent study found that 12% of community-acquired *S. aureus* infections were caused by MRSA strains, and in some regions, this percentage is dramatically higher.

Naimi TS, LeDell KH, Como-Sabetti K, et al. Comparison of community- and health care-associated methicillin-resistant Staphylococcus aureus infection. *JAMA.* 2003;290:2976–2984.
National Nosocomial Infections Surveillance System. National Nosocomial Infections Surveillance (NNIS) System report, data summary from January 1992 through June 2004, issued October 2004. *Am J Infect Control.* 2004;32:470–485.

against *S. aureus*, but in general, these agents should only be used if susceptibilities are known or the use of first-line agents is not possible (Table 10-1). **Rifampin** or synergistic doses of **gentamicin** are sometimes used along with β-lactams or vancomycin in the treatment of endocarditis or osteomyelitis caused by *S. aureus*. Rifampin is thought to facilitate clearance of this bacterium from the surface of prosthetic devices such as artificial heart valves and joints.

S. epidermidis infections are treated similarly to *S. aureus* infections. Nearly all strains are resistant to penicillin and many are resistant to the antistaphylococcal penicillins. Thus, **vancomycin** is often used to treat these infections.

QUESTIONS

1. Two antistaphylococcal penicillins used for intravenous therapy are ________ and ________.
2. *Staphylococcus aureus* strains resistant to antistaphylococcal penicillins are called ________.
3. In addition to being resistant to methicillin, methicillin-resistant *S. aureus* strains are also resistant to all other ________.
4. Methicillin-resistant *S. aureus* strains are usually susceptible to ________.

ADDITIONAL READINGS

David MZ, Daum RS. Community-associated methicillin-resistant Staphylococcus aureus: epidemiology and clinical consequences of an emerging epidemic. *Clin Microb Rev.* 2010;23:616–687.
Lowy FD. Antimicrobial resistance: the example of Staphylococcus aureus. *J Clin Invest.* 2003;111: 1265–1273.
Lowy FD. Staphylococcus aureus infections. *N Engl J Med.* 1998;339:520–532.

Pneumococci

Pneumococci are frequent causes of community-acquired pneumonia, otitis media, sinusitis, and meningitis (Fig. 10-3). These bacteria, which are formally designated *S. pneumoniae*, do not act covertly. Rather than avoid detection and cause disease by subversion, pneumococci boldly and forcefully attack the human body and cause significant amounts of tissue damage. As a result, pneumococcal infections are associated with extensive inflammatory responses that contribute to host tissue injury.

For many years, the treatment of infections caused by *S. pneumoniae* was straightforward: **Penicillin G** or **ampicillin** was given. Physicians now recall those days with nostalgia because the choice of therapy has become more complex. An ever-increasing percentage of pneumococcal strains produce PBPs that are poorly recognized by the natural penicillins and aminopenicillins, resulting in relative resistance. Approximately 40% of *S. pneumoniae* isolates in the United States now have intermediate or high levels of resistance to these agents. In many cases, however, this relative resistance can be overcome by giving higher doses of penicillin or ampicillin, which leads to higher drug concentrations and, as a result, sufficient binding to PBPs to cause bacterial killing.

This situation becomes more complicated when one appreciates that many β-lactams, such as the penicillins, achieve approximately 100-fold higher concentrations in plasma and the lungs than they do in cerebral spinal fluid. Thus, a "penicillin-resistant" strain of *S. pneumoniae* may be killed by the high penicillin concentrations present in the lung but persist in the relatively low concentrations found in the cerebral spinal fluid.

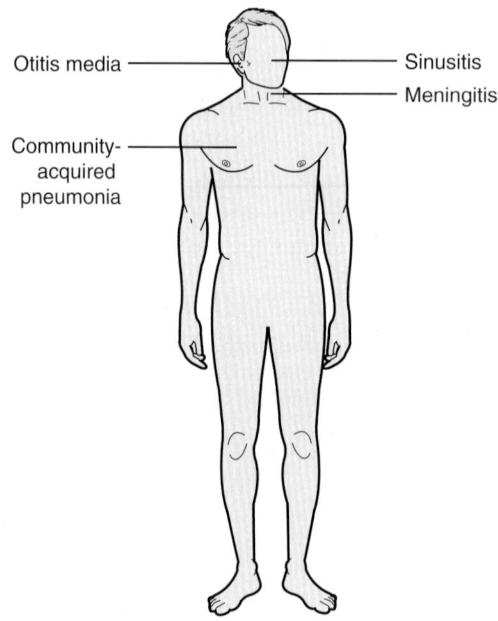

FIGURE 10-3. Sites of *Streptococcus pneumoniae* infections.

Over the same period, resistance to cephalosporins traditionally used to treat pneumococcal infections has increased as well. These cephalosporins include **cefuroxime**, **cefotaxime**, **ceftriaxone**, and **cefepime**. Like penicillin, cephalosporins achieve much higher concentrations in plasma and pulmonary tissues than within the central nervous system. Thus, similar arguments apply to both cephalosporin and penicillin resistance.

So, how is one to treat these infections? In general, the following guidelines apply in the treatment of *S. pneumoniae* infections with penicillin (Table 10-2). Pneumonia, otitis media, sinusitis, and bacteremia caused by all but the most resistant strains of *S. pneumoniae* should be treated with high doses of penicillin. This agent, however, should not be used to treat meningitis caused by strains that have even an intermediate level of resistance. Likewise, third-generation cephalosporins such as cefotaxime and ceftriaxone can be used to treat most kinds of pneumococcal infections regardless of their sensitivities with the exception of meningitis caused by highly resistant strains.

The difficulties in treating infections caused by penicillin-resistant pneumococci are compounded by the fact that these bacteria are also frequently resistant to several other antibiotics. Acquired genetic material that encodes for penicillin resistance also often carries genes that result in loss of susceptibility to many other antibiotics commonly used for pneumococcal infections. These include macrolide-like

Table 10-2 Agents for Treatment of Infections Caused by *Streptococcus Pneumoniae*

Antibiotic Class	Antibiotic
Natural penicillins	Penicillin G
Aminopenicillins	Ampicillin
Also sometimes active	
Clindamycin	
Sulfa drugs	Trimethoprim-sulfamethoxazole
Macrolides	Azithromycin
Tetracyclines	Doxycycline
If penicillin-resistant	
Second-generation cephalosporin	Cefuroxime
Third-generation cephalosporin	Cefotaxime, ceftriaxone
Fourth-generation cephalosporin	Cefepime
Fifth-generation cephalosporin	Ceftaroline
Quinolones	Moxifloxacin, levofloxacin, gemifloxacin
Glycopeptide	Vancomycin
Macrolide-like agents	Telithromycin
Alternatives	
Linezolid	
Carbapenems	Imipenem, meropenem, doripenem
Streptogramins	Quinupristin/dalfopristin

agents (**azithromycin**), tetracyclines (**doxycycline**), **clindamycin**, and sulfa drugs (**trimethoprim-sulfamethoxazole**). For infections caused by highly resistant strains, several options are available (Table 10-2). Certain quinolones (**moxifloxacin, gemifloxacin,** and **levofloxacin**, but not ciprofloxacin), macrolide-like agents (**telithromycin**), and fifth-generation cephalosporins (**ceftaroline**) remain active against penicillin-resistant pneumococci, as does **vancomycin**. Less frequently used alternatives include **linezolid**, carbapenems (**imipenem**, **meropenem**, **doripenem**), or streptogramins (**quinupristin/dalfopristin**).

QUESTIONS

5. Prior to the emergence of resistant strains, *Streptococcus pneumoniae* infections were routinely treated with ________________ or ________________.

6. Currently, many pneumococcal strains are resistant to penicillins because they produce ________________ that are poorly recognized by these agents.

7. Antibiotics frequently used to treat infections caused by penicillin-resistant *S. pneumoniae* strains include ________________, ________________, ________________, and ________________.

8. Penicillin-resistant strains of *S. pneumoniae* are often also resistant to other antibiotics used to treat infections caused by this bacterium, including ________________, ________________, ________________, and ________________.

ADDITIONAL READINGS

Garau J. Treatment of drug-resistant pneumococcal pneumonia. *Lancet Infect Dis*. 2002;2:404–415.

Musher DM, Bartlett JG, Doern GV. A fresh look at the definition of susceptibility of Streptococcus pneumoniae to beta-lactam antibiotics. *Arch Intern Med*. 2001;161:2538–2544.

Tuomanen EI, Austrian R, Masure HR. Pathogenesis of pneumococcal infection. *N Engl J Med*. 1995; 332:1280–1284.

Other Streptococci

S. pneumoniae is only one of many medically important streptococcal species. Bacteria classified as *Streptococcus pyogenes* (also called group A streptococci) are a frequent cause of pharyngitis ("strep throat"), skin and soft tissue infections, and streptococcal toxic shock syndrome (Fig. 10-4). *Streptococcus agalactiae* strains (also called group B streptococci) colonize the female genital tract and cause sepsis and meningitis in neonates and infants less than 3 months of age. Viridans group streptococci, a large heterogenous group of streptococci defined by their hemolysis pattern when grown on blood agar, colonize the human gastrointestinal and urogenital tracts and are the etiologic agents of several severe infections, including infective endocarditis and abscesses.

Traditional treatment of infections caused by these streptococci has consisted of the natural penicillins or aminopenicillins, and many of these bacteria remain susceptible to these agents (Table 10-3). Infections caused by *S. pyogenes* are routinely treated with **penicillin** or **ampicillin**. Alternatives include a first-generation cephalosporin (e.g., **cefazolin**) or a macrolide (e.g., **azithromycin**), although macrolide resistance is becoming more common. In severe invasive group A streptococcal infections, such as necrotizing fasciitis, **clindamycin** is added to a regimen of high-dose penicillin. Theoretically, clindamycin, which inhibits protein translation, blocks production of some of the streptococcal toxins that contribute to the pathogenesis of these diseases. Intravenous immune globulin (IVIG) is also frequently given in these situations because it may contain antibodies that bind and neutralize these toxins. *S. agalactiae* is uniformly sensitive to **penicillin** and **ampicillin**. Synergistic doses of an aminoglycoside such

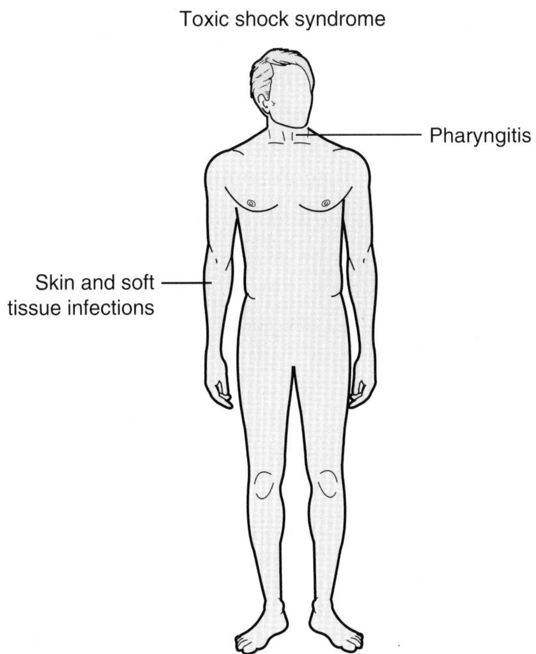

FIGURE 10-4. Sites of *Streptococcus pyogenes* infections.

Table 10-3 Antimicrobial Agents for Treatment of Infections Caused by Streptococcal Species Other than *Streptococcus Pneumoniae*

Antibiotic Class	Antibiotic
Natural penicillins	Penicillin G
Aminopenicillins	Ampicillin
Aminoglycosides are sometimes added for synergy	Gentamicin
Clindamycin is added for severe invasive *Streptococcus pyogenes* infections	
Alternatives	
First-generation cephalosporin	Cefazolin
Macrolide	Azithromycin
If penicillin resistant	
Glycopeptide	Vancomycin
Second-generation cephalosporin	Cefuroxime
Third-generation cephalosporin	Cefotaxime, ceftriaxone

as **gentamicin** are often initially added to regimens for serious infections. Although **penicillin** is still the agent of choice for infections caused by viridans group streptococci, resistance to this agent is increasingly common. As with *S. pneumoniae*, resistance is due to altered PBPs. **Vancomycin** or cephalosporins (e.g., **cefotaxime**) are used to treat these resistant strains. An aminoglycoside (e.g., **gentamicin**) is sometimes added to these agents for synergism.

QUESTIONS

9. Unlike *Streptococcus pneumoniae*, *Streptococcus pyogenes* continues to be nearly universally susceptible to ________________.

10. In the treatment of serious invasive group A streptococcal infections, ________________ should be used in conjunction with penicillin.

11. Viridans group streptococci differ from group A and group B streptococci in that they are often resistant to ________________.

12. In the treatment of infections caused by *Streptococcus agalactiae* and viridans group streptococci, ________________ are sometimes used with penicillins because of synergy between these agents.

ADDITIONAL READINGS

Doern GV, Ferraro MJ, Brueggemann AB, et al. Emergence of high rates of antimicrobial resistance among viridans group streptococci in the United States. *Antimicrob Agents Chemother*. 1996;40:891–894.

Fernandez M, Hickman ME, Baker CJ. Antimicrobial susceptibilities of group B streptococci isolated between 1992 and 1996 from patients with bacteremia or meningitis. *Antimicrob Agents Chemother*. 1998;42:1517–1519.

Richter SS, Heilmann KP, Beekmann SE, et al. Macrolide-resistant Streptococcus pyogenes in the United States, 2002–2003. *Clin Infect Dis*. 2005;41:599–608.

Russell NE, Pachorek RE. Clindamycin in the treatment of streptococcal and staphylococcal toxic shock syndromes. *Ann Pharmacother*. 2000;34:936–939.

Enterococci

Enterococci can be viewed as fickle residents of the human gastrointestinal tract. Normally, they innocuously inhabit this environmental niche, growing and multiplying in the nutritionally rich intestinal contents but causing no problems for their host. If, however, an individual becomes compromised in some way, these traitorous bacteria may turn against him or her and cause serious infections. Compromise may take many forms, including the placement of a vascular or urinary catheter, abdominal surgery, or organ transplantation. Enterococcal disease manifests itself as urinary tract infections, bacteremia, endocarditis, wound infections, or intra-abdominal infections (Fig. 10-5). The enterococcal species most commonly encountered in human disease are *Enterococcus faecalis* and *Enterococcus faecium*.

A truly remarkable aspect of the enterococci is their resistance to many antibiotics (Fig. 10-6). These bacteria are intrinsically resistant to cephalosporins due to the production of altered PBPs. They have the ability to utilize folic acid derivatives from the environment, making them resistant to trimethoprim-sulfamethoxazole. Even penicillins and vancomycin, which are bactericidal against most susceptible bacteria, are only bacteriostatic against enterococci.

The first-line antibiotics used for treatment of enterococcal infections are the penicillins, in particular **penicillin G**, **ampicillin**, and **piperacillin** (Table 10-4). The carbapenems **imipenem**, **meropenem**, and **doripenem** are also sometimes active. Unfortunately, enterococci are increasingly resistant to these antibiotics, often because of production of altered PBPs that do not bind β-lactams. In such strains,

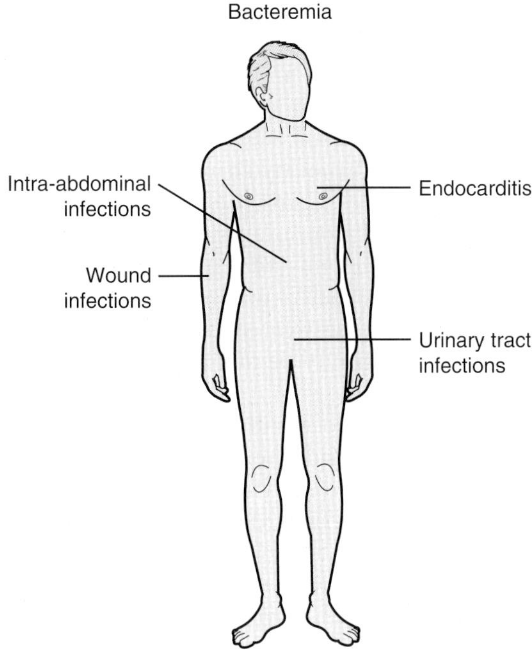

FIGURE 10-5. Sites of enterococcal infections.

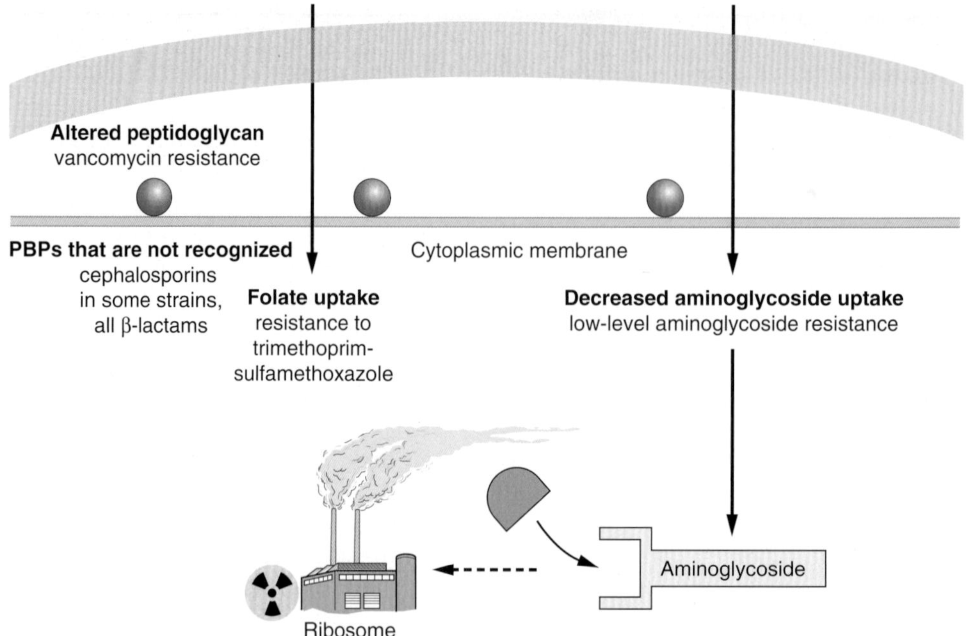

FIGURE 10-6. Mechanisms by which enterococci resist the actions of antibiotics. In some strains, altered peptidoglycan prevents binding by vancomycin. Enterococcal PBPs are not recognized by cephalosporins, and in some strains are not bound by any β-lactam agents. Enterococci do not need to synthesize folate because they assimilate this factor from the host, resulting in resistance to trimethoprim-sulfamethoxazole. Decreased uptake of aminoglycosides causes low-level resistance, whereas aminoglycoside modification and ribosome mutation results in high-level resistance.

vancomycin is used in place of β-lactam antibiotics. Resistance to vancomycin, however, has also become common. Vancomycin-resistant enterococci (VRE) produce peptidoglycan containing an altered peptide side chain. The terminal portion of the peptide side chain is changed from D-alanine–D-alanine to D-alanine–D-lactate. Whereas D-alanine–D-alanine is bound and sequestered by vancomycin, D-alanine–D-lactate is not and thus renders the bacterium resistant to this antibiotic. Unless penicillin susceptible, VRE must be treated with **linezolid**, **daptomycin**, **tigecycline**, or **quinupristin/dalfopristin**. Note that the latter agent is only active against *E. faecium*, not *E. faecalis*.

The interaction between enterococci and aminoglycosides is complex. Enterococci do not normally take up aminoglycosides very well, resulting in universal "low-level" resistance to these agents and rendering them ineffective when used alone against these bacteria. However, aminoglycosides do penetrate these bacteria when used in conjunction with an appropriate antibiotic capable of disrupting the cell wall (e.g., a penicillin or vancomycin) and thus have synergistic activity against enterococci. This synergism converts the activity of penicillins and vancomycin from bacteriostatic to bactericidal. The significance of this change is that bactericidal activity is required for serious enterococcal infections such as endocarditis. Unfortunately, several factors

Table 10-4 Antimicrobial Agents for Treatment of Infections Caused by Enterococci

Antibiotic Class	Antibiotic
Natural penicillins	Penicillin G
Aminopenicillins	Ampicillin
Extended-spectrum penicillins	Piperacillin
Also sometimes active	
Carbapenems	Imipenem, meropenem, doripenem
For serious infections, add an aminoglycoside for synergy	Gentamicin, streptomycin
If penicillin-resistant	
Vancomycin	
If also vancomycin-resistant	
Linezolid	
Tetracycline-like	Tigecycline
Also sometimes active	
Daptomycin	
Quinupristin/dalfopristin (*Enterococcus faecium*)	

limit the usefulness of the synergistic activity of the aminoglycosides. All *E. faecium* strains contain a chromosomally encoded acetyltransferase that modifies tobramycin and prevents it from having even a synergistic effect. Thus, only **gentamicin** and **streptomycin** are usually recommended for use against enterococci. In addition, increasing rates of "high-level" resistance to aminoglycosides among enterococci are now being observed. This occurs when enterococci acquire genetic material that encodes for the production of aminoglycoside-modifying enzymes that abrogate even synergistic activity. Mutations may also occur that result in modification of the aminoglycoside binding site of the enterococcal ribosome, preventing aminoglycoside binding. In either case, synergistic activity is abolished.

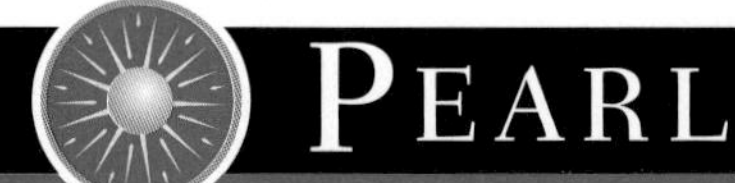

All enterococci are not created equal. *Enterococcus faecium* tends to be much more resistant to antibiotics than *Enterococcus faecalis*. For example, in a recent study, 52% of *E. faecium* strains were resistant to vancomycin and 83% to ampicillin, whereas only 2% of *E. faecalis* strains were resistant to these agents.

Huycke MM, Sahm DF, Gilmore MS. Multiple-drug resistant enterococci: the nature of the problem and an agenda for the future. *Emerg Infect Dis.* 1998;4:239–249.

QUESTIONS

13. The first-line antibiotics for enterococcal infections include the following β-lactams: ________________, ________________, and ________________.

14. Penicillin-resistant enterococci are often treated with ________________.

15. When used alone, cell wall–active agents such as β-lactams and vancomycin are only ________________ for enterococci. To achieve ________________ activity, gentamicin or streptomycin must be added.

16. The following antibiotics are used to treat vancomycin-resistant enterococci: ________________, ________________, ________________, and ________________.

ADDITIONAL READINGS

Chow JW. Aminoglycoside resistance in enterococci. *Clin Infect Dis.* 2000;31:586–589.

Gold HS. Vancomycin-resistant enterococci: mechanisms and clinical observations. *Clin Infect Dis.* 2001;33:210–219.

Landman D, Quale JM. Management of infections due to resistant enterococci: a review of therapeutic options. *J Antimicrob Chemother.* 1997;40:161–170.

Other Gram-Positive Bacteria

LISTERIA MONOCYTOGENES

L. monocytogenes is a gram-positive bacillus that is widespread in nature. It is commonly found in soil and the fecal flora of many animals. Ingestion of a large inoculum of these bacteria can lead to gastroenteritis in otherwise healthy people, whereas the very young, the very old, and the immunocompromised may develop bacteremia that leads to meningitis (Fig. 10-7). Pregnant women are also prone to systemic infections, which may cause fetal demise.

Ampicillin is the antibiotic of choice for infections caused by *L. monocytogenes* (Table 10-5). At first glance, this appears counterintuitive because *L. monocytogenes* is considered an intracellular pathogen and ampicillin penetrates poorly into cells. The likely explanation for this paradox is that although *L. monocytogenes* invades and survives within the cytoplasm of many cell types, in the meninges and cerebral spinal fluid, it is largely extracellular. Ampicillin alone is only bacteriostatic against *L. monocytogenes*. The addition of **gentamicin** results in synergistic bactericidal activity, so this antibiotic is usually used in conjunction with ampicillin. Gentamicin penetrates poorly into cerebral spinal fluid, but the small amounts that do accumulate in this compartment are apparently sufficient to cause synergistic killing. *L. monocytogenes* is intrinsically resistant to some commonly used antibiotics. For example, *L. monocytogenes* is not susceptible to cephalosporins because its PBPs are not bound by these agents. Because cephalosporins are frequently used alone as empiric therapy for meningitis,

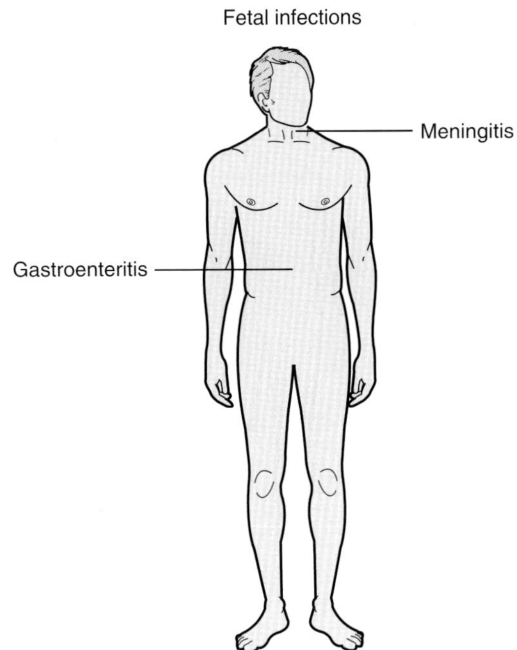

FIGURE 10-7. Sites of *Listeria monocytogenes* infections.

Table 10-5 Antimicrobial Agents for Treatment of Infections Caused by *Listeria Monocytogenes*
Ampicillin + gentamicin
If penicillin allergic
Trimethoprim-sulfamethoxazole

one must remember to add ampicillin to the treatment regimens of patients at risk for *L. monocytogenes* infections. Even vancomycin, which is active against most gram-positive bacteria, may not effectively treat individuals with *L. monocytogenes* meningitis. Patients who cannot tolerate ampicillin should be treated with **trimethoprim-sulfamethoxazole**.

BACILLUS ANTHRACIS

B. anthracis is a gram-positive spore-forming bacillus and the cause of anthrax. Anthrax itself may manifest as one of three forms: inhalational, cutaneous, and gastrointestinal anthrax (Fig. 10-8). In inhalational anthrax, spores are inhaled into the lungs, which causes hemorrhagic mediastinal adenopathy, bloody pleural effusions, and bacteremia. Use of anthrax spores as an agent of bioterrorism occurred in 2001 in the United States and led to 11 cases of confirmed inhalational anthrax. Cutaneous anthrax is characterized by a cutaneous skin ulcer consisting of a central black eschar surrounded

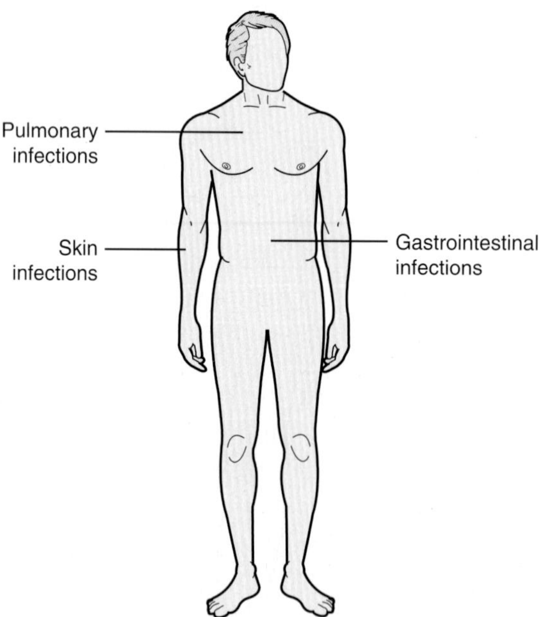

FIGURE 10-8. Sites of *Bacillus anthracis* infections.

Table 10-6 Antimicrobial Agents for Treatment of Infections Caused by *Bacillus Anthracis*

Antibiotic Class	Antibiotic
First-line agents	
Quinolone	Ciprofloxacin
Tetracycline	Doxycycline
For inhalational anthrax, a second agent from the following list should be used along with a first-line agent	
Rifamycin	Rifampin
Glycopeptide	Vancomycin
Natural penicillin	Penicillin
Aminopenicillin	Ampicillin
Chloramphenicol	
Carbapenem	Imipenem
Clindamycin	
Macrolide	Clarithromycin
Postexposure prophylaxis	
Quinolone	Ciprofloxacin

by edema. Gastrointestinal anthrax is relatively rare and most often occurs following ingestion of contaminated meat leading to infection of the bowel and ascites.

Historically, penicillin was used to treat anthrax, but the realization that this bacterium contains an inducible β-lactamase gene has resulted in recent recommendations that penicillin not be used alone for this indication. Currently, ciprofloxacin or doxycycline is the agent of choice for patients with anthrax (Table 10-6). Inhalational anthrax should be treated with one of these agents in conjunction with a second agent, such as **rifampin**, **vancomycin**, **penicillin**, **ampicillin**, **chloramphenicol**, **imipenem**, **clindamycin**, or **clarithromycin**. Because of the potential severity of anthrax, it is felt that the benefits of ciprofloxacin or doxycycline outweigh their risks in children and pregnant women; thus, they are recommended for these two groups of individuals. Because of the severity of inhalational anthrax, individuals potentially exposed to *B. anthracis* spores should be prophylactically treated with ciprofloxacin.

QUESTIONS

17. ________________ is active against *Listeria monocytogenes*, but ________________ is usually given with it to achieve synergistic bacterial killing.

18. *L. monocytogenes* is resistant to ________________, which are frequently used to empirically treat bacterial meningitis.

19. In patients who cannot tolerate penicillins because of allergy, ________________ is used to treat infections caused by *L. monocytogenes*.

20. It is currently recommended that all individuals with anthrax receive one of the following antibiotics: ________________ or ________________.

21. Patients with inhalational anthrax should be treated with at least ________________ antibiotics.

ADDITIONAL READINGS

Bartlett JG, Inglesby TV Jr, Borio L. Management of anthrax. *Clin Infect Dis.* 2002;35:851–858.

Dryden MS, Jones NF, Phillips I. Vancomycin therapy failure in Listeria monocytogenes peritonitis in a patient on continuous ambulatory peritoneal dialysis. *J Infect Dis.* 1991;164:1239.

Hof H, Nichterlein T, Kretschmar M. Management of listeriosis. *Clin Microbiol Rev.* 1997;10:345–357.

Inglesby TV, O'Toole T, Henderson DA, et al. Anthrax as a biological weapon, 2002: updated recommendations for management. *JAMA.* 2002;287:2236–2252.

Swartz MN. Recognition and management of anthrax—an update. *N Engl J Med.* 2001;345:1621–1626.

CHAPTER 11

Gram-Negative Bacteria

"Mail left the wearer vulnerable to crushing blows, and could be pierced by arrows or crossbow bolts. . . . Mail was supplemented by pieces of plate armour from the thirteenth century. . . . By the fifteenth century it is clear that the fully articulated suit of plate-armour had emerged, the wearer's pride in it such that the cloth coverings of earlier periods were abandoned and the armour worn 'white', polished and shining."

—ARMIES AND WARFARE IN THE MIDDLE AGES: THE ENGLISH EXPERIENCE, MICHAEL PRESTWICH

Gram-negative bacteria are characterized by a cell envelope structure that supplements the cross-linked mail-like peptidoglycan cell wall with an additional layer of protection. Just as medieval knights had their mail covered with plate armor, gram-negative bacteria surround the peptidoglycan cell wall with a lipopolysaccharide (LPS)-rich outer membrane. The outer membrane forms a dense barrier that restricts penetration of many antibiotics into the periplasmic space and cytosol of the bacterium. Thus, to be effective against gram-negative bacteria, antibiotics must penetrate one additional layer of protection.

Gram-negative bacteria are among the most common causes of infections in humans. This group includes the Enterobacteriaceae, a large family of bacteria responsible for many gastrointestinal, urinary, and opportunistic infections. The pseudomonad *Pseudomonas aeruginosa* is a frequent cause of hospital-acquired infections and is noteworthy for its resistance to many different classes of antibiotics. *Neisseria* spp., the curved gram-negative bacilli *Helicobacter pylori* and *Campylobacter jejuni*, and the respiratory bacteria *Haemophilus influenzae* and *Bordetella pertussis* are also problematic human pathogens. In this section, we will discuss the treatment of each of these organisms.

Enterobacteriaceae

The Enterobacteriaceae are a large family of gram-negative bacilli, most of which are capable of inhabiting the human gastrointestinal tract. For this reason, they are often referred to as "enteric" gram-negative rods. Many members of this group are part of the normal flora of humans and only cause disease in the context of a compromised host. As such, they are "opportunistic" pathogens. Other members of the Enterobacteriaceae, however, are strict pathogens, and isolation of these bacteria from a stool culture usually indicates a causative role in disease. Some species of bacteria fall into both groups. For example, while most *Escherichia coli* bacteria live harmlessly in the colon, some strains have acquired exogenous genetic material that allows them to cause urinary tract infections or diarrhea even in normal hosts.

ESCHERICHIA COLI, KLEBSIELLA SPP., AND *PROTEUS* SPP.

E. coli, *Klebsiella* spp., and *Proteus* spp. are versatile pathogens that commonly cause community-acquired infections in healthy individuals and also frequently lead to health care–associated infections. Bacteria from all three genera cause community-acquired urinary tract infections, with *E. coli* being the most frequent etiology of this disease (Fig. 11-1). In the normal host, certain strains of *E. coli* are capable of causing gastroenteritis, including traveler's diarrhea and diarrhea associated with hemolytic uremic syndrome. In neonates, it is the leading cause of meningitis. *Klebsiella* spp. cause community-acquired pneumonia in select populations such as alcoholics. In addition, all three genera of pathogens are frequent causes of health care–associated infections such as urinary tract infections in patients with urinary catheters, hospital-acquired pneumonia, bacteremia, wound infections, and intra-abdominal infections.

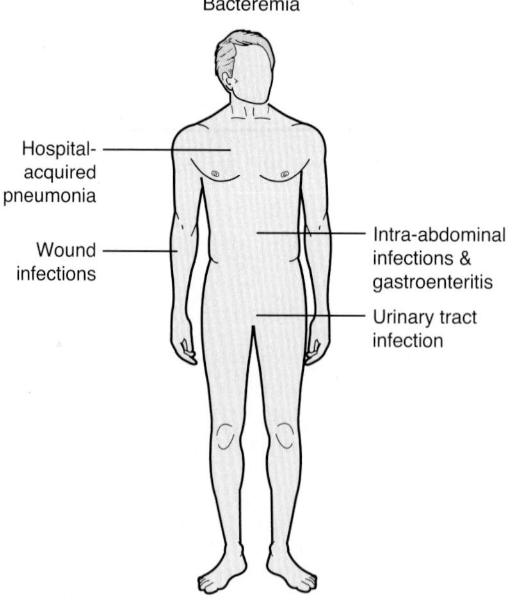

FIGURE 11-1. Common sites of Enterobacteriaceae infections.

One cannot understand treatment of infections caused by the Enterobacteriaceae without understanding β-lactamases. For example, some community-acquired *E. coli* and *Proteus* strains remain susceptible to aminopenicillins such as **ampicillin** (Table 11-1). However, many strains now harbor plasmids encoding the TEM-1 β-lactamase (see "Pearl" box), which allows them to resist killing by ampicillin but not

Table 11-1 Antimicrobial Agents for Treatment of Infections Caused by the Enterobacteriaceae

Antibiotic Class	Antibiotic
***Escherichia coli, Klebsiella* spp., *Proteus* spp.**	
Aminopenicillins (except *Klebsiella* spp. and *Proteus vulgaris*)	Ampicillin
First-generation cephalosporins (except for *P. vulgaris*)	Cefazolin
Sulfa drugs	Trimethoprim-sulfamethoxazole
Quinolones	Ciprofloxacin, levofloxacin, moxifloxacin
If resistant to the above antibiotics	
Third-generation cephalosporins	Cefotaxime, ceftriaxone
Monobactam	Aztreonam
Extended-spectrum penicillins + β-lactamase inhibitor	Piperacillin-tazobactam, ticarcillin-clavulanate
Carbapenems	Imipenem, meropenem, doripenem, ertapenem
+ aminoglycoside in serious infections	Gentamicin, tobramycin, amikacin
***Enterobacter, Serratia, Citrobacter, Providencia, Morganella* spp.**	
Carbapenems	Imipenem, meropenem, doripenem, ertapenem
Sulfa drugs	Trimethoprim-sulfamethoxazole
Quinolones	Ciprofloxacin, levofloxacin, moxifloxacin
Fourth-generation cephalosporins	Cefepime
+ aminoglycoside in serious infections	Gentamicin, tobramycin, amikacin
***Salmonella enterica, Shigella* spp.**	
Quinolones	Ciprofloxacin
Third-generation cephalosporins	Cefotaxime, ceftriaxone
Macrolides	Azithromycin
Some strains remain susceptible to	
Aminopenicillins	Ampicillin
Sulfa drugs	Trimethoprim-sulfamethoxazole
***Yersinia* spp.**	
Aminoglycosides	Gentamicin, streptomycin
Tetracyclines	Doxycycline
Quinolones (*Yersinia enterocolitica*)	Ciprofloxacin
Sulfa drugs (*Y. enterocolitica*)	Trimethoprim-sulfamethoxazole

Pearl

Enterobacteriaceae are particularly adept at producing β-lactamases to defend themselves against β-lactam antibiotics. Thus, a discussion of appropriate therapy for the Enterobacteriaceae necessitates a basic understanding of the types of β-lactamases they produce and the β-lactams they degrade. Four such β-lactamases are TEM-1, AmpC, the extended-spectrum β-lactamases (ESBLs), and *Klebsiella pneumoniae* carbapenemases (KPCs).

TEM-1: This β-lactamase is plasmid encoded and constitutively expressed. It confers absolute resistance to ampicillin and amoxicillin.

AmpC: This β-lactamase is usually chromosomally encoded and inducible. When induced, AmpC β-lactamase confers resistance to penicillin, ampicillin/amoxicillin, and first-generation cephalosporins. Mutant strains that constitutively express large amounts of this enzyme are resistant to all β-lactam antibiotics (including β-lactam/β-lactamase inhibitor combinations such as piperacillin-tazobactam) except carbapenems.

ESBL: β-lactamases of this group are usually plasmid encoded and constitutively expressed. They are especially problematic because strains that produce them may appear susceptible to third-generation cephalosporins but are in fact resistant. These β-lactamases degrade all β-lactams except carbapenems and sometimes β-lactam/β-lactamase inhibitor combinations. In addition, because the plasmids that carry ESBL genes also commonly encode resistance determinants for many other antibiotics, ESBL strains are often resistant to many non–β-lactam antibiotics as well.

KPC: KPCs are a relatively new class of β-lactamases that are increasingly being found in *K. pneumoniae* isolates. These β-lactamases degrade all β-lactams, including carbapenems. The genes encoding KPCs are carried on plasmids that also encode resistance to other antibiotics, making treatment exceedingly difficult. Aminoglycosides, colistin, and tigecycline have been used with some success. The concern is that plasmids encoding KPCs will quickly disseminate to other genera of bacteria; examples of such spread have already been observed.

Hirsch EB, Tam, VH. Detection and treatment options for Klebsiella pneumoniae carbapenemases (KPCs): an emerging cause of multidrug-resistant infections. *J Antimicrob Chemoth.* 2010;65:1119–1125.
Jacoby GA, Munoz-Price LS. The new beta-lactamases. *N Engl J Med.* 2005;352:380–391.
Pitout JDD, Laupland KB. Extended-spectrum β-lactamase-producing Enterobacteriaceae: an emerging public-health concern. *Lancet Infect Dis.* 2008;8:159–166.

first-generation cephalosporins, such as **cefazolin.** In contrast, all strains of *Klebsiella* express a chromosomally encoded β-lactamase that confers resistance to ampicillin. Most community-acquired infections caused by *E. coli*, *Proteus* spp., and *Klebsiella* spp. can be treated with quinolones (**ciprofloxacin**, **levofloxacin**, **moxifloxacin**), **trimethoprim-sulfamethoxazole**, or first-generation cephalosporins (**cefazolin**). One notable exception is *Proteus vulgaris*, which produces a chromosomally encoded β-lactamase that confers resistance to aminopenicillins and the first-generation cephalosporins. Third-generation cephalosporins, such as **cefotaxime** or **ceftriaxone**, are frequently used to treat severe pyelonephritis caused by these bacteria. **Aztreonam** may also be used.

Health care–associated infections are much more difficult to treat because the strains of *E. coli*, *Klebsiella* spp., and *Proteus* spp. that cause them are frequently multidrug resistant.

Potentially useful agents include third-, fourth-, and fifth-generation cephalosporins (e.g., **cefotaxime, ceftriaxone, cefepime, ceftaroline**); extended-spectrum penicillins + β-lactamase inhibitors (**piperacillin-tazobactam, ticarcillin-clavulanate**); and carbapenems (e.g., **imipenem, meropenem, doripenem, ertapenem**), but treatment must be individualized and based on the susceptibilities of each isolate. *E. coli*, *Klebsiella* spp., and *Proteus* spp. are often susceptible to aminoglycosides, such as **gentamicin, tobramycin**, and **amikacin**. However, these agents are usually not used as monotherapy but in conjunction with another agent in life-threatening infections such as sepsis.

Especially powerful β-lactamases, called extended-spectrum β-lactamases (ESBLs) and *Klebsiella pneumoniae* carbapenemases (KPCs), are of particular concern in some isolates of *E. coli* and *Klebsiella*. Strains that express these β-lactamases are resistant to most antibiotics and are very difficult to treat (see "Pearl" box).

ENTEROBACTER, SERRATIA, CITROBACTER, PROVIDENCIA, AND *MORGANELLA* SPP.

Most of these bacteria are capable of colonizing the human gastrointestinal tract without causing disease but can cause pneumonia, urinary tract infections, intra-abdominal infections, wound infections, and bacteremia in compromised or hospitalized patients (Fig. 11-1).

Each of these bacterial species contains an inducible chromosomally encoded AmpC-type β-lactamase that confers resistance to penicillin, ampicillin/amoxicillin, and first-generation cephalosporins (see "Pearl" box). To further complicate matters, mutant strains that constitutively express high levels of this enzyme may be selected during therapy with some β-lactam antibiotics. These mutants are resistant to all β-lactams except the carbapenems (**imipenem, meropenem, doripenem, ertapenem**). Some experts feel that **cefepime** also has activity against these strains. A consequence of such selection is that a strain that initially appears susceptible to certain β-lactam antibiotics may become resistant during the course of therapy, resulting in treatment failure. Although many gram-negative bacteria encode AmpC β-lactamases, this phenomenon of selection of constitutively expressing mutants is particularly problematic in *Enterobacter*, *Serratia*, *Citrobacter*, *Providencia*, and *Morganella* spp. infections when treated with third-generation cephalosporins (see "Remember" box).

REMEMBER

Third-generation cephalosporins should be used with caution with some members of the Enterobacteriaceae. Species of *Enterobacter, Citrobacter, Serratia, Morganella*, and *Providencia* possess inducible chromosomal AmpC β-lactamases that may acquire mutations leading to constitutive high-level expression during the course of therapy with third-generation cephalosporins. For this reason, many experts recommend that third-generation cephalosporins not be used to treat infections caused by these bacteria, even if initial antibiograms indicate susceptibility to these agents. Below is a mnemonic for remembering this special group of bacteria:
Cephalosporins **M**ay **P**rove **S**ub-**E**fficacious (***C**itrobacter*, ***M**organella*, ***P**rovidencia*, ***S**erratia*, ***E**nterobacter*)

Strains of *Enterobacter*, *Serratia*, *Citrobacter*, *Providencia*, and *Morganella* spp. frequently harbor plasmids that confer resistance to other antibiotics as well, and treatment must be tailored to the susceptibilities of each individual strain. Quinolones (**ciprofloxacin**, **levofloxacin**, **moxifloxacin**) and **trimethoprim-sulfamethoxazole** are often effective. As with *E. coli*, *Klebsiella* spp., and *Proteus* spp., aminoglycosides (**gentamicin**, **tobramycin**, **amikacin**) are used in conjunction with another agent in life-threatening infections such as sepsis.

SALMONELLA ENTERICA, SHIGELLA SPP., AND *YERSINIA ENTEROCOLITICA*

Most of the disease burden due to *Salmonella enterica*, *Shigella* spp., and *Yersinia enterocolitica* consists of gastroenteritis in otherwise healthy individuals (Fig. 11-1). In addition, some pathovars of *S. enterica* cause typhoid fever, a serious infection characterized by prolonged bacteremia.

Acute infectious diarrhea caused by *S. enterica* and *Y. enterocolitica* in the immunocompetent host usually does not require antibiotic therapy. Such therapy is recommended, however, if the infection has spread beyond the intestinal tract, if it is severe, or if the patient is immunocompromised. When antibiotics are indicated, *Salmonella* and *Shigella* infections should be treated with quinolones (e.g., **ciprofloxacin**), third-generation cephalosporins (e.g., **cefotaxime, ceftriaxone**), or **azithromycin**. Some strains remain susceptible to the aminopenicillins (**ampicillin**) or **trimethoprim-sulfamethoxazole**. *Y. enterocolitica* is usually susceptible to aminoglycosides (**gentamicin, streptomycin**), tetracyclines (**doxycycline**), quinolones (**ciprofloxacin**), and **trimethoprim-sulfamethoxazole**.

YERSINIA PESTIS

Yersinia pestis is the cause of plague, one of the great infectious scourges of human history. This bacterium has caused several pandemics, one of which is referred to as the Black Death that led to the demise of a quarter to a third of the population of Europe in the 14th century. Although a few cases of endemic plague continue to be seen, the current concern regarding this pathogen is its potential use as an agent of bioterrorism. The treatment of choice is **streptomycin** or **gentamicin** (Table 11-1). **Doxycycline** is also effective.

QUESTIONS

1. Members of the Enterobacteriaceae cause both ________________ -acquired and ________________ ________________-associated infections.
2. Community-acquired urinary tract infections and diarrhea caused by *Escherichia coli* may often be successfully treated with ________________ or a ________________.
3. Extended-spectrum β-lactamases are most often produced by ________________ or ________________.
4. Extended-spectrum β-lactamases confer resistance to all β-lactamases except ________________ and sometimes ________________.

5. When produced in large amounts, AmpC β-lactamases confer resistance to all β-lactams except ________________.
6. In serious infections such as sepsis, an ________________ is often used in conjunction with a standard antibiotic to treat Enterobacteriaceae.
7. Strains of *Salmonella enterica* and *Shigella* spp. cause ________________. These bacteria are susceptible to ________________, ________________, and ________________.

ADDITIONAL READINGS

Livermore DM. Beta-lactamases in laboratory and clinical resistance. *Clin Microbiol Rev*. 1995;8:557–584.

Nataro JP, Kaper JB. Diarrheagenic Escherichia coli. *Clin Microbiol Rev*. 1998;11:142–201.

O'Hara CM, Brenner FW, Miller JM. Classification, identification, and clinical significance of Proteus, Providencia, and Morganella. *Clin Microbiol Rev*. 2000;13:534–546.

Pitout JD, Sanders CC, Sanders WE Jr. Antimicrobial resistance with focus on beta-lactam resistance in gram-negative bacilli. *Am J Med*. 1997;103:51–59.

Podschun R, Ullmann U. Klebsiella spp. as nosocomial pathogens: epidemiology, taxonomy, typing methods, and pathogenicity factors. *Clin Microbiol Rev*. 1998;11:589–603.

Sanders WE Jr, Sanders CC. Enterobacter spp. pathogens poised to flourish at the turn of the century. *Clin Microbiol Rev*. 1997;10:220–241.

Yu VL. Serratia marcescens: historical perspective and clinical review. *N Engl J Med*. 1979;300: 887–893.

Pseudomonas

The genus *Pseudomonas* contains many species of gram-negative bacilli found in the environment, some of which occasionally cause serious infections in compromised individuals. By far the most medically important of these opportunistic pathogens is *P. aeruginosa*. This bacterium is a frequent cause of hospital-acquired infections, especially pneumonia, urinary tract infections, and wound infections (Fig. 11-2). In addition, the airways of most individuals with cystic fibrosis are chronically infected with *P. aeruginosa* by the time they are adults.

Treatment of *P. aeruginosa* infections is complicated by the array of resistance mechanisms that it harbors (Fig. 11-3). This bacterium has a relatively impermeable outer membrane containing highly selective porins, produces multiple efflux pumps, and has a chromosome containing an inducible β-lactamase. For these reasons, aminopenicillins, macrolides, and most cephalosporins are ineffective against this bacterium. Nonetheless, several treatment options are available (Table 11-2). The extended-spectrum penicillin **piperacillin** does penetrate the outer membrane porins but at a relatively low rate. Therefore, this agent must be given in high doses to cause killing. Some members of the third-generation cephalosporins (e.g., **ceftazidime**), fourth-generation cephalosporins (e.g., **cefepime**), monobactams (**aztreonam**), carbapenems (e.g., **imipenem**, **meropenem**, **doripenem**), quinolones (e.g., **ciprofloxacin**, **levofloxacin**), and aminoglycosides (e.g., **gentamicin**, **tobramycin**, and **amikacin**) are active against *P. aeruginosa*. However, not all drugs within a class are equivalent with regard to their antipseudomonal activity. For example, piperacillin is more active than ticarcillin, ciprofloxacin is more active than the other quinolones, and tobramycin is

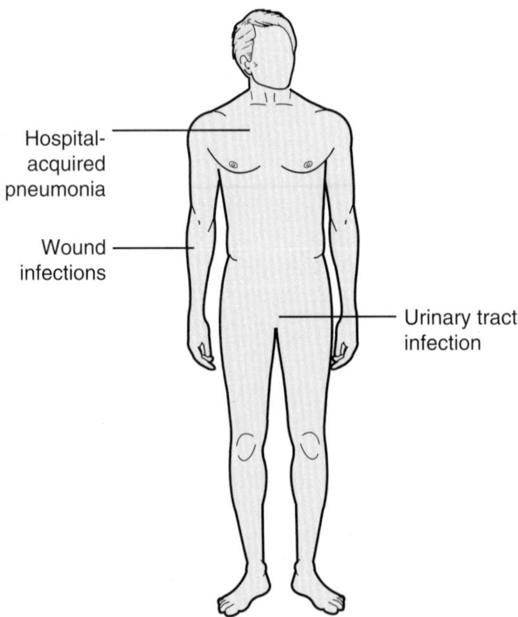

FIGURE 11-2. Sites of *Pseudomonas aeruginosa* infections.

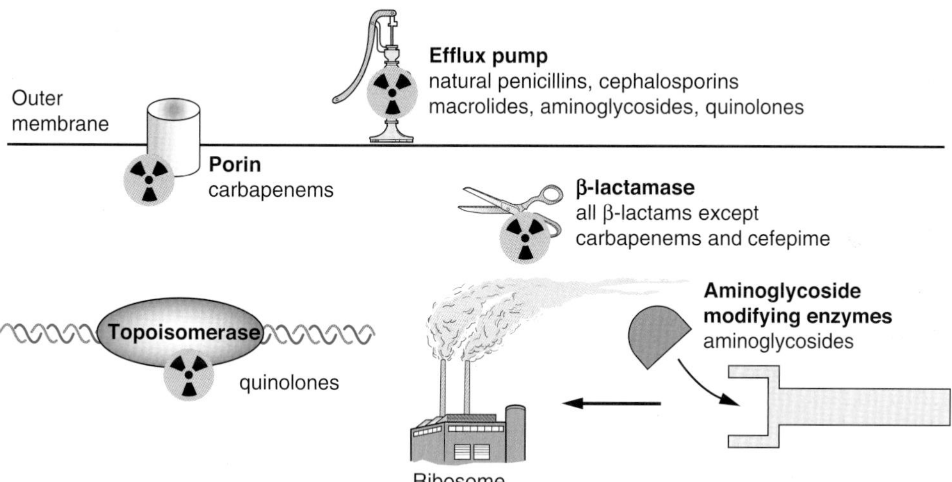

FIGURE 11-3. Intrinsic and acquired resistance mechanisms of *Pseudomonas aeruginosa*. Intrinsic resistance mechanisms are present in all strains of *P. aeruginosa*. Mutations and the acquisition of exogenous genetic material allow certain strains to acquire resistance to additional antibiotics through enhancement of intrinsic resistance mechanisms and production of new resistance determinants. The radioactivity symbol represents the acquisition of mutations that alter the production of the indicated protein(s).

more active than gentamicin. Among the carbapenems, ertapenem should not be used to treat *P. aeruginosa* infections. **Colistin** is increasingly being used to treat infections caused by isolates resistant to other antibiotics.

Unfortunately, *P. aeruginosa* is also especially adept at acquiring resistance to most antibiotics, so it is not reliably susceptible to any of these agents. Acquired resistance occurs by various mechanisms (Fig. 11-3). Mutations resulting in hyperproduction of the chromosomal β-lactamase result in resistance to all β-lactams except the carbapenems and cefepime. Likewise, mutations can cause the overproduction of efflux pumps, which may result in resistance to penicillins, cephalosporins, aminoglycosides, and quinolones. Mutations in the gene encoding one of the outer membrane porins may prevent penetration of the carbapenems, and production of altered topoisomerases may result in loss of sensitivity to quinolones. Aminoglycoside resistance may also occur following acquisition of genes that encode for the production of factors that acetylate or adenylate the aminoglycoside itself, preventing it from binding the ribosome.

Table 11-2 Antimicrobial Agents for Treatment of Infections Caused by *Pseudomonas Aeruginosa*

Antibiotic Class	Antibiotic
Extended-spectrum penicillins	Piperacillin
Third-generation cephalosporins	Ceftazidime
Fourth-generation cephalosporins	Cefepime
Carbapenems	Imipenem, meropenem, doripenem
Monobactams	Aztreonam
Quinolones	Ciprofloxacin, levofloxacin
Aminoglycosides	Gentamicin, tobramycin, amikacin
Colistin	
Combination therapy for serious infections	
Antipseudomonal β-lactam + aminoglycoside	e.g., ceftazidime + tobramycin
Extended-spectrum penicillin + antipseudomonal quinolone	e.g., piperacillin + ciprofloxacin

As a result of intrinsic and acquired resistance, *P. aeruginosa* strains are frequently not susceptible to one or more antibiotics. For example, recent surveys indicate that 15% to 25% of strains are resistant to piperacillin, 20% to 30% to ceftazidime, and 40% to 45% to aztreonam. Thus, no antibiotic regimen is uniformly effective against *P. aeruginosa*, and therapy must be guided by the susceptibility profiles of individual strains.

Even more disconcerting is the emergence of resistance *during* appropriate treatment of *P. aeruginosa* infections, which obviously leads to treatment failure. To prevent this phenomenon, severe *P. aeruginosa* infections are usually treated with two antibiotics simultaneously. Certain combinations have a synergistic effect on killing. In other words, use of these agents together results in significantly greater killing than would be anticipated given the effects of each agent alone. These combinations include an antipseudomonal β-lactam with an aminoglycoside and perhaps an antipseudomonal β-lactam in conjunction with an antipseudomonal quinolone.

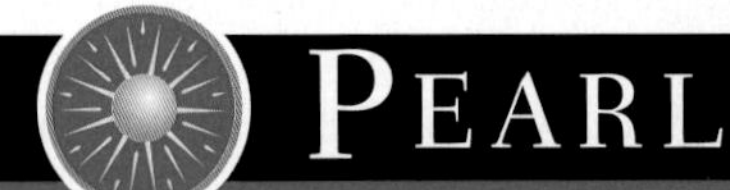

Tazobactam does not have activity against common β-lactamases of *Pseudomonas aeruginosa*. As a result, strains of *P. aeruginosa* that are resistant to piperacillin are usually also resistant to piperacillin-tazobactam.

Acar JF, Goldstein FW, Kitzis MD. Susceptibility survey of piperacillin alone and in the presence of tazobactam. *J Antimicrob Chemoth.* 1993;31(suppl A):23–28.

QUESTIONS

8. The following commonly used cephalosporins have antipseudomonal activity: ________________ and ________________.

9. ________________ is more active than ticarcillin against *Pseudomonas aeruginosa*.

10. Severe *P. aeruginosa* infections are usually treated with ________________ antibiotics concurrently.

11. Certain combinations of antibiotics exhibit synergistic killing of *P. aeruginosa*. These include ________________ + ________________ and ________________ + ________________.

ADDITIONAL READINGS

Bonomo RA, Szabo D. Mechanisms of multidrug resistance in Acinetobacter species and Pseudomonas aeruginosa. *Clin Infect Dis*. 2006;43(suppl 2):S49–S56.

Cunha BA. Pseudomonas aeruginosa: resistance and therapy. *Semin Respir Infect*. 2002;17:231–239.

Hauser AR, Sriram P. Severe Pseudomonas aeruginosa infections: tackling the conundrum of drug resistance. *Postgrad Med*. 2005;117:41–48.

Lambert PA. Mechanisms of antibiotic resistance in Pseudomonas aeruginosa. *J R Soc Med*. 2002; 95(suppl 41):22–26.

Neisseria

The genus *Neisseria* includes two commonly encountered and medically important species: *Neisseria meningitidis* and *Neisseria gonorrhoeae*. *N. meningitidis* is a much feared cause of meningitis and sepsis (Fig. 11-4). Infections can progress at a remarkably rapid rate and lead to death of young, healthy individuals. *N. gonorrhoeae* causes the sexually transmitted disease gonorrhea. Infection with this bacterium usually leads to localized disease manifestations such as cervicitis, urethritis, and pelvic inflammatory disease. The organism, however, may spread via the bloodstream to joints and the skin, resulting in disseminated gonococcal disease.

Strains of *N. meningitidis* usually are sensitive to **penicillin**, which remains the treatment of choice for this organism (Table 11-3). Resistance to penicillin has been reported, however, so the susceptibility of individual strains should be checked. Third-generation cephalosporins, such as **ceftriaxone** and **cefotaxime**, achieve high levels in cerebral spinal fluid and are universally effective against *N. meningitidis*. **Chloramphenicol** is an alternative for patients who cannot tolerate β-lactam antibiotics. Because meningitis and sepsis caused by this bacterium may be rapidly fatal, prophylaxis is given to close contacts of cases to prevent acquisition of disease. **Ciprofloxacin**, **rifampin**, or **ceftriaxone** is used for this purpose.

In the past, *N. gonorrhoeae* infections were also routinely treated with penicillin. However, the gradual emergence of strains harboring resistance-conferring traits has resulted in the ineffectiveness of penicillin for most cases of gonorrhea. These traits include plasmids that encode β-lactamases, mutations that result in increased efflux

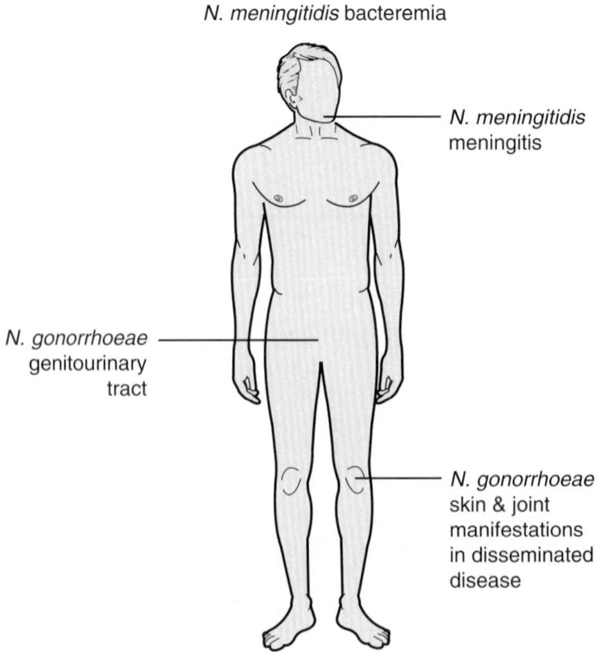

FIGURE 11-4. Sites of *Neisseria* spp. infections.

Table 11-3 **Antimicrobial Agents for Treatment of Infections Caused by *Neisseria Meningitidis***

Antibiotic Class	Antibiotic
Natural penicillins	Penicillin G
Third-generation cephalosporins	Ceftriaxone, cefotaxime
Postexposure prophylaxis	
Quinolone	Ciprofloxacin
Rifamycin	Rifampin
Third-generation cephalosporins	Ceftriaxone

and decreased penetration through porins, and modification of penicillin-binding proteins (PBPs). Fortunately, these mechanisms have not resulted in resistance to the third-generation cephalosporins. Thus, current recommendations for the treatment of uncomplicated gonorrhea in adults call for the use of **ceftriaxone** or **cefixime** (Table 11-4). Note that gonorrhea is frequently complicated by coinfection with *Chlamydia trachomatis*, so empiric treatment for *Chlamydia* is recommended for anyone diagnosed with *N. gonorrhoeae* disease.

QUESTIONS

12. The treatment of choice for *Neisseria meningitidis* infections is ________________.

13. The treatments of choice for uncomplicated *Neisseria gonorrhoeae* infections in adults are ________________ or ________________.

14. Because of the frequency of coinfection, antibiotics for ________________ should also be given to anyone being treated for gonorrhoea.

ADDITIONAL READINGS

Centers for Disease Control and Prevention. Sexually transmitted diseases treatment guidelines, 2006. *MMWR Recomm Rep*. 2006;55:1–94.

Deguchi T, Saito I, Tanaka M, et al. Fluoroquinolone treatment failure in gonorrhea. Emergence of a Neisseria gonorrhoeae strain with enhanced resistance to fluoroquinolones. *Sex Transm Dis*. 1997;24:247–250.

Lyss SB, Kamb ML, Peterman TA, et al. Chlamydia trachomatis among patients infected with and treated for Neisseria gonorrhoeae in sexually transmitted disease clinics in the United States. *Ann Intern Med*. 2003;139:178–185.

Tunkel AR, Hartman BJ, Kaplan SL, et al. Practice guidelines for the management of bacterial meningitis. *Clin Infect Dis*. 2004;39:1267–1284.

Table 11-4 **Antimicrobial Agents for Treatment of Infections Caused by *Neisseria Gonorrhoeae***

Antibiotic Class	Antibiotic
Third-generation cephalosporins	Ceftriaxone, cefixime

Curved Gram-Negative Bacteria

C. jejuni, *H. pylori*, and *Vibrio cholerae* all share a similar morphology, that of a curved gram-negative rod. In addition, these bacteria all infect the human gastrointestinal tract. However, they each differ in their disease manifestations and the antimicrobial regimens used to treat them.

CAMPYLOBACTER JEJUNI

C. jejuni is one of the most common causes of acute bacterial gastroenteritis in the world. This organism colonizes many types of wild and domesticated animals; humans become infected following ingestion of contaminated food or water. Clinical manifestations include diarrhea, fever, and abdominal pain (Fig. 11-5).

Antibiotic treatment is indicated for only a subset of patients infected with *C. jejuni*. These include individuals with high fevers, bloody or profuse diarrhea, or prolonged symptoms, or those who are immunocompromised. Preferred treatments are macrolides (**erythromycin**, **azithromycin**, **clarithromycin**) or quinolones (**ciprofloxacin**), although resistance rates to ciprofloxacin are increasing. Alternatives include tetracyclines (**tetracycline**, **doxycycline**), aminoglycosides (**gentamicin**, **tobramycin**, **amikacin**), **amoxicillin plus clavulanic acid**, or **chloramphenicol** (Table 11-5).

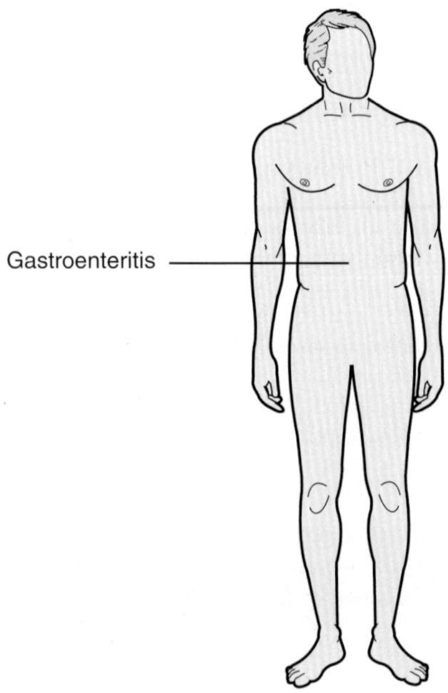

FIGURE 11-5. Sites of *Campylobacter jejuni* infections.

Table 11-5 **Antimicrobial Agents for Treatment of Infections Caused by *Campylobacter Jejuni***

Antibiotic Class	Antibiotic
Treatment of choice	
Macrolides	Erythromycin, azithromycin, clarithromycin
Quinolones	Ciprofloxacin
Alternatives	
Tetracyclines	Tetracycline, doxycycline
Aminoglycosides	Gentamicin, tobramycin, amikacin
Aminopenicillin + β-lactamase inhibitor	Amoxicillin + clavulanic acid
Chloramphenicol	

HELICOBACTER PYLORI

The discovery of the role of *H. pylori* in peptic ulcer disease is one of the great paradigm shifts in medicine in which an infectious etiology was identified for a disease formerly thought to be idiopathic in origin. *H. pylori* inhabits the human stomach, where it is associated with inflammation that predisposes to peptic ulcer disease (Fig. 11-6). In the absence of antimicrobial therapy, infections tend to last for years, often for the lifetime of the individual.

H. pylori is susceptible to several antibiotics in vitro. These include **amoxicillin**, **clarithromycin**, **metronidazole**, and **tetracycline** (Table 11-6). In addition, **bismuth**

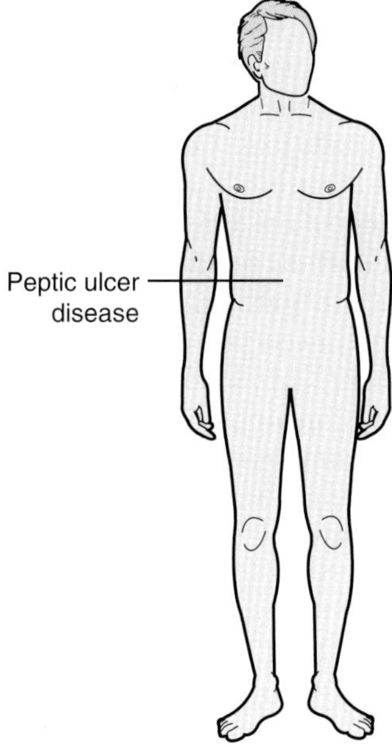

FIGURE 11-6. Sites of *Helicobacter pylori* infections.

Table 11-6 Antimicrobial Agents for Treatment of Infections Caused by *Helicobacter Pylori*

Antibiotic Class	Antibiotic
Aminopenicillins	Amoxicillin
Macrolides	Clarithromycin
Metronidazole	
Tetracyclines	Tetracycline
Bismuth subsalicylate	
Recommended regimens	
Amoxicillin + clarithromycin + proton pump inhibitor	
Metronidazole + clarithromycin + proton pump inhibitor	
Bismuth subsalicylate + metronidazole + tetracycline + proton pump inhibitor	

subsalicylate, more commonly known in the United States as Pepto-Bismol, is active against this bacterium. The bismuth component of this preparation disrupts the integrity of the *H. pylori* cell wall. Despite these in vitro susceptibilities, *H. pylori* is relatively difficult to eradicate with antibiotic therapy. Several factors may contribute to its recalcitrance. It is prone to develop resistance to antimicrobial agents, an especially problematic trait given that this organism causes chronic infections. A strain of *H. pylori* chronically inhabiting the stomach experiences the same cumulative antibiotic exposure as its host, and each exposure increases the risk of resistance. In addition, the acidic environment of the stomach limits the efficacy of certain antibiotics, allowing *H. pylori* bacteria to survive for longer periods during therapy and further predisposing to antimicrobial resistance. Therefore, it is not surprising that 20% to 40% of isolates are resistant to metronidazole and 10% are resistant to clarithromycin. Resistance to metronidazole results from mutations in the nitroreductase gene, which encodes a protein that reduces metronidazole to its active form. Mutations in one of the genes encoding a component of the 50S ribosomal subunit prevent binding of clarithromycin to the ribosome. For these reasons, eradication rates in infected individuals treated with a single antibiotic are quite low.

To counteract *H. pylori*'s predilection to develop resistance, combination regimens are used to treat this bacterium (Table 11-6). These regimens each consist of at least two antimicrobial agents in conjunction with an antisecretory agent that blocks acid production. The antisecretory component of the regimen increases gastric pH, which allows for optimal activity of some antimicrobial agents and may also limit ongoing tissue damage due to acid exposure.

VIBRIO CHOLERAE

V. cholerae continues to be of global significance and causes pandemics of the diarrheal illness cholera. Patients with cholera often have profuse watery diarrhea that

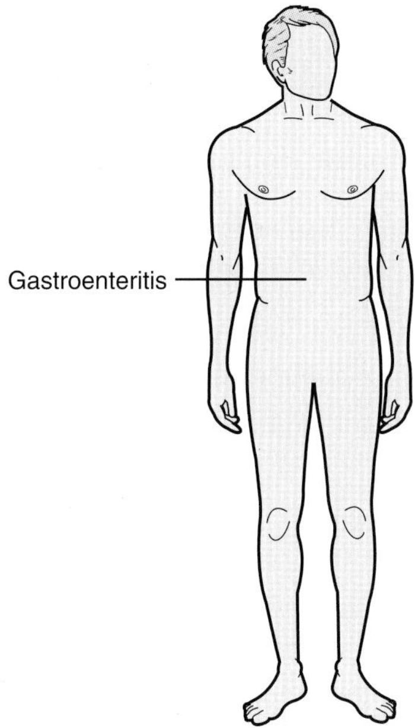

FIGURE 11-7. Sites of *Vibrio cholerae* infections.

may lead to dehydration and death in a matter of hours (Fig. 11-7). Antibiotics play an important role in decreasing the volume of stool and the duration of diarrhea in these patients. In the past, **tetracycline** and **doxycycline** were the agents of choice for cholera, but resistance is becoming increasingly common and occurs when strains acquire a plasmid that coexpresses resistance determinants to multiple antibiotics. Other active agents include a quinolone (**ciprofloxacin**), macrolide (**erythromycin, azithromycin**), or **trimethoprim-sulfamethoxazole** (Table 11-7), although resistance to trimethoprim-sulfamethoxazole is becoming more common.

Table 11-7 Antimicrobial Agents for Treatment of Infections Caused by *Vibrio Cholerae*

Antibiotic Class	Antibiotic
Active agents	
Tetracyclines	Tetracycline, doxycycline
Sulfa drugs	Trimethoprim-sulfamethoxazole
Quinolones	Ciprofloxacin
Macrolides	Erythromycin, azithromycin

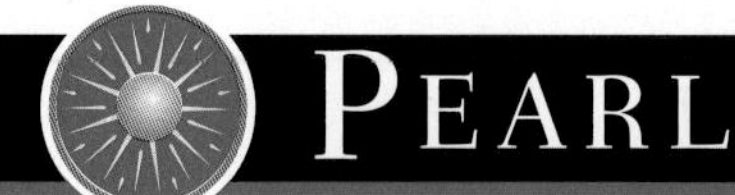

In addition to peptic ulcer disease, *Helicobacter pylori* infection has been associated with a form of gastric malignancy called mucosa-associated lymphoid tissue (MALT) lymphoma. Interestingly, eradication of *H. pylori* has been associated with long-term remission of these cancers. This represents an example of the successful use of antibiotics to treat cancer!

Stolte M, Bayerdorffer E, Morgner A, et al. Helicobacter and gastric MALT lymphoma. *Gut.* 2002;50(suppl 3): III19–III24.

QUESTIONS

15. Antimicrobial therapy for *Campylobacter jejuni* infections should ____________ be given for uncomplicated diarrhea in a normal host.

16. First-line agents for the treatment of *C. jejuni* infections include ____________ and ____________.

17. *Helicobacter pylori* is prone to developing resistance to antibiotics, so treatment regimens consisting of ____________ agents are recommended.

18. Treatment of *H. pylori* infections consists of two parts: an ____________ component and an ____________ component.

19. Traditionally, ____________ and ____________ were the antibiotics of choice for cholera, but resistance is now becoming increasingly common.

20. Other antibiotics used to treat cholera include ____________, ____________, ____________, and ____________.

ADDITIONAL READINGS

Bhattacharya SK. An evaluation of current cholera treatment. *Expert Opin Pharmacother*. 2003;4: 141–146.

Guerrant RL, Van Gilder T, Steiner TS, et al. Practice guidelines for the management of infectious diarrhea. *Clin Infect Dis*. 2001;32:331–351.

Howden CW, Hunt RH. Guidelines for the management of Helicobacter pylori infection. Ad Hoc Committee on Practice Parameters of the American College of Gastroenterology. *Am J Gastroenterol*. 1998;93:2330–2338.

Lariviere LA, Gaudreau CL, Turgeon FF. Susceptibility of clinical isolates of Campylobacter jejuni to twenty-five antimicrobial agents. *J Antimicrob Chemother*. 1986;18:681–685.

Megraud F. Resistance of Helicobacter pylori to antibiotics and its impact on treatment options. *Drug Resist Update*. 2001;4:178–186.

Walsh JH, Peterson WL. The treatment of Helicobacter pylori infection in the management of peptic ulcer disease. *N Engl J Med*. 1995;333:984–991.

Yamamoto T, Nair GB, Albert MJ, et al. Survey of in vitro susceptibilities of Vibrio cholerae O1 and O139 to antimicrobial agents. *Antimicrob Agents Chemother*. 1995;39:241–244.

Other Gram-Negative Bacteria

Many other gram-negative bacterial species are also common causes of infections in humans. Here, we will discuss four of them: *H. influenzae*, *B. pertussis*, *Moraxella catarrhalis*, and *Acinetobacter* spp.

HAEMOPHILUS INFLUENZAE

H. influenzae is a small pleomorphic (of variable morphology) gram-negative bacterium that is associated with mild as well as life-threatening infections. This organism causes otitis media, sinusitis, community-acquired pneumonia, conjunctivitis, meningitis, epiglottitis, and septic arthritis (Fig. 11-8). *H. influenzae* strains with type B capsules are especially virulent and historically were a major cause of invasive infections such as meningitis. However, they are becoming less common with the widespread use of the conjugate vaccine composed in part of type B capsular antigen.

For years, ampicillin or amoxicillin was routinely used to treat infections caused by *H. influenzae*. However, approximately 30% of strains now harbor plasmids that encode a β-lactamase that degrades these agents. Fortunately, this β-lactamase is inhibited by clavulanate and sulbactam, so aminopenicillin/β-lactamase inhibitor

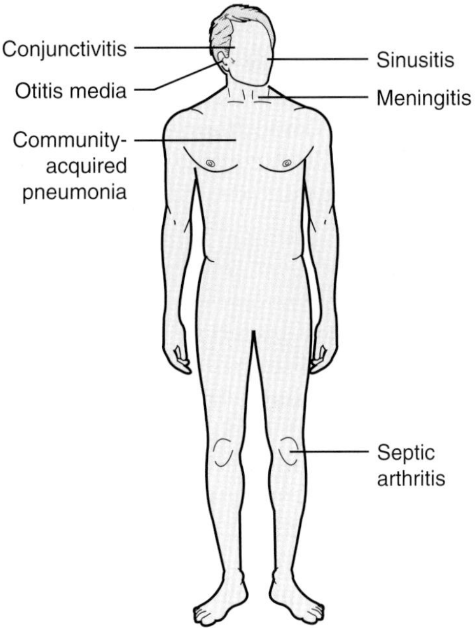

FIGURE 11-8. Sites of *Haemophilus influenzae* infections.

Table 11-8 Antimicrobial Agents for Treatment of Infections Caused by *Haemophilus Influenzae*

Antibiotic Class	Antibiotic
Treatment of choice	
Aminopenicillins + β-lactamase inhibitor	Amoxicillin/clavulanate, ampicillin/sulbactam
Second-generation cephalosporins	Cefuroxime
Third-generation cephalosporins	Ceftriaxone, cefotaxime
Also active	
Tetracyclines	Tetracycline, doxycycline
Macrolide-like agents	Azithromycin, telithromycin
Quinolones	Ciprofloxacin, levofloxacin, moxifloxacin, gemifloxacin
Carbapenems	Imipenem, meropenem, doripenem, ertapenem
Sometimes active	
Sulfa drugs	Trimethoprim-sulfamethoxazole
Prophylaxis for serotype B	
Rifamycins	Rifampin

combinations (**amoxicillin plus clavulanate**, **ampicillin plus sulbactam**) remain effective (Table 11-8). Likewise, second- and third-generation cephalosporins (**cefuroxime**, **ceftriaxone**, **cefotaxime**) are stable in the presence of this β-lactamase. Other useful antibiotics include quinolones (**ciprofloxacin**, **levofloxacin**, **moxifloxacin**, **gemifloxacin**), macrolide-like agents (**azithromycin**, **telithromycin**), tetracyclines (**tetracycline**, **doxycycline**), and carbapenems (**imipenem**, **meropenem**, **doripenem**, **ertapenem**). **Trimethoprim-sulfamethoxazole** is also active, although resistance is increasing. Close contacts of patients infected with serotype B *H. influenzae* should receive prophylaxis with **rifampin**.

BORDETELLA PERTUSSIS

B. pertussis is a small coccobacillary bacterium that causes pertussis, or whooping cough (Fig. 11-9). In children, this disease is characterized by a series of short, rapid coughs followed by a gasp for air, causing a "whoop." Although traditionally viewed as a disease of children, whooping cough is increasingly being recognized as a frequent cause of cough lasting several weeks or longer in adults.

Antimicrobial treatment of pertussis is controversial but is usually recommended early in disease because it may shorten the course of the illness and limit transmission. Macrolides (**azithromycin**, **clarithromycin**, **erythromycin**) are the drugs of choice for both children and adults based on their in vitro activity and the results of clinical trials (Table 11-9). Other active agents include the quinolones (**ciprofloxacin**, **levofloxacin**, **moxifloxacin**), **telithromycin**, **trimethoprim-sulfamethoxazole**, and the tetracyclines (**tetracycline**, **doxycycline**). Postexposure

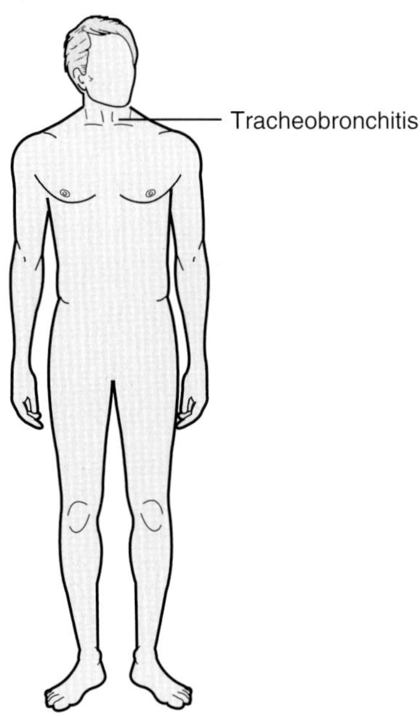

FIGURE 11-9. Sites of *Bordetella pertussis* infections.

prophylaxis with a macrolide should be considered in close contacts of contagious individuals with pertussis.

MORAXELLA CATARRHALIS

M. catarrhalis is a gram-negative diplococcus that commonly causes otitis media, pneumonia, and sinusitis (Fig. 11-10). Nearly all strains produce a β-lactamase that

Table 11-9 Antimicrobial Agents for Treatment of Infections Caused by *Bordetella Pertussis*

Antibiotic Class	Antibiotic
Treatment of choice	
Macrolides	Azithromycin, clarithromycin, erythromycin
Other active agents	
Sulfa drugs	Trimethoprim-sulfamethoxazole
Quinolone*	Ciprofloxacin, levofloxacin, moxifloxacin
Tetracyclines*	Tetracycline, doxycycline
Macrolide-like agents	Telithromycin
Postexposure prophylaxis	
Macrolides	Azithromycin, clarithromycin, erythromycin

*Quinolones and tetracyclines are contraindicated in children and pregnant women.

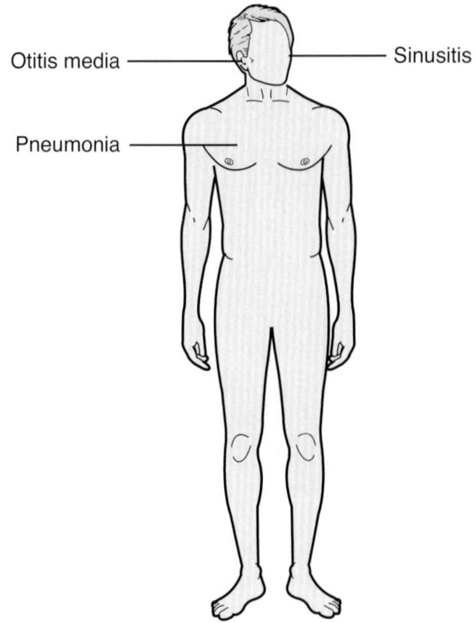

FIGURE 11-10. Sites of *Moraxella catarrhalis* infections.

confers resistance to amoxicillin and ampicillin. Antibiotics with some efficacy against this bacterium include the extended-spectrum penicillins (**piperacillin**), β-lactam/β-lactamase inhibitor combinations (**amoxicillin plus clavulanate**, **ampicillin plus sulbactam**), second- and third-generation cephalosporins (**cefuroxime**, **ceftriaxone**, **cefotaxime**), aminoglycosides (**gentamicin**, **tobramycin**, **amikacin**), **trimethoprim-sulfamethoxazole**, tetracyclines (**tetracycline**, **doxycycline**), macrolides (**azithromycin**, **chlarithromycin**), and quinolones (**ciprofloxacin**, **levofloxacin**, **moxifloxacin**) (Table 11-10).

Table 11-10 Antimicrobial Agents for Treatment of Infections Caused by *Moraxella Catarrhalis*

Antibiotic Class	Antibiotic
Extended-spectrum penicillins	Piperacillin
Aminopenicillins + β-lactamase inhibitor	Amoxicillin/clavulanate, ampicillin/sulbactam
Second-generation cephalosporins	Cefuroxime
Third-generation cephalosporins	Ceftriaxone, cefotaxime
Macrolides	Azithromycin, clarithromycin
Aminoglycosides	Gentamicin, tobramycin, amikacin
Sulfa drugs	Trimethoprim-sulfamethoxazole
Quinolones	Ciprofloxacin, levofloxacin, moxifloxacin
Tetracyclines	Tetracycline, doxycycline

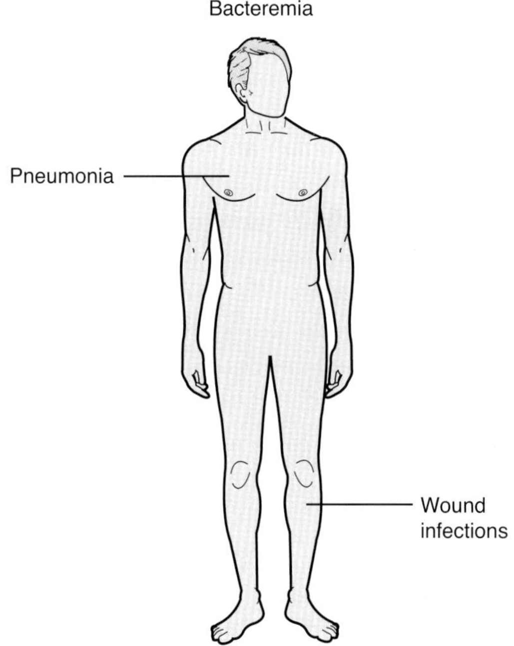

FIGURE 11-11. Sites of *Acinetobacter baumannii* infections.

ACINETOBACTER

Acinetobacter spp. are gram-negative rod-shaped and coccobacillary bacteria that cause several hospital- and community-acquired infections. These include pneumonia, bacteremia, and wound infections (Fig. 11-11). Treatment can be problematic because many strains are highly antibiotic resistant. Interestingly, the β-lactamase inhibitor **sulbactam** has intrinsic bactericidal activity against this bacterium, and as expected, **ampicillin-sulbactam** has proven effective in treating infections caused by these organisms (Table 11-11). Likewise, carbapenems (**imipenem**, **meropenem**, **doripenem**), **rifampin**, and **amikacin** may be active. However, resistance to each of these agents is increasing. **Colistin** and **tigecycline** are sometimes used for strains resistant to other antibiotics.

Table 11-11 **Antimicrobial Agents for Treatment of Infections Caused by *Acinetobacter* Spp.**

Antibiotic Class	Antibiotic
Aminopenicillins + β-lactamase inhibitor	Ampicillin/sulbactam
Carbapenems	Imipenem, meropenem, doripenem
Rifamycins	Rifampin
Aminoglycosides	Amikacin
Colistin	
Tetracycline-like agents	Tigecycline

Questions

21. The use of ampicillin and amoxicillin for treatment of *Haemophilus influenzae* infections is now limited by the production of a ________________ by many strains.

22. The agents of choice for *H. influenzae* infections are ________________, ________________, ________________, or ________________.

23. The agents of choice for *Bordetella pertussis* infections are ________________, ________________, and ________________.

24. Other antibiotics active against *B. pertussis* include ________________, ________________, ________________, and ________________.

25. Nearly all strains of *Moraxella catarrhalis* produce a ________________ that confers resistance to β-lactams.

26. The β-lactamase inhibitor ________________ has activity against *Acinetobacter baumannii.*

Additional Readings

Doern GV, Brueggemann AB, Pierce G, et al. Antibiotic resistance among clinical isolates of Haemophilus influenzae in the United States in 1994 and 1995 and detection of beta-lactamase-positive strains resistant to amoxicillin-clavulanate: results of a national multicenter surveillance study. *Antimicrob Agents Chemother*. 1997;41:292–297.

Gordon KA, Fusco J, Biedenbach DJ, et al. Antimicrobial susceptibility testing of clinical isolates of Bordetella pertussis from northern California: report from the SENTRY Antimicrobial Surveillance Program. *Antimicrob Agents Chemother*. 2001;45:3599–3600.

Hewlett EL, Edwards KM. Clinical practice. Pertussis—not just for kids. *N Engl J Med*. 2005;352: 1215–1222.

Munoz-Price LS, Weinstein RA. Acinetobacter infection. *N Engl J Med*. 2008;358:1271–1281.

Murphy TF. Respiratory infections caused by non-typeable Haemophilus influenzae. *Curr Opin Infect Dis*. 2003;16:129–134.

Murphy TF, Parameswaran GI. Moraxella catarrhalis, a human respiratory tract pathogen. *Clin Infect Dis*. 2009;49:124–131.

Verduin CM, Hol C, Fleer A, et al. Moraxella catarrhalis: from emerging to established pathogen. *Clin Microbiol Rev*. 2002;15:125–144.

Vila J, Pachon J. Therapeutic options for Acinetobacter baumannii infections. *Expert OpinPharmacother*. 2008;9:587–599.

von Konig CH. Use of antibiotics in the prevention and treatment of pertussis. *Pediatr Infect Dis J*. 2005;24:S66–S68.

CHAPTER 12

Anaerobic Bacteria

"The trebuchet was a lever on a fulcrum, and proved very effective although it was costly and cumbersome. Heavy weights were suspended from the forward end and these, when the rear portion was released, swung it into the air with its missile. . . . In 1345 a captured messenger was launched back into Auberoche."

—SIEGES OF THE MIDDLE AGES, PHILIP WARNER

Just as medieval attackers shattered the defensive walls of castles using trebuchets and other assault weapons, many anaerobes injure the human body by elaborating powerful toxins. Some of these toxins, such as those made by several clostridial species, are among the most potent bacterial toxins known.

Anaerobes are bacteria unable to grow in the physiologic concentrations of oxygen. Many of these organisms are normal inhabitants of the human oral cavity, gastrointestinal tract, and female genital tract. Infections often occur following disruption of mucosal surfaces in regions where large numbers of anaerobic bacteria reside. *Bacteroides*, *Porphyromonas*, and *Prevotella* spp. are anaerobic gram-negative bacteria that are frequently encountered in such scenarios. Other anaerobic bacteria are found in the environment and cause infections following inadvertent inoculation into the human body. *Clostridium* spp. that cause tetanus, botulism, and gas gangrene are examples of such anaerobic bacteria. In this section, we will discuss these organisms, with particular emphasis on effective antimicrobial therapies used to treat the infections they cause.

Clostridia

Clostridia spp. are gram-positive spore-forming anaerobic bacilli. They cause several well-known and feared diseases in humans, such as tetanus, botulism, and gas gangrene. In addition, one member of this group, *Clostridium difficile*, is an important cause of iatrogenic gastrointestinal infections. Although these diseases are quite distinct, they have in common that each is mediated by a potent toxin or toxins.

Clostridium tetani is the etiologic agent of tetanus (Fig. 12-1). This disease is characterized by persistent tonic spasm usually involving the masseter muscles ("lockjaw") and the musculature of the trunk. Symptoms follow inoculation of *C. tetani* spores into a deep wound. The devitalized tissue creates an anaerobic environment that allows germination of the spores and subsequent release of tetanus toxin. This toxin is transported to the brain and spinal cord through nerve axons and cause generalized muscle spasms and autonomic dysfunction. Treatment of tetanus consists of intensive supportive care with a focus on the respiratory and neuromuscular system. Antitoxin is given to neutralize circulating tetanus toxin. **Metronidazole** and **penicillin** are the antimicrobial agents of choice, with some data indicating that metronidazole is associated with better outcomes (Table 12-1).

Classically, botulism is acquired by ingestion of food contaminated with *Clostridium botulinum* spores, although it can also follow contamination of wounds (Fig. 12-1). *C. botulinum*, like *C. tetani*, produces a neurotoxin that causes systemic effects. Botulinum toxin, however, leads to cranial neuropathies and weakness rather than muscular spasm. Thus, the signs and symptoms of botulism differ significantly from those of tetanus. Patients with botulism also require intensive supportive care and the administration of antitoxin. **Penicillin** is the therapy of choice, and **metronidazole** is a useful alternative (Table 12-1).

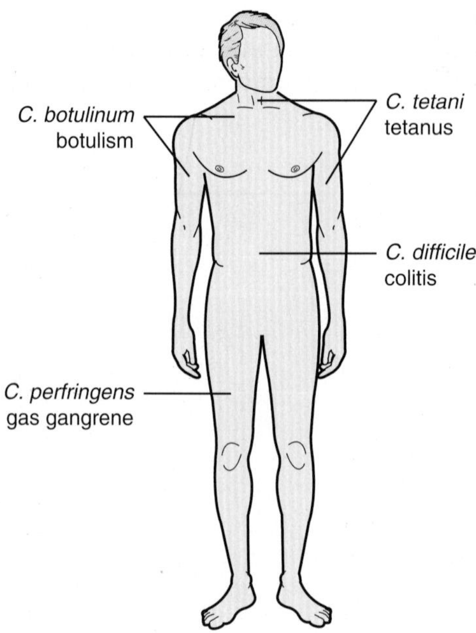

FIGURE 12-1. Sites of infections caused by *Clostridium* spp.

Table 12-1 Antimicrobial Agents for Treatment of Infections Caused by *Clostridium* Spp.

Antibiotic Class	Antibiotic
Treatment of choice	
Natural penicillins	Penicillin G*
Metronidazole	

* Exception: *Clostridium difficile* infections should not be treated with penicillin. Oral vancomycin or oral metronidazole should be used.

Clostridium perfringens is the cause of gas gangrene, a life-threatening and rapidly progressive infection of the soft tissues, muscles, and deeper structures of the body (Fig. 12-1). Therapy consists of surgical debridement in conjunction with antimicrobial therapy. **Penicillin** plus either **clindamycin**, **tetracycline**, or **metronidazole** is usually used (Table 12-1).

Unlike the other members of the clostridia genus, *C. difficile* causes disease that is not associated with trauma or ingestion but rather with antibiotic use. The normal flora of the human colon appears to be sufficient to prevent high levels of colonization by *C. difficile*. Following administration of antibiotics, however, many components of the normal flora are suppressed, allowing overgrowth by *C. difficile*. In this regard, clindamycin appears to be particularly problematic. Infection by this bacterium is associated with a wide spectrum of disease, from minimal diarrhea to fulminant and life-threatening pseudomembranous colitis (Fig. 12-1). Treatment includes stopping the causative antibiotic if possible and administering an anticlostridial antibiotic. The agent of choice is oral **metronidazole** for mild to moderate disease. Oral **vancomycin**, which is not appreciably absorbed but achieves high levels in the gastrointestinal tract, is recommended for severe disease (Table 12-1).

PEARL

The antibiotics most often associated with the development of *Clostridium difficile* disease are clindamycin, ampicillin, and the cephalosporins. Whereas ampicillin and cephalosporins cause a large proportion of *C. difficile* disease because these antibiotics are so frequently prescribed, the association with clindamycin appears to be more specific. Like most species of anaerobic bacteria, *C. difficile* is generally susceptible to clindamycin. However, strains of *C. difficile* that cause hospital outbreaks of diarrhea and colitis tend to be resistant to this antibiotic. Thus, in addition to suppressing the normal flora, clindamycin may actually select for *C. difficile* bacteria in the colon.

Johnson S, Samore MH, Farrow KA, et al. Epidemics of diarrhea caused by a clindamycin-resistant strain of Clostridium difficile in four hospitals. *N Engl J Med.* 1999;341:1645–1651.

QUESTIONS

1. *Clostridium* spp. are ________________, ________________-forming, gram-________________ bacilli.
2. For most clostridial infections, ________________ and ________________ are the agents of choice.
3. *Clostridium difficile* colitis is treated with oral ________________ or oral ________________.

ADDITIONAL READINGS

Ahmadsyah I, Salim A. Treatment of tetanus: an open study to compare the efficacy of procaine penicillin and metronidazole. *Br Med J (Clin Res Ed)*. 1985;291:648–650.

Alexander CJ, Citron DM, Brazier JS, et al. Identification and antimicrobial resistance patterns of clinical isolates of Clostridium clostridioforme, Clostridium innocuum, and Clostridium ramosum compared with those of clinical isolates of Clostridium perfringens. *J Clin Microbiol.* 1995;33:3209–3215.

Cohen SH, Gerding DN, Johnson S, et al. Clinical practice guidelines for Clostridium difficile infections in adults: 2010 update by the Society for Healthcare Epidemiology of America (SHEA) and the Infectious Diseases Society of America (IDSA). *Infect Control Hosp Epidemiol.* 2010;31:431–455.

Darke SG, King AM, Slack WK. Gas gangrene and related infection: classification, clinical features and aetiology, management and mortality. A report of 88 cases. *Br J Surg*. 1977;64:104–112.

Sobel J. Botulism. *Clin Infect Dis*. 2005;41:1167–1173.

Anaerobic Gram-Negative Bacilli

The oral cavity, gastrointestinal tract, and vagina of humans are colonized to high levels by several anaerobic gram-negative bacilli, including *Bacteroides* (most importantly, the *Bacteroides fragilis* group), *Prevotella*, and *Porphyromonas* spp. Under appropriate circumstances, these bacteria can contribute to periodontal disease, pleuropulmonary infections, pelvic inflammatory disease, and intra-abdominal abscesses (Fig. 12-2). It has been postulated that their virulence is enhanced by other bacterial species, and thus these organisms are usually associated with polymicrobial infections.

Anaerobic gram-negative bacilli, particularly the *B. fragilis* group of bacteria, frequently produce β-lactamases that destroy many of the penicillins and cephalosporins. Carbapenems and some cephalosporins (the cephamycins cefotetan and cefoxitin), however, are usually stable with these β-lactamases. Likewise, these enzymes are inactivated by β-lactamase inhibitors.

Treatment of anaerobic infections is often empirical and based on the observation that anaerobic gram-negative bacilli are nearly uniformly susceptible to β-lactam/β-lactamase inhibitor combinations (**ampicillin-sulbactam**, **piperacillin-tazobactam**, **ticarcillin-clavulanate**), carbapenems (**imipenem**, **meropenem**, **doripenem**, **ertapenem**), and **metronidazole** (Table 12-2). **Chloramphenicol** is also highly effective, but its use is limited by its toxicity. Other agents with relatively good activity against anaerobic gram-negative bacilli are **clindamycin**, **piperacillin**, **tigecycline**, and certain members of the cephalosporin (**cefotetan**, **cefoxitin**) and quinolone (**moxifloxacin**) classes.

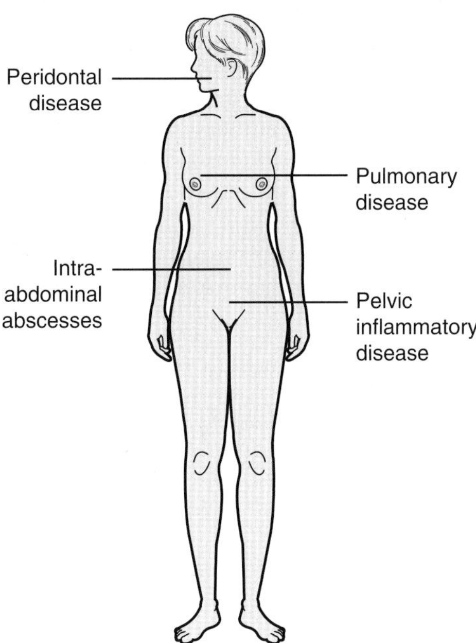

FIGURE 12-2. Sites of infections caused by anaerobic gram-negative bacilli.

Table 12-2 Antimicrobial Agents for Treatment of Infections Caused by *Bacteroides*, *Prevotella*, and *Porphyromonas* Spp.

Antibiotic Class	Antibiotic
First-line agents	
β-lactam/β-lactamase inhibitor combinations	Ampicillin-sulbactam, piperacillin-tazobactam, ticarcillin-clavulanate
Carbapenems	Imipenem, meropenem, doripenem, ertapenem
Metronidazole	
Second-line agents	
Clindamycin	
Second-generation cephalosporins	Cefotetan, cefoxitin
Extended-spectrum penicillins	Piperacillin
Quinolones	Moxifloxacin
Tetracycline-like agents	Tigecycline
Chloramphenicol	

QUESTIONS

4. ________________, ________________, and ________________ spp. are clinically important anaerobic gram-negative bacilli.
5. The four types of antibiotics that have excellent activity against anaerobic gram-negative bacilli are ________________, ________________, ________________, and ________________.
6. Other antibiotics that have good activity against anaerobic gram-negative bacilli include ________________, ________________, ________________, ________________, and certain members of the ________________.

ADDITIONAL READINGS

Aldridge KE, Ashcraft D, Cambre K, et al. Multicenter survey of the changing in vitro antimicrobial susceptibilities of clinical isolates of Bacteroides fragilis group, Prevotella, Fusobacterium, Porphyromonas, and Peptostreptococcus species. *Antimicrob Agents Chemother*. 2001;45: 1238–1243.

Snydman DR, Jacobus NV, McDermott LA, et al. National survey on the susceptibility of Bacteroides fragilis group: report and analysis of trends for 1997–2000. *Clin Infect Dis*. 2002; 35(suppl 1):S126–S134.

Vedantam G, Hecht DW. Antibiotics and anaerobes of gut origin. *Curr Opin Microbiol*. 2003;6:457–461.

CHAPTER 13

Atypical Bacteria

"On the next day Cestius, at the head of a large force of picked men and all the archers, began to assault the Temple from the north. The Jews resisted from the roof of the colonnade, and repeatedly drove back those who approached the wall, but at length they were overwhelmed by the hail of missiles and withdrew. The front rank of the Romans then rested their shields against the wall, and on these the second row rested theirs and so on, till they formed a protective covering known to them as a 'tortoise.' When the missiles fell on this they glanced off harmlessly, so that the soldiers received no hurt as they undermined the wall. . . ."

—The Jewish War, Josephus

As mentioned previously, several bacteria do not conveniently fall into the categories of gram-positive bacteria, gram-negative bacteria, anaerobic bacteria, spirochete, or mycobacteria. These organisms will be discussed here and referred to as "atypical bacteria" because many of them are hard to visualize by routine methods such as Gram staining or are difficult to grow on laboratory media. Although this classification is not perfect, it does allow for a way of thinking about this diverse group of bacteria regarding antimicrobial therapy. The following bacteria will be discussed in this group: *Chlamydia* spp., *Mycoplasma* spp., *Legionella pneumophila*, *Brucella* spp., *Francisella tularensis*, and *Rickettsia* spp.

Many of the bacteria in this group kill or damage human cells by actually living and multiplying within them. In this way, they are similar to the medieval miners who tunneled under formidable defensive walls to allow an assault on the castle from within. A practical implication of this intracellular lifestyle is that the antibiotics used to treat infections caused by these bacteria usually must penetrate well into host cells.

Chlamydia

Bacteria of the genus *Chlamydia* are obligate intracellular organisms that have an interesting biphasic life cycle. These bacteria exist either as an inert but transmissible extracellular form called an elementary body (EB) or a metabolically active and multiplicative intracellular form called a reticulate body (RB). The *Chlamydia* genus formerly consisted of three clinically important species: *Chlamydia trachomatis*, *Chlamydia pneumoniae*, and *Chlamydia psittaci*. However, recent observations have suggested that the latter two species are actually quite distinct from *C. trachomatis*. As a result, they have now been relegated to their own genus called *Chlamydophila*.

Chlamydia trachomatis is the cause of one of the most common sexually transmitted diseases and also a leading cause of blindness in some parts of the world. *Chlamydophila pneumoniae* is a common etiology of community-acquired pneumonia, and *Chlamydophila psittaci* causes psittacosis, a rare type of pneumonia that is acquired from exotic birds (Fig. 13-1).

Because *Chlamydia* and *Chlamydophila* spp. are metabolically active only within host cells, antibiotics that penetrate to high levels within cells are required to treat infections caused by these bacteria. Agents of choice include some macrolides (**azithromycin**, **erythromycin**), tetracyclines (**doxycycline**, **tetracycline**), and some quinolones (Table 13-1). Whereas **ofloxacin** and **levofloxacin** are recommended for the treatment of infections caused by *Chlamydia trachomatis*, **moxifloxacin** and **gemifloxacin** have the best activity against *Chlamydophila pneumoniae*. **Telithromycin** is also active against *Chlamydophila pneumoniae*. *Chlamydia* and *Chlamydophila* spp. lack peptidoglycan, so β-lactams are in general ineffective, but for unclear reasons,

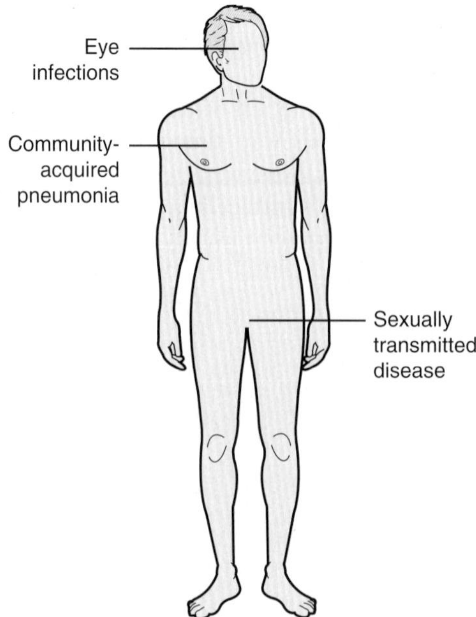

FIGURE 13-1. Sites of infections caused by *Chlamydia trachomatis* and *Chlamydophila* spp.

Table 13-1 Antimicrobial Agents for Treatment of Infections Caused by *Chlamydia* and *Chlamydophila* Spp.

Antibiotic Class	Antibiotic
Tetracyclines	Tetracycline, doxycycline
Macrolide-like agents	Azithromycin, erythromycin, telithromycin (*Chlamydophila pneumoniae*)
Quinolones	Ofloxacin (*Chlamydia trachomatis*), levofloxacin (*Chlamydia trachomatis*), moxifloxacin(*Chlamydophila pneumoniae*), gemifloxacin (*Chlamydophila pneumoniae*)
During pregnancy	
Macrolide-like agents	Azithromycin, erythromycin
Aminopenicillins	Amoxicillin

amoxicillin retains some activity. Because of its long history of safe use during pregnancy, it is often used in this situation for *Chlamydia trachomatis* infections. Note that **clindamycin** has some activity against *Chlamydia trachomatis* and is used in some antibiotic regimens for the treatment of pelvic inflammatory disease.

QUESTIONS

1. The three classes of antibiotics with the best activity against *Chlamydia trachomatis* are ________________, ________________, and ________________.
2. *Chlamydia* and *Chlamydophila* spp. do not make peptidoglycan and are therefore resistant to many ________________, although for unclear reasons, ______________ has some activity against *Chlamydia trachomatis*.

ADDITIONAL READINGS

Adimora AA. Treatment of uncomplicated genital Chlamydia trachomatis infections in adults. *Clin Infect Dis*. 2002;35(suppl 2):S183–S186.

Hammerschlag MR. Pneumonia due to Chlamydia pneumoniae in children: epidemiology, diagnosis, and treatment. *Pediatr Pulmonol*. 2003;36:384–390.

Kirchner JT. Psittacosis. Is contact with birds causing your patient's pneumonia? *Postgrad Med*. 1997;102:181–182, 187–188, 193–194.

Workowski KA, Berman S, Centers for Disease Control and Prevention. Sexually transmitted diseases treatment guidelines, 2010. *MMWR Recomm Rep*. 2010;59:1–110.

Mycoplasma

Members of the *Mycoplasma* genus share the property of being among the smallest known free-living organisms. Although several species are capable of causing disease in humans, *Mycoplasma pneumoniae* is the most commonly encountered. These bacteria, which can only grow when intimately associated with host cells or on highly supplemented laboratory media, are a frequent cause of community-acquired pneumonia (Fig. 13-2). Effective treatments include a macrolide (**azithromycin**, **clarithromycin**, **erythromycin**) or a tetracycline (**doxycycline**, **tetracycline**) (Table 13-2). Other active agents include quinolones (**levofloxacin**, **moxifloxacin**, **gemifloxacin**) and **telithromycin**. Mycoplasmas lack cell walls, so β-lactams have no activity against them.

Questions

3. The three classes of antibiotics with best activity against *Mycoplasma pneumoniae* are ________________, ________________, and ________________.
4. *M. pneumoniae* bacteria lack a cell wall, so ________________ are not active against them.

Additional Readings

Mandell LA, Bartlett JG, Dowell SF, et al. Update of practice guidelines for the management of community-acquired pneumonia in immunocompetent adults. *Clin Infect Dis*. 2003;37:1405–1433.

Taylor-Robinson D, Bébéar C. Antibiotic susceptibilities of mycoplasmas and treatment of mycoplasmal infections. *J Antimicrob Chemother*. 1997;40:622–630.

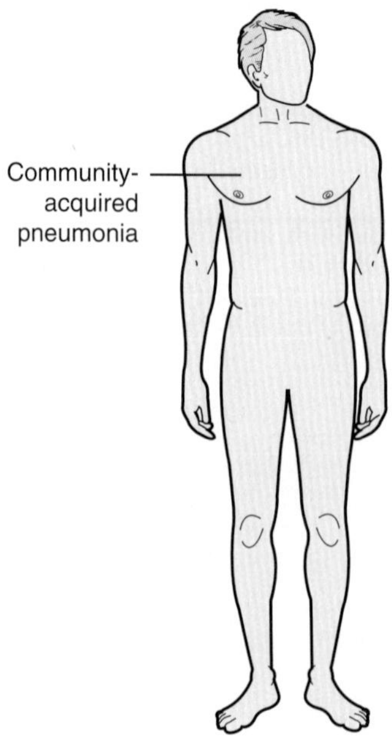

FIGURE 13-2. Sites of infections caused by *Mycoplasma pneumoniae*.

Table 13-2 Antimicrobial Agents for Treatment of Infections Caused by *Mycoplasma Pneumoniae*

Antibiotic Class	Antibiotic
Macrolide-like agents	Azithromycin, clarithromycin, erythromycin, telithromycin
Tetracyclines	Tetracycline, doxycycline
Quinolones	Levofloxacin, moxifloxacin, gemifloxacin

Legionella

Legionella spp. are environmental bacteria that inhabit natural and man-made water systems. Several species of *Legionella* are capable of causing disease in humans, but *L. pneumophila* is the most common. These bacteria cause Legionnaires disease, a severe form of pneumonia following inhalation or aspiration of this environmental organism, as well as Pontiac fever, which is a milder form of the disease that lacks respiratory features (Fig. 13-3). *Legionella* may cause either community- or hospital-acquired pneumonia. Once in the lung, *Legionella* organisms are taken up by macrophages and multiply within them. The net result of this process is the development of pneumonia that is frequently severe and often accompanied by systemic signs and symptoms, including high fever, chills, nausea, vomiting, diarrhea, and confusion. Laboratory studies may show evidence of hepatic or renal dysfunction and hyponatremia.

Because *Legionella* resides within macrophages during infection, treatment consists of antibiotics that penetrate into and are active within these phagocytes. Such antibiotics include the macrolides, tetracyclines, and quinolones. Agents of choice are **azithromycin**, **levofloxacin**, and **moxifloxacin** (Table 13-3). Other active agents include **ciprofloxacin**, **gemifloxacin**, **clarithromycin**, **telithromycin**, **erythromycin**, and **doxycycline**.

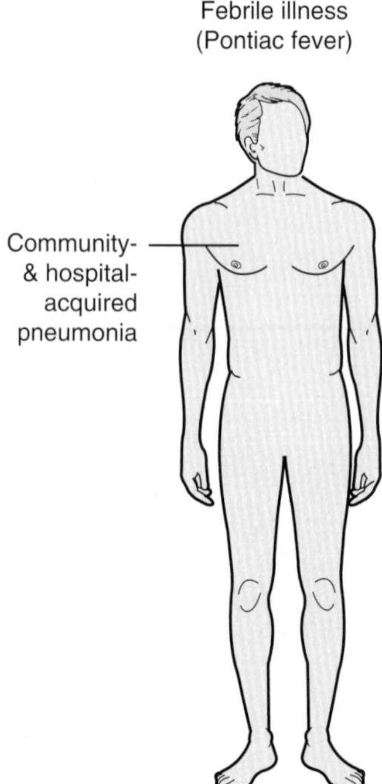

FIGURE 13-3. Sites of infections caused by *Legionella* spp.

Table 13-3 Antimicrobial Agents for Treatment of Infections Caused by *Legionella* Spp.

Antibiotic Class	Antibiotic
First-line agents	
Macrolides	Azithromycin
Quinolones	Levofloxacin, moxifloxacin
Second-line agents	
Macrolide-like agents	Erythromycin, clarithromycin, telithromycin
Quinolones	Ciprofloxacin, gemifloxacin
Tetracyclines	Doxycycline

QUESTIONS

5. The agents of choice for *Legionella* infections are ________________, ________________, and ________________.
6. During infection, *Legionella* bacteria reside primarily within ________________, so antibiotics must penetrate into these cells to kill these bacteria.

ADDITIONAL READINGS

Blázquez Garrido RM, Espinosa Parra FJ, Alemany Francés L, et al. Antimicrobial chemotherapy for Legionnaires disease: levofloxacin versus macrolides. *Clin Infect Dis*. 2005;40:800–806.

Roig J, Rello J. Legionnaires' disease: a rational approach to therapy. *J Antimicrob Chemother*. 2003;51:1119–1129.

Sabrià M, Pedro-Botet ML, Gómez J, et al. Fluoroquinolones vs macrolides in the treatment of Legionnaires disease. *Chest*. 2005;128:1401–1405.

Yu VL, Greenberg RN, Zadeikis N, et al. Levofloxacin efficacy in the treatment of community-acquired legionellosis. *Chest*. 2004;125:2135–2139.

Brucella

Brucella spp. are small gram-negative coccobacilli and cause brucellosis, a disease of animals that is occasionally transmitted to humans. Species most commonly associated with human disease include *Brucella melitensis*, *Brucella abortus*, *Brucella suis*, and *Brucella canis*. Close contact with animals and ingestion of unpasteurized milk or cheese are risk factors for acquisition. Symptoms include fever, sweats, malaise, anorexia, and fatigue (Fig. 13-4). Brucellosis is difficult to diagnose and, if untreated, may last for weeks or months. Prolonged infections tend to cause localized manifestations such as osteoarthritis, sacroiliitis, or epididymo-orchitis.

During infection, these *Brucella* bacteria survive and multiply within phagocytic cells. Therefore, the antibiotic regimens for brucellosis contain doxycycline, an agent that penetrates well into cells. The preferred regimens are **doxycycline** plus **rifampin** or **doxycycline** plus either **streptomycin** or **gentamicin** (Table 13-4). Quinolones (**ciprofloxacin**, **levofloxacin**, **moxifloxacin**) are also effective when used in conjunction with other agents such as **rifampin**, but experience is more limited. **Trimethoprim-sulfamethoxazole** plus **rifampin** is recommended for children and **trimethoprim-sulfamethoxazole** plus **rifampin** or **rifampin** alone for pregnant women, in whom doxycycline and quinolones are contraindicated. Infections must be treated for extended periods (e.g., 6 weeks), and relapses may occur.

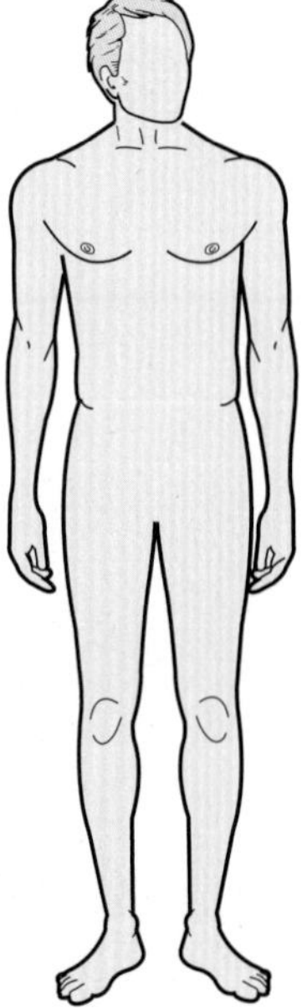

FIGURE 13-4. Sites of infections caused by *Brucella* spp.

Table 13-4 Antimicrobial Agents for Treatment of Infections Caused by *Brucella* Spp.

Antibiotic Class	Antibiotic
First-line regimens	
Tetracyclines + rifamycins	Doxycyline + rifampin
Tetracyclines + aminoglycosides	Doxycyline +gentamicin, Doxycyline + streptomycin
Alternative agents	
Sulfa drugs	Trimethoprim-sulfamethoxazole
Quinolones	Ciprofloxacin, levofloxacin, moxifloxacin

QUESTIONS

7. The four antibiotics most commonly used in treatment regimens for brucellosis are ________________, ________________, ________________ and ________________.
8. Combination therapy is usually used to treat brucellosis. Three common regimens are doxycycline + ________________, doxycycline + ________________, and doxycycline + ________________.
9. Because doxycycline and quinolones are not recommended for pregnant women, ________________ ± ________________ is used for these individuals when they acquire brucellosis.

ADDITIONAL READINGS

Ariza J, Gudiol F, Pallares R, et al. Treatment of human brucellosis with doxycycline plus rifampin or doxycycline plus streptomycin. A randomized, double-blind study. *Ann Intern Med.* 1992;117:25–30.
Franco MP, Mulder M, Gilman RH, et al. Human brucellosis. *Lancet Infect Dis.* 2007;7:775–786.
Pappas G, Akritidis N, Bosilkovski M, et al. Brucellosis. *N Engl J Med.* 2005;352:2325–2336.

HISTORY

Brucellosis has been blamed by some for one of the worst peacetime naval disasters, the collision between the HMS Victoria and the HMS Camperdown in 1893 off the coast of Syria. This collision resulted in the sinking of the Victoria, the flagship of the British Mediterranean Fleet, and the death of 358 of her crew. Some authorities believe that the commanders of these ships were suffering from brucellosis, which was endemic in parts of the Mediterranean region at that time. This may have led to impairment of their judgment and performance, leading to the collision.

Vassallo DJ. The centenary of the sinking of the Mediterranean Fleet flagship, HMS Victoria. What was the role of Malta fever? *J R Nav Med Serv.* 1993;79:91–99.

Francisella tularensis

Francisella tularensis, a gram-negative coccobacillus that primarily infects animals, causes tularemia. Humans acquire the infection from animals either directly through contact with contaminated animals or animal products, or indirectly through the bite of an insect, exposure to contaminated water or mud, or inhalation of aerosolized organisms. Because aerosolized *F. tularensis* is highly transmissible and may result in severe disease, this organism is currently classified as a bioterrorism agent.

Tularemia presents as one of several syndromes: ulceroglandular, glandular, typhoidal, pneumonic, oropharyngeal, and oculoglandular disease (Fig. 13-5). In ulceroglandular disease, patients typically have a skin lesion at the site of inoculation and tender regional lymphadenopathy involving one or more draining lymph nodes. Glandular tularemia is similar except that there is no apparent portal of entry. Patients with typhoidal tularemia present with a febrile illness and sepsis. Those with pneumonic disease have the signs and symptoms of pneumonia. In oropharyngeal tularemia, individuals have an ulcerative pharyngitis with enlarged cervical lymph nodes. Finally, oculoglandular disease is characterized by conjunctival erythema following inoculation of the organism into the eye.

Although *F. tularensis* is a facultative intracellular bacterium, use of **streptomycin** has yielded the best results in the treatment of tularemia (Table 13-5). The reasons for this are unclear but may indicate that antimicrobial killing of the extracellular phase of infection is sufficient for cure. **Gentamicin** is frequently used in place of streptomycin because it is more readily available, although outcomes may not be quite as good. **Tetracycline**, **doxycycline**, and **chloramphenicol** are acceptable alternatives.

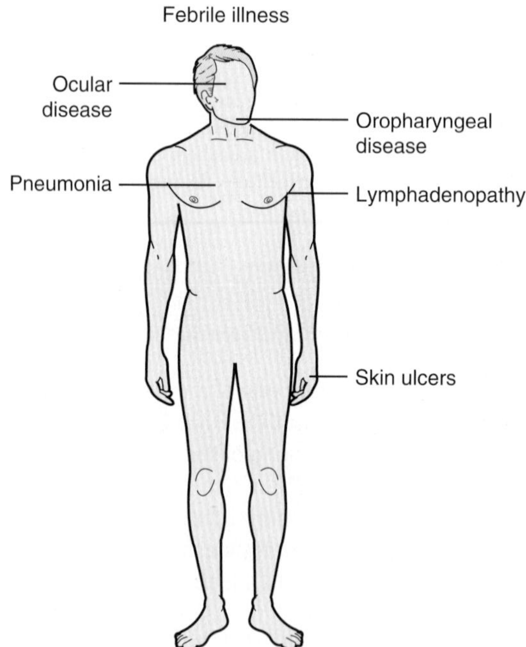

FIGURE 13-5. Sites of infections caused by *Francisella tularensis*.

Table 13-5 Antimicrobial Agents for Treatment of Infections Caused by *Francisella Tularensis*

Antibiotic Class	Antibiotic
First-line agent	
Aminoglycosides	Streptomycin
Alternatives	
Aminoglycosides	Gentamicin
Tetracyclines	Tetracycline, doxycycline
Chloramphenicol	

QUESTIONS

10. The antibiotic of choice for tularemia is ______________.

11. Because it is more readily available, ______________ is often substituted for streptomycin in the treatment of tularemia.

12. Other antibiotics useful in the treatment of tularemia include ______________, ______________, and ______________.

ADDITIONAL READINGS

Ellis J, Oyston PC, Green M, et al. Tularemia. *Clin Microbiol Rev*. 2002;15:631–646.

Enderlin G, Morales L, Jacobs RF, et al. Streptomycin and alternative agents for the treatment of tularemia: review of the literature. *Clin Infect Dis*. 1994;19:42–47.

Evans ME, Gregory DW, Schaffner W, et al. Tularemia: a 30-year experience with 88 cases. *Medicine (Baltimore)*. 1985;64:251–269.

Rickettsia

A large number of *Rickettsia* spp. are capable of causing disease in humans. These bacteria are small, have a gram-negative–like cell envelope structure, and are obligate intracellular pathogens. While the particular features of the rickettsial diseases differ somewhat, most consist of fever, headache, and rash, and most are acquired from arthropod vectors (Fig. 13-6). Many of these diseases will also have a characteristic black eschar at the site where the organism was inoculated by the vector. Examples of rickettsial diseases include Rocky Mountain spotted fever (*Rickettsia rickettsii*), Mediterranean spotted fever (*Rickettsia conorii*), rickettsialpox (*Rickettsia akari*), epidemic typhus (*Rickettsia prowazekii*), murine typhus (*Rickettsia typhi*), and scrub typhus (caused by the closely related bacterium *Orientia tsutsugamushi*).

Most rickettsial diseases are treated with **doxycycline**, which penetrates well into cells where the obligate intracellular *Rickettsia* bacteria reside (Table 13-6). This antibiotic is even recommended for children with some rickettsial diseases because the short course required for treatment is unlikely to harm bone or teeth. **Tetracycline** may also be used. Although not as effective as the tetracyclines, **chloramphenicol** is a useful alternative for pregnant women. **Ciprofloxacin** may also be used to treat Rocky Mountain spotted fever, Mediterranean spotted fever, and rickettsialpox.

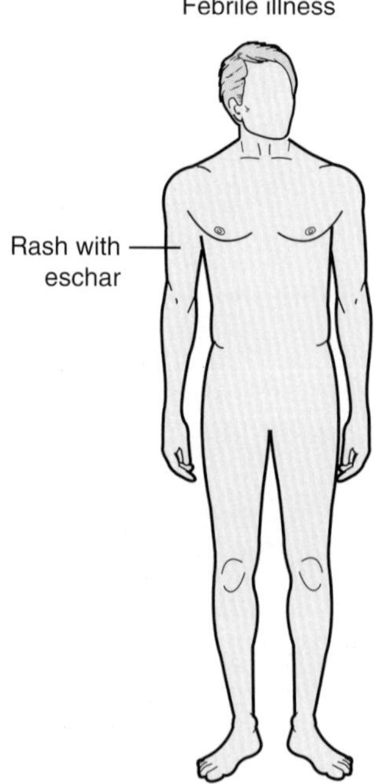

FIGURE 13-6. Sites of infections caused by *Rickettsia* spp.

Table 13-6 Antimicrobial Agents for Treatment of Infections Caused by *Rickettsia*

Antibiotic Class	Antibiotic
First-line agent	
Tetracyclines	Doxycycline, tetracycline
Alternatives	
Chloramphenicol	
Quinolones	Ciprofloxacin

QUESTIONS

13. The treatment of choice for rickettsial infections is ________________.
14. Other agents with activity against *Rickettsia* spp. are ________________, ________________, and ________________.

ADDITIONAL READINGS

Maender JL, Tyring SK. Treatment and prevention of rickettsial and ehrlichial infections. *Dermatol Ther*. 2004;17:499–504.

Parola P, Paddock CD, Raoult D. Tick-borne rickettsioses around the world: emerging diseases challenging old concepts. *Clin Microbiol Rev*. 2005;18:719–756.

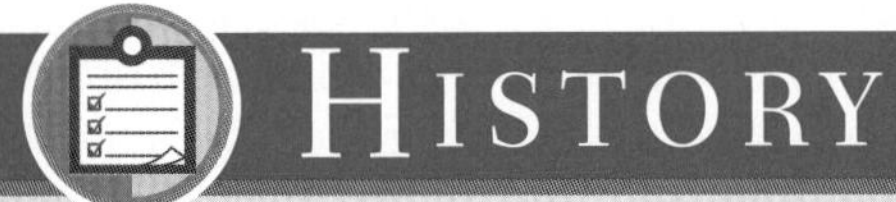

HISTORY

It has been speculated that louse-borne rickettsial diseases greatly weakened Napoleon's army during its retreat from Russia. Recently, investigators have verified this by detecting the DNA of *Rickettsia prowazekii* in dental pulp from the remains of soldiers buried in Lithuania.

Raoult D, Dutour O, Houhamdi L, et al. Evidence for louse-transmitted diseases in soldiers of Napoleon's grand army in Vilnius. *J Infect Dis*. 2006;193:112–120.

CHAPTER 14

Spirochetes

"So they sent Robert Fitz Hildebrand, a man of low birth indeed but also of tried military qualities, and, what disgraces and sullies the prime and the fame of soldiers, he was likewise a lustful man, drunken and unchaste. On arriving with a fine body of knights he obtained a most cordial reception, became extremely intimate with William, and could go in and out of his castle as he liked. Then, stung by desire, he seduced his wife, and afterwards, when a vile and abominable plan had been formed by agreement between him and the wife, he fettered William very tightly and imprisoned him in a dungeon, and enjoying his castle, wealth, and wife he likewise abandoned and rejected the countess, who had proudly sent him there, and made a pact with the king and the bishop. Nor did that reckless seducer escape punishment, as I have already said, for daring to devise such a villainous and treacherous plot, since, God most justly avenging his injustice, a worm was born at the time when the traitorous corrupter lay in the unchaste bosom of the adulteress and crept through his vitals, and slowly eating away his entrails it gradually consumed the scoundrel, and at length, in affliction of many complaints and the torment of many dreadful sufferings, it brought him to his end by a punishment he richly deserved."

—Gesta Stephani, edited and translated by K. R. Potter

Spirochetes are spiral- or corkscrew-shaped bacteria. Several types of bacteria within this group are medically important, but two in particular are commonly encountered by clinicians. These are *Treponema pallidum*, the cause of the sexually transmitted disease syphilis, and *Borrelia burgdorferi*, the etiologic agent of Lyme disease. *Leptospira interrogans* causes a less common but potentially serious disease called leptospirosis. In this section, these bacteria and the antimicrobial treatment of the infections they cause will be discussed.

Treponema pallidum

Syphilis is a sexually transmitted disease that is caused by the spirochete *Treponema pallidum*. Acute infection, known as primary syphilis, is usually manifested by the presence of a chancre at the site of inoculation (Fig. 14-1). The chancre spontaneously heals, but several weeks later, the signs and symptoms of secondary syphilis may develop. These include skin rashes, mucous patches, fever, malaise, and lymphadenopathy. The manifestations of secondary syphilis usually resolve but are prone to recur. However, at some point, individuals usually enter a disease phase known as *latent syphilis*, during which there is no overt evidence of infection. Latent syphilis is divided into two parts: *early latent syphilis*, which is defined as infection having occurred within the previous year, and *late latent syphilis*, which is defined as latent syphilis in which infection has been present for longer than 1 year. This distinction is important because antibiotic treatment regimens differ for these two phases of illness. Long after the initial infection, some individuals will develop clinical illness that presents as chronically progressive disease and is referred to as late or tertiary syphilis. Tertiary syphilis usually manifests as cardiovascular abnormalities or gumma formation in the skin or internal organs. To further complicate matters, invasion of the central nervous system by *T. pallidum* may occur during any stage of syphilis. This results in neurosyphilis, which may take the form of meningeal or meningovascular disease, ocular involvement, general paresis, tabes dorsalis, or gummatous central nervous system disease.

Because *T. pallidum* cannot be grown in vitro, most of what is known about its susceptibility to antibiotics is based on human trials. These indicate that **penicillin** is quite effective against this organism (Table 14-1). The route of administration and the duration of treatment vary with the stage and type of syphilis as well as host factors. For example, primary, secondary, and early latent syphilis are treated with a single

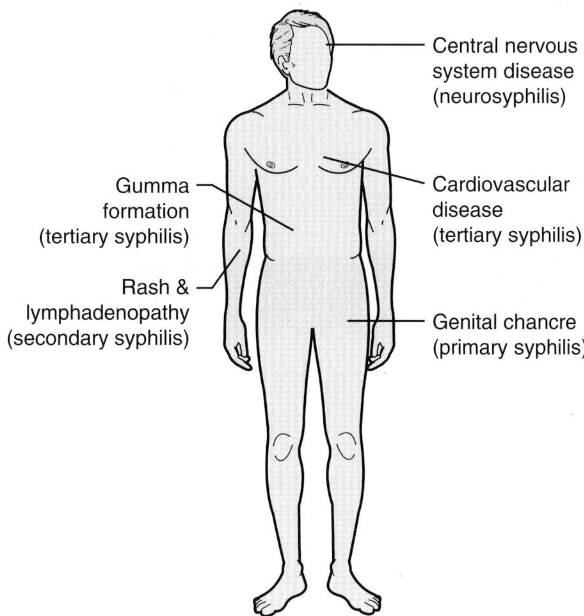

FIGURE 14-1. Sites of infections caused by *Treponema pallidum*.

Table 14-1 Antimicrobial Agents for Treatment of Infections Caused by *Treponema pallidum*

Antibiotic Class	Antibiotic
Agent of choice	
Natural penicillins	Penicillin G (including benzathine penicillin)
Alternatives	
Tetracyclines	Tetracycline, doxycycline
Third-generation cephalosporins	Ceftriaxone

intramuscular injection of benzathine penicillin (see "Pearl" box). In contrast, late latent and tertiary syphilis are treated with three injections of benzathine penicillin given at 1-week intervals. Neurosyphilis is treated with 10 to 14 days of intravenous penicillin G. Alternatives for patients with allergies to penicillin include **tetracycline**, **doxycycline**, or **ceftriaxone**. Supportive data for the use of these alternative agents are lacking for certain clinical situations; as a result, desensitization and subsequent treatment with penicillin is considered optimal therapy in some penicillin-allergic patients, such as pregnant women.

Questions

1. The antibiotic of choice for syphilis is ________________.
2. The route of administration and the duration of treatment for syphilis depend on the ________________ of disease.
3. Intramuscular ________________ ________________ allows for slow release of penicillin into the circulation over several days.

Additional Readings

Centers for Disease Control and Prevention, Workowski KA, Berman JM. Sexually transmitted diseases treatment guidelines, 2006. *MMWR Recomm Rep*. 2006;55:1–94.

Golden MR, Marra CM, Holmes KK. Update on syphilis: resurgence of an old problem. *JAMA*. 2003;290:1510–1514.

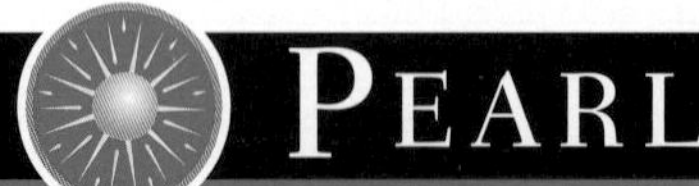

Pearl

Benzathine penicillin is a repository form of penicillin consisting of the benzathine tetrahydrate salt of penicillin G. In vivo, the compound is hydrolyzed to slowly release penicillin G. Thus, low but long-lasting levels of penicillin can be achieved following a single intramuscular dose. Depending on the dose, levels can be detected from 1 to 4 weeks following injection. Thus, this form of penicillin is useful in treating bacteria that are exquisitely sensitive to penicillin (i.e., have low minimal inhibitory concentrations) but require prolonged exposure. *Treponema pallidum* is one example of such an organism.

Kaplan EL, Berrios X, Speth J, et al. Pharmacokinetics of benzathine penicillin G: serum levels during the 28 days after intramuscular injection of 1,200,000 units. *J Pediatr.* 1989;115:146–150.

Borrelia burgdorferi

Borrelia burgdorferi causes Lyme disease, the most common vector-borne illness in the United States and Europe. Similar to syphilis, Lyme disease occurs in stages. Stage 1 disease occurs shortly after inoculation of the bacterium into the host via a tick bite. This results in a characteristic annular skin rash known as erythema migrans, which occurs at the site of the tick bite (Fig. 14-2). Stage 2 disease occurs days to weeks later, when the organism has disseminated. Patients may have secondary skin rashes, lymphadenopathy, meningitis and neurologic findings, or evidence of cardiac involvement. Months to years later, patients may develop stage 3 disease, which is characterized by arthritis or chronic neurologic abnormalities such as cognitive impairment.

The treatment of choice for most manifestations of Lyme disease in people 8 years of age or older and in nonpregnant women is oral **doxycycline** (Table 14-2). The best studied alternative agent is **amoxicillin**. Other alternatives include oral **cefuroxime** or oral **erythromycin**. Individuals with neurologic or serious cardiac involvement should be treated with an intravenous antibiotic such as **ceftriaxone** or **penicillin G**. In vitro and in vivo observations indicate that rifampin, quinolones, aminoglycosides, and first-generation cephalosporins are ineffective against this organism.

QUESTIONS

4. The antibiotic of choice for Lyme disease is ________________.
5. Other antibiotics used for the treatment of stage 1 Lyme disease include ________________, ________________, and ________________.
6. Lyme disease with neurologic or serious cardiac involvement should be treated with intravenous ________________ or ________________.

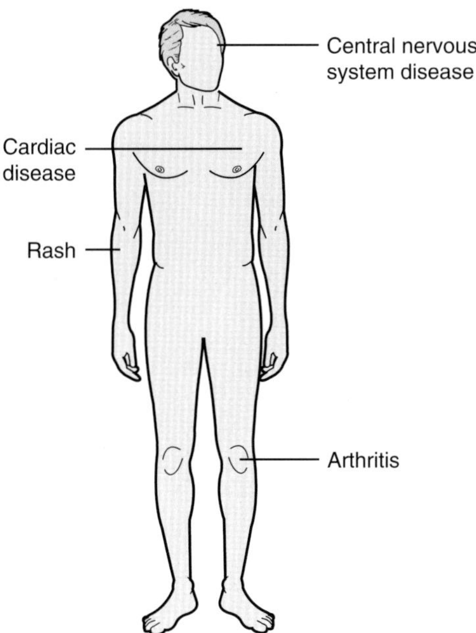

FIGURE 14-2. Sites of infections caused by *Borrelia burgdorferi*.

Table 14-2 Antimicrobial Agents for Treatment of Infections Caused by *Borrelia burgdorferi*

Antibiotic Class	Antibiotic
First-line agent	
Tetracyclines	Doxycycline
Second-line agent	
Aminopenicillins	Amoxicillin
Alternatives	
Second-generation cephalosporins	Cefuroxime
Macrolide	Erythromycin
Neurologic abnormalities and serious cardiac involvement	
Third-generation cephalosporins	Ceftriaxone
Natural penicillins	Penicillin G

ADDITIONAL READINGS

Steere AC. Lyme disease. *N Engl J Med.* 2001;345:115–125.

Wormser GP, Nadelman RB, Dattwyler RJ, et al. Practice guidelines for the treatment of Lyme disease. The Infectious Diseases Society of America. *Clin Infect Dis.* 2000;31(suppl 1):1–14.

Leptospira interrogans

Leptospira interrogans is a thin spirochete that causes the zoonotic infection leptospirosis. This bacterium is shed in the urine of many types of domestic and wild animals; acquisition by humans occurs following direct or indirect exposure to contaminated water, mud, or animal tissues. Individuals with leptospirosis may present with disease severity ranging from subclinical illness to multiorgan failure leading to death. Those with severe disease often have a biphasic illness consisting of initial fever, headaches, conjunctival suffusion, and myalgias followed by defervescence and subsequent recrudescence with liver, renal, or meningeal involvement (Fig. 14-3).

Mild leptospirosis is usually treated with oral antibiotics, such as **doxycycline** or **amoxicillin**. Moderate or severe disease is treated with intravenous agents such as **penicillin G**, **ceftriaxone**, or **ampicillin** (Table 14-3).

QUESTIONS

7. Like the other spirochetes, *Leptospira interrogans* is susceptible to penicillin/amoxicillin and ________________.
8. ________________ and ________________ are the agents of choice for mild leptospirosis.
9. For severe leptospirosis, intravenous ________________, ________________, or ________________ is recommended.

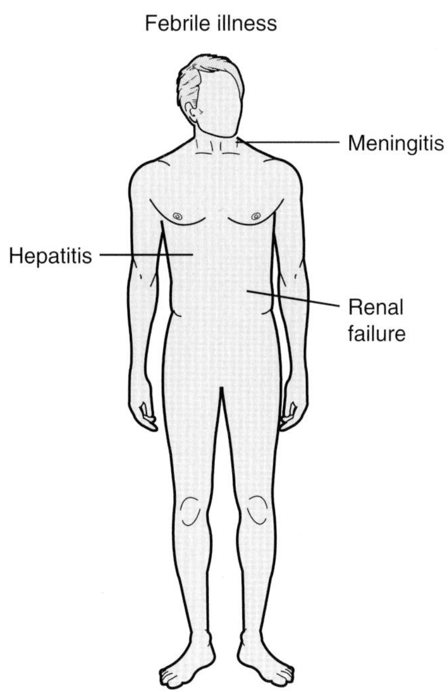

FIGURE 14-3. Sites of infections caused by *Leptospira interrogans*.

Table 14-3 Antimicrobial Agents for Treatment of Infections Caused by *Leptospira interrogans*

Antibiotic Class	Antibiotic
Mild disease	
Tetracyclines	Doxycycline
Aminopenicillins	Amoxicillin
Moderate and severe disease	
Natural penicillins	Penicillin G
Aminopenicillins	Ampicillin
Third-generation cephalosporins	Ceftriaxone

ADDITIONAL READINGS

Bharti AR, Nally JE, Ricaldi JN, et al. Leptospirosis: a zoonotic disease of global importance. *Lancet Infect Dis*. 2003;3:757–771.

Levett PN. Leptospirosis. *Clin Microbiol Rev*. 2001;14:296–326.

CHAPTER 15

Mycobacteria

"'My dear lords, you are very gallant knights with much experience of war, and you know that the King of France whom we serve sent us to this place (Calais) to hold the town and castle for as long as our honour and his interests might require it. We have done everything in our power, but now our help has failed us and you are pressing us so hard that we have nothing left to eat. We must all die or go mad with hunger if the noble king whom you serve does not take pity on us. So I ask you, dear lords, to beg him humbly to have mercy on us and allow us to go away just as we are, taking for himself the town and citadel and all the things in them. He will find enough to satisfy him.'"

—CHRONICLES, JEAN FROISSART

The mycobacteria are, in general, slow-growing organisms that cause chronic diseases. Often, individuals afflicted with mycobacterial infections succumb after prolonged infections that slowly and progressively weaken the body and result in emaciation and debilitation. In this regard, mycobacterial disease is akin to a protracted siege on the body rather than an all-out assault that rapidly overruns its defenses.

The *mycobacteria* are a group of organisms that produce cell envelopes rich in lipids and fatty acids. One fatty acid, mycolic acid, is particularly abundant and makes up 60% of the cell wall mass of these bacteria. Although mycobacteria have a gram-positive cell envelope structure, their high lipid content does not allow penetration of Gram stain, preventing visualization of these organisms by this technique. Rather, a method called "acid-fast" staining must be used to detect them.

In this section, we will discuss *Mycobacterium tuberculosis*, the cause of tuberculosis; *Mycobacterium avium* complex (MAC), a frequent cause of disseminated disease in individuals with AIDS; and *Mycobacterium leprae*, the etiologic agent of leprosy. Although the unique lipid-rich cell envelopes of mycobacteria allow these pathogens to cause severe disease, they are also their Achilles heels in that certain antibiotics, such as isoniazid and pyrazinamide, target production of these molecules. Thus, these agents tend to be quite specific for mycobacteria. Other agents used to treat mycobacteria, such as rifampin and streptomycin, have more general antimicrobial mechanisms and can also be used to treat other bacteria.

Mycobacterium tuberculosis

Mycobacterium tuberculosis is the etiologic agent of tuberculosis, which, on a global level, is second only to AIDS as a cause of death by a single infectious agent. Inhalation of these bacteria may lead directly to overt disease or more commonly results in latent infection, in which the individual is asymptomatic but still harbors the mycobacteria. In latent infection, the bacteria may overcome the host's containment at a later time, resulting in reactivation disease. This most frequently occurs during the 2-year period following initial infection or when the host's immune system becomes weakened as a result of increasing age or other forms of immunosuppression. Reactivation disease predominantly affects the lungs, but virtually any organ may be involved (Fig. 15-1). In pulmonary disease, the lung apices are classically affected, and cavitary formation is common. Extrapulmonary disease may involve lymph nodes, the pleural space, bone, the genitourinary system, or the central nervous system. Disseminated disease, referred to as "miliary tuberculosis," also occurs. Regardless of the organ systems involved, disease tends to be chronic, debilitating, and associated with formation of necrotizing granulomas.

M. tuberculosis is prone to develop resistance to antimicrobial agents. As a result, most drug regimens contain multiple agents. A typical initial regimen is **isoniazid**, **rifampin**, **pyrazinamide**, and **ethambutol** (Table 15-1). All four drugs are continued for 2 months, after which the regimen is usually narrowed to isoniazid plus rifampin if the infecting strain is susceptible to these agents. Isoniazid and rifampin are

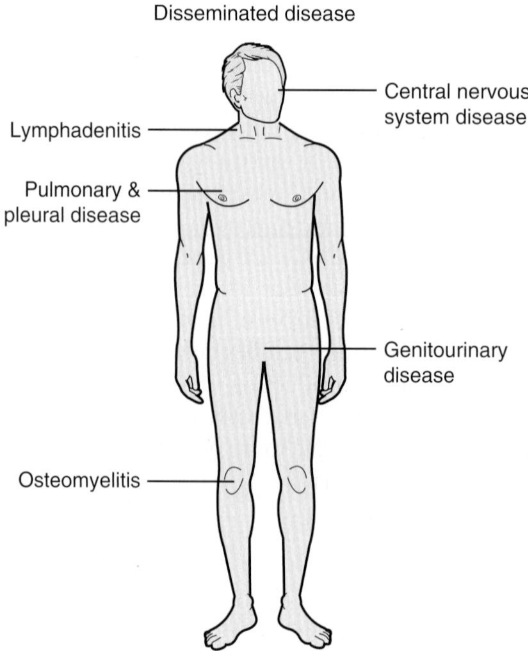

FIGURE 15-1. Sites of infections caused by *Mycobacterium tuberculosis*.

Table 15-1 Antimicrobial Agents for Treatment of Infections Caused by *Mycobacterium tuberculosis*

Active Disease
(Isoniazid + rifampin + pyrazinamide + ethambutol) × 2 months, followed by (isoniazid + rifampin) × 4 months
Latent Infection
Isoniazid × 9 months

then continued for an additional 4 months to complete therapy. **Rifapentine** is sometimes substituted for rifampin in the continuation phase of therapy for nonimmunocompromised patients because it may be given only once per week instead of daily. **Rifabutin** is frequently substituted for rifampin in patients simultaneously being treated for HIV infection because it interferes less with the metabolism of antiretroviral agents.

If the infecting strain is resistant to isoniazid and rifampin, the patient is said to have multidrug-resistant (MDR) tuberculosis. Treatment of MDR tuberculosis is difficult and often requires the use of several second-line agents, such as streptomycin, amikacin, cycloserine, ethionamide, capreomycin, *p*-aminosalicylic acid, or a quinolone. These agents tend to be less active than first-line agents and their use is associated with an increased frequency of adverse effects. Current recommendations for the treatment of MDR tuberculosis are that at least three previously unused drugs to which the mycobacterial strain is susceptible in vitro be administered. Therapy should be continued for a minimum of 18 months.

Because individuals with latent infections (as opposed to active disease) have a much lower bacterial burden, the likelihood of spontaneous mutations that lead to antibiotic resistance is much lower. Thus, these individuals can be successfully treated with a single agent, usually **isoniazid** for 9 months. Individuals suspected of being latently infected with an isoniazid-resistant strain can be treated with **rifampin** for 4 months.

HISTORY

Tuberculosis is indeed a very old disease. Polymerase chain reaction amplification of samples from mummified remains has confirmed its presence in ancient Egypt and in the Americas before the arrival of Columbus.

Mackowiak PA, Blos VT, Aguilar M, et al. On the origin of American tuberculosis. *Clin Infect Dis.* 2005;41:515–518.
Zink AR, Sola C, Reischl U, et al. Characterization of Mycobacterium tuberculosis complex DNAs from Egyptian mummies by spoligotyping. *J Clin Microbiol.* 2003;41:359–367.

QUESTIONS

1. Because *Mycobacterium tuberculosis* is prone to develop resistance to antimicrobial agents, most initial treatment regimens for active disease consist of ________________ drugs.
2. The most commonly used treatment regimen for active tuberculosis consists of ________________, ________________, ________________, and ________________.
3. Second-line agents for the treatment of tuberculosis include ________________, ________________, ________________, ________________, ________________, ________________, and ________________.
4. Latent tuberculosis is usually treated with ________________ alone.

ADDITIONAL READINGS

Blumberg HM, Burman WJ, Chaisson RE, et al. American Thoracic Society/Centers for Disease Control and Prevention/Infectious Diseases Society of America: treatment of tuberculosis. *Am J Respir Crit Care Med.* 2003;167:603–662.

Di Perri G, Bonora S. Which agents should we use for the treatment of multidrug-resistant Mycobacterium tuberculosis? *J Antimicrob Chemother.* 2004;54:593–602.

Espinal MA, Laszlo A, Simonsen L, et al. Global trends in resistance to antituberculosis drugs. World Health Organization-International Union against Tuberculosis and Lung Disease Working Group on Anti-Tuberculosis Drug Resistance Surveillance. *N Engl J Med.* 2001;344:1294–1303.

Jasmer RM, Nahid P, Hopewell PC. Clinical practice. Latent tuberculosis infection. *N Engl J Med.* 2002;347:1860–1866.

Mycobacterium avium Complex

Mycobacterium avium complex (MAC) consists of two closely related mycobacterial species: *M. avium* and *Mycobacterium intracellulare*. These pathogens can cause pulmonary disease in adults, especially in those with predisposing lung abnormalities (Fig. 15-2). In contrast, cervical lymphadenitis caused by MAC most often occurs in children. Disseminated disease is almost exclusively seen in severely immunocompromised individuals, especially those with AIDS. As with illnesses caused by other mycobacterial species, each of these diseases is chronic in nature and tends to have an insidious onset.

MAC disease, like tuberculosis, must be treated with multiple agents for prolonged periods to prevent the emergence of resistance and accomplish clinical cure. In addition, immunocompromised individuals must be placed on maintenance therapy for life or until immune reconstitution is achieved to prevent relapse. The recommended treatment regimen for MAC disease consists of **clarithromycin** plus **ethambutol** (Table 15-2). **Rifabutin** is often added to this regimen if pulmonary disease is present or if the patient is severely immunocompromised. Alternative agents include **azithromycin**, **ciprofloxacin**, **levofloxacin**, or **amikacin.** Because of the high incidence of disease in individuals with AIDS who have CD4 counts less than 50 cells/μL, prophylactic antibiotics are recommended. Weekly administered **azithromycin** is usually used for this purpose.

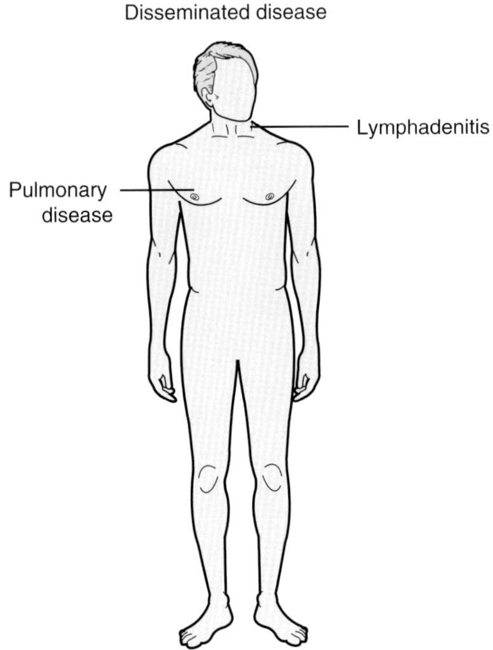

FIGURE 15-2. Sites of infections caused by *Mycobacterium avium* complex.

Table 15-2 Antimicrobial Agents for Treatment of Infections Caused by *Mycobacterium avium Complex*

Antibiotic Class	Antibiotic
Clarithromycin + ethambutol ± rifabutin	
Alternative Agents	
Macrolides	Azithromycin
Quinolones	Ciprofloxacin, levofloxacin
Aminoglycosides	Amikacin
Prophylaxis	
Macrolides	Azithromycin

Questions

5. Infections caused by *Mycobacterium avium* complex require prolonged treatment with ________________ or ________________ antibiotics.
6. Most treatment regimens for *M. avium* complex infections include ____________ and ________________.
7. Severely immunocompromised individuals infected with HIV are often given ________________ as prophylaxis to prevent *M. avium* complex infection.

Additional Readings

Benson CA, Kaplan JE, Masur H, et al. Treating opportunistic infections among HIV-infected adults and adolescents: recommendations from CDC, the National Institutes of Health, and the HIV Medicine Association/Infectious Diseases Society of America. *Clin Infect Dis*. 2005;40:S131–S235.

Masur H, Kaplan JE, Holmes KK. Guidelines for preventing opportunistic infections among HIV-infected persons—2002. Recommendations of the U.S. Public Health Service and the Infectious Diseases Society of America. *Ann Intern Med*. 2002;137(pt 2):435–478.

Mycobacterium leprae

Mycobacterium leprae causes one of the oldest and most stigmatized of human diseases: leprosy or Hansen's disease. Recognition of leprosy dates back to biblical times, when inflicted individuals were shunned for fear of spreading the dreaded disease. This illness is chronic and is characterized by infiltrative skin lesions and progressive neuropathy that may lead to disfigurement (Fig. 15-3). It is now clear that leprosy can have a spectrum of disease manifestations, from tuberculoid to lepromatous. In tuberculoid leprosy, examination of affected tissues shows evidence of a robust immune response but few bacteria. In lepromatous leprosy, bacteria are numerous and appear to elicit little or no immune response.

Three antibiotics are widely used in the treatment of leprosy: **dapsone**, **rifampin**, and **clofazimine** (Table 15-3). As is seen with other mycobacterial infections, the emergence of resistance occurs when a single antibiotic is used, so combination therapy is recommended, at least initially. Leprosy regimens usually include dapsone plus rifampin with or without clofazimine, but the frequency of administration and the duration of therapy differ with the type of leprosy. For example, lepromatous leprosy is usually treated for a year or more, whereas tuberculoid leprosy can be treated for only 6 months. Alternative agents, for which there is less clinical experience, include **minocycline**, **ofloxacin**, and **clarithromycin**.

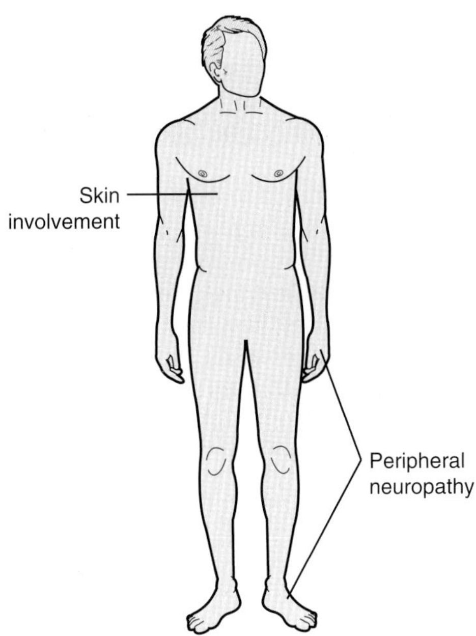

FIGURE 15-3. Sites of infections caused by *Mycobacterium leprae*.

Table 15-3 Antimicrobial Agents for Treatment of Infections Caused by *Mycobacterium leprae*

Antibiotic Class	Antibiotic
Dapsone + rifampin ± clofazimine	
Alternative Agents	
Tetracyclines	Minocycline
Quinolones	Ofloxacin
Macrolides	Clarithromycin

QUESTIONS

8. Like other mycobacterial infections, leprosy requires treatment with ________________ antibiotics for ________________ periods.

9. Most treatment regimens for leprosy include ________________ and ________________.

10. In treating leprosy, some experts recommend that ________________ be used in conjunction with dapsone and rifampin.

ADDITIONAL READINGS

Britton WJ, Lockwood DN. Leprosy. *Lancet*. 2004;363:1209–1219.

van Saane P, Timmerman H. Pharmacochemical aspects of leprosy. Recent developments and prospects for new drugs. *Pharm Weekbl Sci*. 1989;11:3–8.

HISTORY

Beginning in 1866 and continuing for the next 103 years, people living in Hawaii and diagnosed with leprosy were exiled to arguably the most famous leprosy colony in the world: Molokai. It is estimated that more than eight thousand people were forcibly moved to this island in an attempt to limit the spread of leprosy among the people of Hawaii. In the early days of the colony, inhabitants were provided only minimal food and shelter and virtually no medical care. As a consequence, the mortality rate for individuals during their first 5 years at Molokai was nearly 50%.

Tayman J. *The Colony. The Harrowing True Story of the Exiles of Molokai.* New York, NY: Scribner; 2006.

PART 

Empiric Therapy

"I must say that to die with one's sword still sheathed is most regrettable."

—The Book of Five Rings, Miyamoto Musashi

Choosing the correct antibiotic is relatively straightforward when the causative bacterium has been identified, but what does one do when the microbiologic etiology of an infection is unknown? In severely ill patients, waiting for culture results is not possible, so antibiotics must be administered empirically. That is, antibiotics are prescribed based on what is known about the usual bacterial causes of such infections and their anticipated susceptibilities.

In the preceding chapter, we discussed the major pathogenic bacteria and the infectious syndromes they cause. We then listed the antibiotics that were effective against each of these bacteria. In this section, we will discuss the major infectious syndromes and list the bacteria that commonly cause them. Based on this information and what we learned in the preceding section, we will then list the antimicrobial agents that will adequately target most of the likely etiologic bacteria for each disease.

Rather than being arbitrary, recommended empiric antibiotic choices make sense when one understands the common bacterial causes of infectious syndromes and the antibiotics that are active against these bacteria. Thus, by the end of this section, you should be able to easily list the appropriate antibiotic regimens for the treatment of these common infectious diseases.

A word of caution: Although in this section we will focus on choosing antibiotics with activity against the expected bacterial pathogens for each disease, in clinical practice, other factors enter into these decisions. Local patterns of antibiotic resistance must be taken into account, as should the history of infections and the agents used to treat them in each individual patient. Cost is an important factor in choosing antibiotics. A patient's allergic profile and comorbidities must also be considered. Finally, agents that have proved to be effective in clinical trials are given preference over agents that are indicated on theoretical grounds alone.

CHAPTER 16

Pneumonia

In the war between bacteria and the human body, the lungs are a common battlefield. Frequent bacterial incursions from the nonsterile oropharynx and nasopharynx are facilitated by the straight, short, and open conduits of the trachea and bronchi. Fortunately, many bacteria that successfully enter the lungs are quickly and imperceptibly eradicated. However, all too often, the protective mechanisms of the respiratory tract are overwhelmed, and the features of pneumonia become apparent. The patient develops fever, chills, rigors, cough, pleurisy, and, sometimes, dyspnea. On physical examination, tachycardia, tachypnea, and abnormalities on chest auscultation are noted. Laboratory abnormalities include an elevated peripheral blood leukocyte count, often with a left shift representing immature neutrophils being marginated into the blood. Chest radiographs show pulmonary infiltrates.

Pneumonia occurs in two major forms: community-acquired pneumonia (CAP) and hospital-acquired pneumonia (HAP). As suggested by their names, these entities are defined by where the infectious agent is acquired. Whereas CAP typically occurs in individuals residing in their homes, HAP afflicts those who are in a hospital. The importance of this distinction is that the circumstances under which the pneumonia was acquired dictate to a large extent the type of pathogens that may cause it and, therefore, the most appropriate empiric therapy. Note that an increasingly large number of individuals fall between these two extremes; they reside in nursing homes or long-term care facilities, or they are frequently exposed to medical personnel or medical settings such as dialysis centers. When these individuals develop pneumonia, they are said to have health care–associated pneumonia (HCAP) and should be treated similarly to those with HAP.

COMMUNITY-ACQUIRED PNEUMONIA

Acute CAP has been divided into two categories: typical and atypical. Although these classifications are useful in understanding the etiology of pneumonia, significant overlap occurs between them, and the clinical presentations of typical and atypical pneumonia are not distinct enough to be useful in decisions about therapy.

Typical CAP usually presents with the sudden onset of fever, chills, pleuritic chest pain, and a productive cough. Afflicted individuals are usually older than 50 years of age. Radiographic examination shows a lobar or subsegmental infiltrate. The usual suspects in cases of typical CAP are *Streptococcus pneumoniae* and *Haemophilus influenzae* (Table 16-1). Other aerobic gram-negative bacteria and *Staphylococcus aureus* are less common.

In contrast, atypical CAP is often preceded by a mild respiratory illness manifested by pharyngitis and rhinorrhea. The pneumonia is often, but not always, mild and is accompanied by a nonproductive cough. Patients are frequently younger than those with

Table 16-1 Bacterial Causes of Community-Acquired Pneumonia

Bacteria	Incidence
Streptococcus pneumoniae	42%
Mycoplasma pneumoniae	19%
Chlamydophila pneumoniae	10%
Haemophilus influenzae	9%
Other aerobic gram-negative bacteria	7%
Legionella spp.	4%

Jones RN. Microbial etiologies of hospital-acquired bacterial pneumonia and ventilator-associated bacterial pneumonia. *Clin Infect Dis*. 2010;51(suppl 1):581–587.

typical CAP, and chest radiographs may show interstitial infiltrates instead of lobar or subsegmental infiltrates. *Legionella* spp., *Mycoplasma pneumoniae*, and *Chlamydophila pneumoniae* are frequent bacterial causes of atypical pneumonia (Table 16-1). Viral infections such as influenza also cause this type of pneumonia.

Optimal empiric therapy for CAP is controversial but in all cases is based on the most common etiologic bacteria, host predisposing factors, and the severity of illness (Fig. 16-1 and Table 16-2).

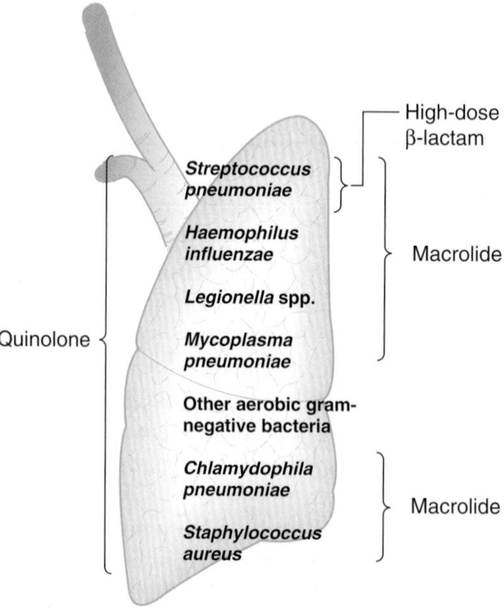

FIGURE 16-1. Activities of agents used to treat community-acquired pneumonia.

Table 16-2 Empiric Antimicrobial Therapy for Community-Acquired Pneumonia

Antibiotic Class	Antibiotic
Mild disease (outpatient therapy)	
Previously healthy (no risk factors for penicillin-resistant *Streptococcus pneumoniae*)	
• Oral macrolide	Azithromycin, clarithromycin, erythromycin
or	
• Oral tetracycline	Doxycycline
Risk factors for penicillin-resistant *Streptococcus pneumoniae*	
• Oral quinolone	Moxifloxacin, levofloxacin, gemifloxacin
or	
• Oral β-lactam given in high doses	Amoxicillin, amoxicillin/clavulanate, cefuroxime
plus	
Oral macrolide	Azithromycin, clarithromycin, erythromycin
Moderately severe disease (patient admitted to a medical ward)	
• Quinolone	Moxifloxacin, levofloxacin
or	
• Macrolide	Azithromycin, clarithromycin, erythromycin
plus	
β-Lactam	Cefotaxime, ceftriaxone, high-dose ampicillin
Severe disease (patient admitted to an intensive care unit)	
• β-Lactam	Cefotaxime, ceftriaxone, high-dose ampicillin/sulbactam
plus either	
Macrolide	Azithromycin
or	
Antistreptococcal quinolone	Moxifloxacin, levofloxacin
If* Pseudomonas aeruginosa *is suspected, add:	
• Two antipseudomonal agents	
If methicillin-resistant* Staphylococcus aureus *is suspected, add:	
• Glycopeptide	Vancomycin
or	
• Linezolid	

For individuals with mild disease that can be treated in the outpatient setting, experts recommend an oral macrolide (**azithromycin**, **clarithromycin**, **erythromycin**) or **doxycycline** unless the patient has comorbidities or is otherwise at risk for infection with penicillin-resistant *S. pneumoniae*. In this case, treatment should be with (1) an oral antistreptococcal quinolones (**moxifloxacin**, **levofloxacin**,

gemifloxacin) or (2) an oral β-lactam agent (**amoxicillin**, **amoxicillin/clavulanate**, **cefuroxime**) given in high doses plus a macrolide (**azithromycin**, **clarithromycin**, **erythromycin**). Macrolides and doxycycline are effective against atypical pathogens, *H. influenzae*, and some strains of *S. pneumoniae*. In contrast, the strength of the β-lactams is their activity against *S. pneumoniae*. When given in high doses, β-lactam antibiotics achieve levels within the lung that are sufficient to kill all strains of *S. pneumoniae* except those that are highly resistant to these agents. The β-lactams amoxicillin/clavulanate and cefuroxime also have excellent activity against *H. influenzae*. Given the complementary strengths of these agents, experts feel that they should be used together to treat CAP in patients at risk for penicillin-resistant *S. pneumoniae*. Oral antistreptococcal quinolones are highly effective against penicillin-resistant *S. pneumoniae*, *H. influenzae*, and atypical pathogens and are also efficacious for the treatment of CAP in the outpatient setting if there is concern for penicillin-resistant *S. pneumoniae*. Obviously, quinolones and doxycycline should be avoided in small children.

For patients with moderately severe CAP requiring admission to the hospital, intravenous therapy is usually given. It is recommended that these patients receive either (1) a combination of a macrolide (**azithromycin**, **clarithromycin**, **erythromycin**) and β-lactam (**cefotaxime**, **ceftriaxone**, high-dose **ampicillin**) or (2) monotherapy with an antistreptococcal quinolone (**moxifloxacin**, **levofloxacin**). Either of these regimens is effective against *S. pneumoniae* (including most penicillin-resistant strains), *H. influenzae*, *Legionella* spp., and atypical pathogens.

Patients with severe CAP requiring admission to an intensive care unit should receive a combination of a β-lactam (**cefotaxime**, **ceftriaxone**, **ampicillin/sulbactam**) plus either **azithromycin** or an antistreptococcal quinolone (**moxifloxacin**, **levofloxacin**). If risk factors for *Pseudomonas aeruginosa* infection are present (e.g., a history of bronchiectasis, steroid use, or broad-spectrum antibiotic therapy), regimens should include two antipseudomonal agents. Likewise, if risk factors for community-acquired methicillin-resistant *Staphylococcus aureus* (MRSA) are present, an appropriate antistaphylococcal agent (**vancomycin**, **linezolid**) should be added.

HOSPITAL-ACQUIRED PNEUMONIA

HAP is divided into early-onset (occurring within the first 5 days following admission) and late-onset (occurring after 5 days of hospitalization) disease. Early-onset HAP often resembles CAP in that the etiologic pathogens are acquired in the community. These pathogens are *Streptococcus pneumoniae*, *H. influenzae*, methicillin-sensitive *Staphylococcus aureus*, and antibiotic-sensitive enteric gram-negative bacilli (Table 16-3). In contrast, late-onset HAP is caused by bacteria acquired in the hospital, such as *P. aeruginosa*, *Acinetobacter* spp., antibiotic-resistant enteric gram-negative bacilli, and MRSA. In some hospitals, *Legionella pneumophila* also causes a significant proportion of these pneumonias. Bacteria acquired in the hospital are often resistant to multiple antibiotics and are associated with poorer clinical outcomes in patients with HAP. For these reasons, the treatments of early- and late-onset HAP differ.

Exceptions to the distinction between early- and late-onset HAP are those patients who have early-onset HAP (or CAP) but who have been recently (within

Table 16-3 Bacterial Causes of Hospital-Acquired Pneumonia (HAP)

Bacteria	Incidence
Early-onset HAP (without risk factors for multidrug-resistant organisms)	
Methicillin-sensitive *Staphylococcus aureus*	29%–35%
Haemophilus influenzae	23%–33%
Enterobacteriaceae	5%–25%
Streptococcus pneumoniae	7%–23%
Late-onset HAP (or HAP with risk factors for multidrug-resistant organisms)	
Pseudomonas aeruginosa	39%–64%
Acinetobacter spp.	6%–26%
Enterobacteriaceae	16%–31%
Methicillin-resistant *Staphylococcus aureus*	0%–20%

Rello J, Ausina V, Ricart M, et al. Impact of previous antimicrobial therapy on the etiology and outcome of ventilator-associated pneumonia. *Chest.* 1993;104:1230–1235; Rello J, Sa-Borges M, Correa H, et al. Variations in etiology of ventilator-associated pneumonia across four treatment sites: implications for antimicrobial prescribing practices. *Am J Respir Crit Care Med.* 1999;160:608–613.

the preceding 3 months) hospitalized, who reside in a nursing home or an extended care facility, or who have otherwise been exposed to the health care environment, or those who have received prolonged antimicrobial therapy. Such individuals are said to have HCAP and may have acquired antibiotic-resistant bacteria normally associated with the hospital setting and thus should be treated as if they have late-onset HAP.

The choice of initial empiric therapy for HAP is particularly important because inappropriate treatment regimens (e.g., antibiotics that are not effective against the causative bacteria) are associated with increased mortality, even when subsequently adjusted after culture data become available. Obviously, a risk factor for inappropriate antimicrobial therapy is infection by a multidrug-resistant organism because these organisms are more likely to be resistant to empirically prescribed treatment regimens.

Because the bacteria that cause early-onset HAP are similar to those that cause CAP (Table 16-3), the antimicrobial therapies for these two syndromes are similar. Empiric antibiotic therapy for early-onset HAP (without risk factors for multidrug-resistant organisms) consists of **ceftriaxone**, quinolone (**levofloxacin**, **moxifloxacin**, **ciprofloxacin**), **ampicillin/sulbactam**, or **ertapenem** (Table 16-4 and Fig. 16-2). Treatment of late-onset HAP or pneumonia in patients with other risk factors for multidrug-resistant organisms is more complex. To maximize the likelihood of giving at least one agent that is effective against the highly resistant bacteria that cause this type of pneumonia, combination therapy using antibiotics from at least two different classes is recommended. In addition, these agents should have activity against *P. aeruginosa*, one of the most common causes of late-onset HAP. Useful regimens include an antipseudomonal cephalosporin (**ceftazidime**, **cefepime**), carbapenem (**imipenem**, **meropenem**) or **piperacillin/tazobactam** in combination with a quinolone

Table 16-4 Empiric Antimicrobial Therapy for Hospital-Acquired Pneumonia (HAP)

Antibiotic Class	Antibiotic
Early-onset HAP (without risk factors for multidrug-resistant organisms)	
• Cephalosporin	Ceftriaxone
or	
• Quinolone	Levofloxacin, moxifloxacin, ciprofloxacin
or	
• Aminopenicillin/β-lactamase	Ampicillin/sulbactam
or	
• Carbapenem	Ertapenem
Late-onset HAP (or HAP with risk factors for multidrug-resistant organisms)	
• Antipseudomonal cephalosporin	Ceftazidime, cefepime
or	
• Carbapenem	Imipenem, meropenem
or	
• Extended-spectrum penicillin/ β-lactamase inhibitor	Piperacillin/tazobactam
plus	
Quinolone	Ciprofloxacin, levofloxacin
or	
Aminoglycoside	Gentamicin, tobramycin, amikacin
If suspicion of methicillin-resistant* Staphylococcus aureus, *add:	
• Glycopeptide	Vancomycin
or	
• Linezolid	

(**ciprofloxacin**, **levofloxacin**), or aminoglycoside (**gentamicin**, **tobramycin**, **amikacin**) (Table 16-4 and Fig. 16-3). In patients suspected of being infected with MRSA, **linezolid** or **vancomycin** should be added. Such patients would be those with gram-positive cocci in a tracheal aspirate sample or those in an intensive care unit with a high incidence of MRSA.

Several issues should be kept in mind when choosing antibiotics from this list for individual patients. First, it is best to use agents that the patient has not recently received because prior exposure to an antibiotic increases the risk of resistance. Second, local resistance patterns should be used to guide the choice of an agent. Finally, antibiotics should be chosen to minimize the chance of an allergic or adverse drug reaction. For example, if possible, the prolonged use of aminoglycosides should be avoided in elderly patients and those with chronic renal insufficiency because of the risk of nephrotoxicity.

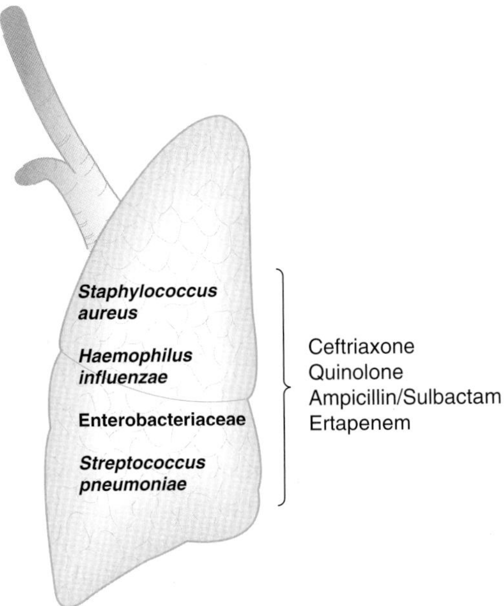

FIGURE 16-2. Activities of agents used to treat early-onset hospital-acquired pneumonia.

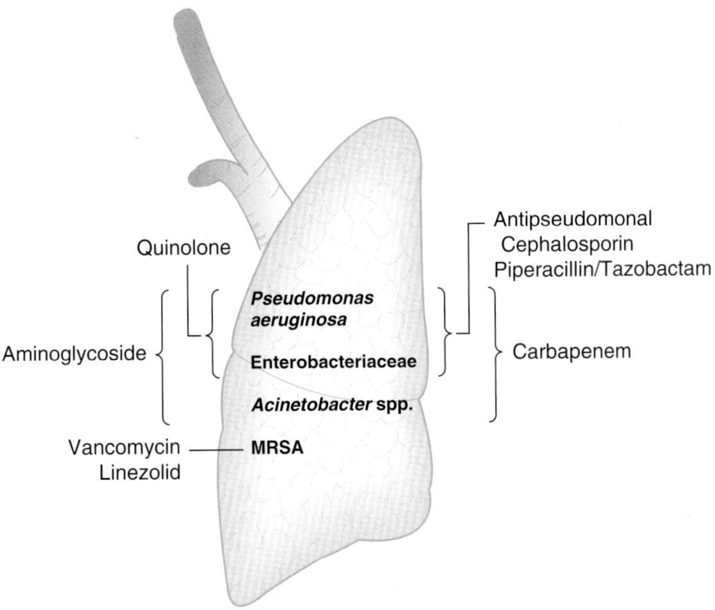

FIGURE 16-3. Activities of agents used to treat late-onset hospital-acquired pneumonia and hospital-acquired pneumonia with risk factors for multidrug-resistant organisms.

QUESTIONS

1. Bacterial pathogens that cause atypical community-acquired pneumonia (CAP) include ________________, ________________, and ________________.
2. The three drug classes most commonly used to treat CAP are the ________________, ________________, and ________________.
3. Empiric treatment for severe CAP is a ________________ plus either ________________ or a ________________.
4. The bacterial causes of hospital-acquired pneumonia (HAP) can be divided into two groups: (a) bacteria that cause ________________ HAP and (b) bacteria that cause ________________ HAP or HAP in an individual with other risk factors for multidrug-resistant pathogens.
5. Treatment of early-onset HAP (in a patient without risk factors for multidrug-resistant organisms) is with one of the following: ________________, ________________, ________________, or ________________.
6. Treatment of HAP in a patient with risk factors for multidrug-resistant organisms includes one agent from each of two groups of antibiotics: (group 1) an antipseudomonal ________________, a ________________ with *Pseudomonas* activity, or ________________; plus (group 2) a ________________ or an ________________. If methicillin-resistant *Staphylococcus aureus* is suspected, ________________ or ________________ should be added.

ADDITIONAL READINGS

Chastre J, Fagon JY. Ventilator-associated pneumonia. *Am J Respir Crit Care Med.* 2002;165:867–903.

Halm EA, Teirstein AS. Clinical practice. Management of community-acquired pneumonia. *N Engl J Med.* 2002;347:2039–2045.

Mandell LA, Wunderink RG, Anzueto A, et al. Infectious Diseases Society of America/American Thoracic Society consensus guidelines on the management of community-acquired pneumonia. *Clin Infect Dis.* 2007;44(suppl 2):S27–S72.

Niederman MS, Craven DE, Bonten MJ, et al. Guidelines for the management of adults with hospital-acquired, ventilator-associated, and healthcare-associated pneumonia. *Am J Respir Crit Care Med.* 2005;171:388–416.

Waterer GW, Rello J, Wunderink RG. Management of community-acquired pneumonia in adults. *Am J Respir Crit Care Med.* 2011;183:157–164.

CHAPTER 17

Urinary Tract Infections

The urinary system is another portal between the outside environment and the interior of the human body, and it is frequently exploited by bacterial pathogens to cause infection. The vulnerability of this aspect of human anatomy is underscored by the incidence of urinary tract infections (UTIs); it is estimated that approximately 10% of women have a UTI each year. These infections may be relatively benign, involving only the urethra and the bladder, in which case they are referred to as *acute cystitis*. Alternatively, they may be more severe and involve the kidneys in the form of pyelonephritis. Individuals with acute bacterial cystitis often present with symptoms of dysuria, urinary frequency, and hematuria. The additional symptoms of fevers, chills, nausea, vomiting, and flank pain suggest pyelonephritis. Laboratory analysis shows pyuria, hematuria, and bacteriuria.

UTIs are classified as "uncomplicated" or "complicated." Uncomplicated UTIs are those that occur in young, healthy, nonpregnant women; complicated UTIs are all other UTIs. The typical complicated UTI would be an infection in a woman with diabetes or with a structural abnormality of her urinary system or who acquired her infection in the hospital. The differentiation between complicated and uncomplicated infections is important because it affects both the spectrum of bacteria involved and the duration of antibiotic treatment.

In uncomplicated acute cystitis and pyelonephritis, the causative bacteria are predictable. In most cases, *Escherichia coli* will be the etiologic organism (Table 17-1 and Figs. 17-1 and 17-2). *Staphylococcus saprophyticus*, *Proteus mirabilis*, *Klebsiella* spp., and other Enterobacteriaceae are also sometimes cultured. Unlike their hospital-acquired counterparts, these community-acquired bacteria are usually susceptible to most antibiotics. In complicated UTIs, bacteria that are more antibiotic resistant, such as *Pseudomonas aeruginosa*, *Enterobacter* spp., *Serratia* spp., *Citrobacter* spp., and *Staphylococcus aureus*, assume a more prominent role, as do enterococci (Table 17-1 and Fig. 17-3).

Recommended empirical treatment of acute uncomplicated cystitis is a 5-day course of **nitrofurantoin** (Table 17-2). A 3-day course of oral **trimethoprim-sulfamethoxazole** was formerly the treatment of choice; but because of increasing resistance, it is now only recommended if local resistance rates of uropathogens do not exceed 20% and this agent has not been used to treat a UTI in the preceding 3 months. Both nitrofurantoin and trimethoprim-sulfamethoxazole are effective against many of the *E. coli*, other Enterobacteriaceae, and *S. saprophyticus* strains that cause these infections.

The same bacteria that cause uncomplicated cystitis also cause uncomplicated pyelonephritis (Fig. 17-2). The treatment recommendations, however, are different because nitrofurantoin does not achieve the high serum levels necessary to treat pyelonephritis-associated bacteremia and because the consequences of inappropriate

Table 17-1 Bacterial Causes of Urinary Tract Infections

Bacteria	Incidence
Uncomplicated	
Escherichia coli	53%–79%
Proteus mirabilis	4%–5%
Staphylococcus saprophyticus	3%
Klebsiella spp.	2%–3%
Other Enterobacteriaceae	3%
Complicated	
E. coli	26%–29%
Enterococci	13%–17%
Pseudomonas aeruginosa	9%–16%
Klebsiella spp.	8%–10%
Other Enterobacteriaceae	9%–11%

Bronsema DA, Adams JR, Pallares R, et al. Secular trends in rates and etiology of nosocomial urinary tract infections at a university hospital. *J Urol.* 1993;150:414–416; Gaynes R, Edwards JR. Overview of nosocomial infections caused by gram-negative bacilli. *Clin Infect Dis.* 2005;41:848–854; Goldstein FW. Antibiotic susceptibility of bacterial strains isolated from patients with community-acquired urinary tract infections in France. Multicentre Study Group. *Eur J Clin Microbiol Infect Dis.* 2000;19:112–117; Kahlmeter G. An international survey of the antimicrobial susceptibility of pathogens from uncomplicated urinary tract infections: the ECO.SENS Project. *J Antimicrob Chemother.* 2003;51:69–76.

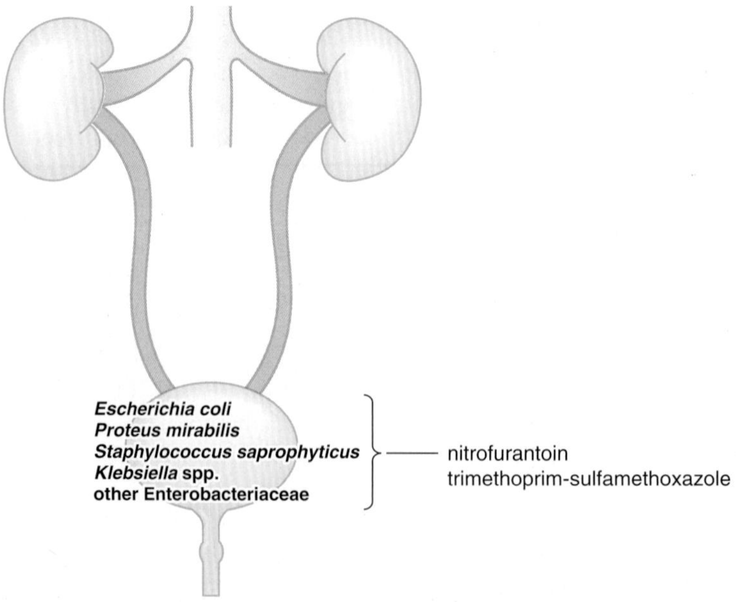

FIGURE 17-1. Activities of agents used to treat uncomplicated acute cystitis.

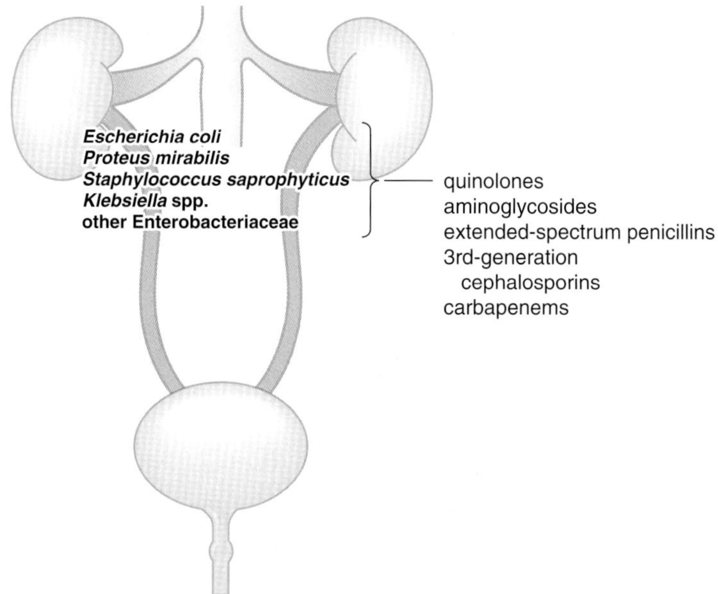

FIGURE 17-2. Activities of agents used to treat uncomplicated acute pyelonephritis.

treatment of resistant organisms with trimethoprim-sulfamethoxazole are more severe with pyelonephritis. Recommended treatment regimens depend on the severity of the disease, with oral agents being used for mild disease and intravenous therapy for severe disease (Table 17-2). For mild disease, oral quinolones (**ciprofloxacin**, **levofloxacin**) are often used empirically. Therapy for severe disease is with a parenteral quinolone (**ciprofloxacin**, **levofloxacin**); an aminoglycoside (**gentamicin**, **tobramycin**, **amikacin**), with or without **ampicillin**; an extended-spectrum penicillin (**piperacillin**, **ticarcillin**), with or without an aminoglycoside; a third-generation cephalosporin (**ceftriaxone**, **cefotaxime**), with or without an aminoglycoside; or a carbapenem (**imipenem**, **meropenem**, **doripenem**, **ertapenem**). Antimicrobial treatment for acute pyelonephritis should be continued for 7 to 14 days. Note that moxifloxacin is not approved for use in the treatment of UTIs.

Antibiotic therapy for complicated UTIs must be effective against the more resistant organisms that sometimes cause these infections (Fig. 17-3 and Table 17-2). Typical regimens include a quinolone (**ciprofloxacin**, **levofloxacin**), **cefepime**, carbapenem (**imipenem**, **meropenem**, **doripenem**, **ertapenem**), or extended-spectrum penicillin/β-lactamase inhibitor combination (**piperacillin/tazobactam**, **ticarcillin/clavulanate**). If gram-positive bacteria are seen on Gram stain of the urine (suggesting the presence of enterococci), **ampicillin** or **amoxicillin** should be added. Treatment is usually continued for 7 to 14 days or longer.

Questions

1. The most common cause of uncomplicated acute cystitis is ________________.
2. Recommended empiric antibiotic therapy for acute cystitis in a young healthy woman who is not pregnant is ________________ or ________________.

Table 17-2 Empiric Antimicrobial Therapy for Urinary Tract Infections

Antibiotic Class	Antibiotic
Uncomplicated acute cystitis	
• Nitrofurantoin	
• Oral trimethoprim-sulfamethoxazole	
Uncomplicated acute pyelonephritis	
• Quinolones	Ciprofloxacin, levofloxacin
• Aminoglycosides ± ampicillin	Gentamicin, tobramycin, amikacin
• Extended-spectrum penicillin ± aminoglycoside	Piperacillin
• Third-generation cephalosporins ± aminoglycoside	Ceftriaxone, cefotaxime
Complicated urinary tract infections	
• Quinolones	Ciprofloxacin, levofloxacin
• Fourth-generation cephalosporins	Cefepime
• Carbapenems	Imipenem, meropenem, doripenem
• Extended-spectrum penicillin/β-lactamase combination	Piperacillin/tazobactam, ticarcillin/clavulanate
If gram-positive bacteria are seen in urine, add:	
• Aminopenicillin	Ampicillin, amoxicillin

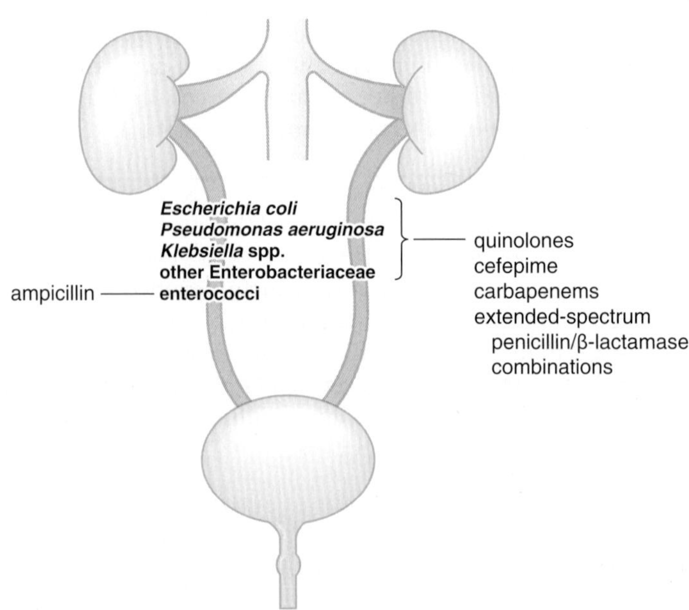

FIGURE 17-3. Activities of agents used to treat complicated urinary tract infections.

3. If gram-positive bacteria are seen in the urine of a patient with a complicated urinary tract infection, one must be concerned about ________________ as the etiologic organisms.
4. Patients with diabetes, with structural abnormalities of their urinary systems, who acquired their infection in the hospital, or who have other conditions that predispose to infection by a broader range of bacteria, are said to have ________________ urinary tract infections.
5. Antibiotic treatment of complicated urinary tract infections is with ________________, ________________, ________________, or a ________________.

ADDITIONAL READINGS

Fihn SD. Clinical practice. Acute uncomplicated urinary tract infection in women. *N Engl J Med.* 2003;349:259–266.

Gupta K, Hooton TM, Naber KG, et al. Executive summary: international clinical practice guidelines for the treatment of acute uncomplicated cystitis and pyelonephritis in women: A 2010 update by the Infectious Diseases Society of America and the European Society for Microbiology and Infectious Diseases. *Clin Infect Dis.* 2011;52:561–564.

Hooton TM, Besser R, Foxman B, et al. Acute uncomplicated cystitis in an era of increasing antibiotic resistance: a proposed approach to empirical therapy. *Clin Infect Dis.* 2004;39:75-80.

Rubenstein JN, Schaeffer AJ. Managing complicated urinary tract infections: the urologic view. *Infect Dis Clin North Am.* 2003;17:333–351.

CHAPTER 18

Pelvic Inflammatory Disease

Pelvic inflammatory disease (PID) is the unfortunate consequence of the failure of successive barriers of the female reproductive system to check the invasion of sexually transmitted microbes. In PID, bacteria migrate from the cervix into the uterus and subsequently to the fallopian tubes, ovaries, and peritoneal cavity. Persistent inflammation may lead to abscess formation and scarring of these structures, which predisposes to infertility and ectopic pregnancy.

The patient with PID typically presents with abnormal bleeding, dyspareunia, vaginal discharge, lower abdominal pain, fever, and chills. Physical examination is often remarkable for fever, abnormal cervical or vaginal mucopurulent discharge, uterine or adnexal tenderness, and cervical motion tenderness. Laboratory examination may show an elevated peripheral white blood cell count, the presence of white blood cells in vaginal secretions, and elevated erythrocyte sedimentation rate and C-reactive protein measurements.

The pathogenesis of PID involves a complex interaction between sexually transmitted bacteria and normal flora, particularly anaerobes (Table 18-1 and Fig. 18-1). As such, it is a polymicrobial infection. The sexually transmitted bacteria that are most often implicated are *Neisseria gonorrhoeae* and *Chlamydia trachomatis*. Components of the vaginal flora frequently isolated from PID lesions include the anaerobic *Bacteroides* and *Peptostreptococcus* spp. as well as facultative bacteria such as *Escherichia coli*, *Gardnerella vaginalis*, *Haemophilus influenzae*, and group B streptococci. Currently, the extent to which each of these contributes to the progression of PID is unclear.

Empiric treatment of PID must take into account the spectrum of organisms that contribute to this infection as well as the severity of illness (Table 18-2 and Fig. 18-1). All regimens should be effective against *N. gonorrhoeae* and *C. trachomatis*. Currently, the role of anaerobic bacteria in PID is controversial, but some experts feel that therapy should also be directed against these organisms. Individuals who have only mild-to-moderate disease should be treated as outpatients with oral antibiotics. Recommended regimens include a single intramuscular dose of a cephalosporin (e.g., **ceftriaxone**,

Table 18-1 Bacterial Causes of Pelvic Inflammatory Disease

Bacteria	Incidence
Neisseria gonorrhoeae	27%–56%
Chlamydia trachomatis	22%–31%
Anaerobic and facultative bacteria	20%–78%

Jossens MO, Schachter J, Sweet RL. Risk factors associated with pelvic inflammatory disease of differing microbial etiologies. *Obstet Gynecol.* 1994;83:989–997; Sweet RL. Role of bacterial vaginosis in pelvic inflammatory disease. *Clin Infect Dis.* 1995;20(suppl 2):S271–S275.

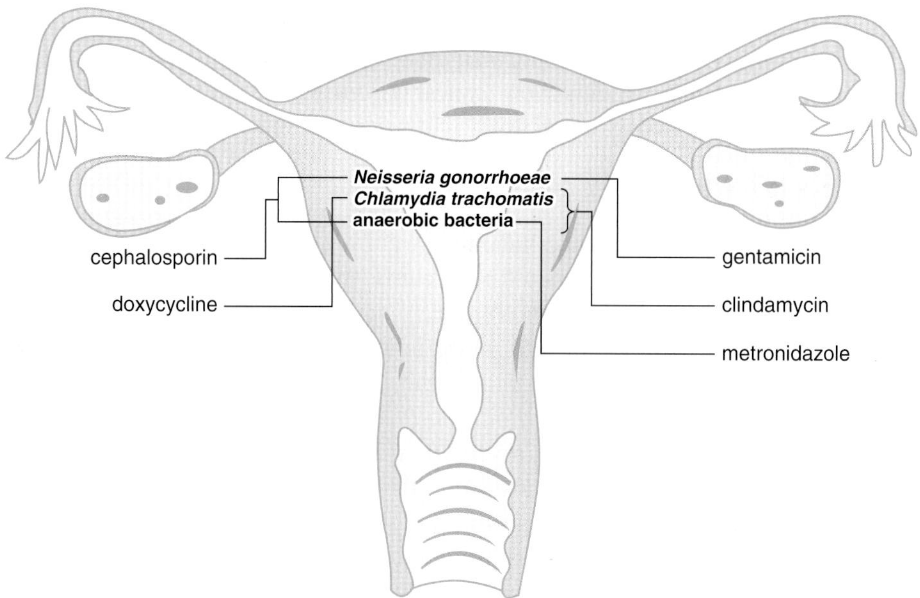

FIGURE 18-1. Activities of agents used to treat pelvic inflammatory disease.

cefoxitin + probenecid, **cefotaxime**) along with a 14-day course of oral doxycycline with or without **metronidazole**. (Concurrent administration of probenecid with cefoxitin delays excretion of this antibiotic, prolonging therapeutic serum levels.) Those who are severely ill should be admitted to the hospital and treated initially with intravenous agents. Common initial regimens include (1) a cephalosporin with anaerobic activity (e.g., **cefotetan**, **cefoxitin**) plus **doxycycline** or (2) **clindamycin** plus **gentamicin**. The latter regimen is efficacious because gentamicin is effective

Table 18-2 Empiric Antimicrobial Therapy for Pelvic Inflammatory Disease

Mild-to-moderate disease	
• Single IM dose of cephalosporin	Ceftriaxone, cefoxitin + probenecid, cefotaxime
+ Oral doxycycline	
± Oral metronidazole	
Severe disease*	
• Cephalosporin	Cefotetan, cefoxitin
+ Doxycycline	
or	
• Clindamycin	
+ Aminoglycoside	Gentamicin

*Twenty-four hours after clinical improvement, intravenous antibiotics may be discontinued and a total 14-day course of therapy completed with oral doxycycline or clindamycin. *IM*, intramuscular.

against the gram-negative *N. gonorrhoeae* and clindamycin has some activity against *C. trachomatis* as well as against many anaerobes. Intravenous antibiotics can be discontinued 24 hours after patients show clinical improvement, and a total course of 14 days of therapy completed with oral doxycycline or oral clindamycin.

QUESTIONS

1. Antibiotic treatment of pelvic inflammatory disease should include agents with activity against sexually transmitted bacteria such as ________________ and ________________ and perhaps also ________________ bacteria.
2. The treatment regimen for mild pelvic inflammatory disease is a single intramuscular dose of a ________________ plus ________________ with or without ________________.
3. Two treatment regimens for severe pelvic inflammatory disease are (1) a ________________ with anaerobic activity plus ________________ and (2) ________________ plus ________________.
4. In the pelvic inflammatory disease antibiotic regimen consisting of cefotetan plus doxycycline, cefotetan is effective against ________________ as well as ________________ bacteria, whereas doxycycline is effective against ________________.

ADDITIONAL READINGS

Beigi RH, Wiesenfeld HC. Pelvic inflammatory disease: new diagnostic criteria and treatment. *Obstet Gynecol Clin North Am*. 2003;30:777–793.

Centers for Disease Control and Prevention. Sexually transmitted diseases treatment guidelines, 2010. *MMWR Recomm Rep*. 2010;59:1–110.

Newkirk GR. Pelvic inflammatory disease: a contemporary approach. *Am Fam Physician*. 1996; 53:1127–1135.

Ross JD. Pelvic inflammatory disease: how should it be managed? *Curr Opin Infect Dis*. 2003;16:37–41.

CHAPTER 19

Meningitis

The overwhelming pathogenic potential of bacteria is arguably most apparent in acute bacterial meningitis. This illness often evolves rapidly and is uniformly fatal in the absence of antimicrobial therapy. Even with modern medicine's sophisticated diagnostic techniques and array of highly potent antibiotics, approximately one in four adults with acute bacterial meningitis die. Obviously, there is little margin for error in choosing appropriate antibiotic therapy for this disease.

Individuals with acute bacterial meningitis present with headache, fever, neck stiffness, altered mental status, photophobia, nausea, vomiting, and seizures. Physical examination is often remarkable for nuchal rigidity and sometimes for neurologic deficits. Of critical diagnostic importance is examination of the cerebral spinal fluid (CSF). Patients with meningitis will have an elevated white blood cell count and protein concentration with a decreased glucose level in their CSF. In addition, bacteria are often visualized by Gram stain in a specimen of this fluid.

The typical bacterial causes of acute meningitis vary with the age of the patient (Table 19-1). In neonates, *Streptococcus agalactiae* and *Escherichia coli* predominate. Now that the *Haemophilus influenzae* type B vaccine is widely used, *Streptococcus pneumoniae* and *Neisseria meningitidis* have become the most common bacteria isolated from small children. *N. meningitidis* is the major cause of acute bacterial meningitis in older children and young adults, whereas *S. pneumoniae* is seen with greatest frequency in older adults. In a minority of the very young, of older individuals, and of those who are immunocompromised, *Listeria monocytogenes* will be identified as the cause of acute bacterial meningitis. Aerobic gram-negative bacilli are also a concern in older individuals.

An understanding of the pathogenesis of acute bacterial meningitis aids one in choosing appropriate therapy. In this disease, bacteria multiply in the CSF, which often lacks antibodies and complement. Because of these deficiencies in the immune response, antibiotics that merely inhibit bacterial growth (i.e., those that are bacteriostatic) are not sufficient for cure. Rather, antibiotics must actually kill the bacteria (i.e., have bactericidal activity) to sterilize the CSF. In addition, the antibiotics must efficiently cross the blood–brain barrier to reach the CSF in concentrations sufficient for killing. As a result, many antibiotics are administered at higher doses to patients with meningitis relative to patients with other infections. Finally, a significant portion of the tissue damage associated with bacterial meningitis is thought to result from the inflammation provoked by the large numbers of bacteria in the CSF and meninges; this inflammatory response may be enhanced by the rapid lysis of these bacteria when they are initially exposed to bactericidal antibiotics. For this reason, some experts recommend the concomitant administration of corticosteroids with antimicrobial agents in some situations.

Table 19-1	Bacterial Causes of Acute Bacterial Meningitis
Age	**Bacterium**
0–3 months	*Streptococcus agalactiae* *Escherichia coli* *Listeria monocytogenes*
3 months to 18 years	*Neisseria meningitidis* *Streptococcus pneumoniae* *Haemophilus influenzae*
18–50 years	*S. pneumoniae* *N. meningitidis*
>50 years	*S. pneumoniae* *L. monocytogenes* Aerobic gram-negative bacilli

Quagliarello VJ, Scheld WM. Treatment of bacterial meningitis. *N Engl J Med.* 1997;336:708–716.

In the absence of a diagnostic Gram stain of CSF, antimicrobial therapy for acute bacterial meningitis must be empiric (Table 19-2 and Fig. 19-1). Third-generation cephalosporins (**cefotaxime**, **ceftriaxone**) are the backbone of most empiric antimicrobial regimens because they are bactericidal, penetrate relatively well into the CSF, and are effective against most strains of *S. pneumoniae*, *N. meningitidis*, and *H. influenzae*. However, the percentage of *S. pneumoniae* strains resistant to cephalosporins is increasing in many parts of the world. Although cephalosporins achieve high levels in the lungs and are effective therapy for pneumonia caused by all but the most resistant strains, they fail to reach levels sufficient for killing of moderately resistant strains in the CSF. Thus, it is now recommended that **vancomycin** be used in conjunction with a cephalosporin

Table 19-2	Empiric Antimicrobial Therapy for Acute Bacterial Meningitis (Nondiagnostic Gram Stain of Cerebral Spinal Fluid)
Antibiotic Class	**Antibiotic**
• Third-generation cephalosporin **plus** Glycopeptide	Cefotaxime, ceftriaxone Vancomycin
If patient <3 months or >50 years of age Add Aminopenicillin	 Ampicillin
If patient compromised • Glycopeptide **plus** Cephalosporin **with or without** Aminopenicillin	 Vancomycin Ceftazidime Ampicillin

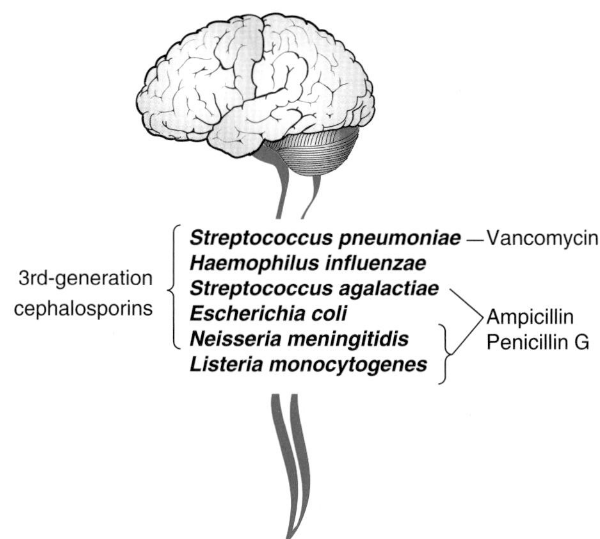

FIGURE 19-1. Activities of agents used to treat acute bacterial meningitis.

as empiric therapy for acute bacterial meningitis. **Ampicillin** should be added in infants younger than 3 months of age and in adults older than 50 years to provide coverage of *L. monocytogenes* and *S. agalactiae*. (Note that *L. monocytogenes* is one of the few gram-positive bacteria against which vancomycin is not effective—hence, the need for ampicillin.) In compromised patients such as those who develop meningitis following neurosurgery or those who have CSF shunts or are receiving high doses of steroids, treatment should be broadened to cover staphylococci or antibiotic-resistant gram-negative bacilli.

In infants younger than 3 months of age, the Gram stain CSF findings are not often diagnostic, and these patients should all receive at least a third-generation cephalosporin plus vancomycin until culture results are available. However, in adults, the results of a Gram stain specimen of CSF should guide the initial choice of antibiotics for acute bacterial meningitis. Because of the requirement for bactericidal activity and efficient penetration into the CSF, only a subset of potentially useful antibiotics is suitable for treating meningitis (Table 19-3). Gram-positive cocci in pairs in the CSF of an adult patient suggest *S. pneumoniae*, which should be treated with a third-generation cephalosporin (**cefotaxime**, **ceftriaxone**) plus **vancomycin** to ensure effective therapy against penicillin-resistant strains. In contrast, gram-positive cocci in a specimen from an infant younger than 3 months of age suggest *S. agalactiae*, for which **ampicillin** plus **gentamicin** should be given. Gram-negative diplococci indicate *N. meningitidis*, which should be treated with **penicillin G** or **ampicillin**. Small pleomorphic gram-negative bacilli are consistent with *H. influenzae*, which is treated with a third-generation cephalosporin (**cefotaxime**, **ceftriaxone**). Larger gram-negative bacilli, especially in a neonate, suggest *E. coli*, which is treated with a third-generation cephalosporin (**cefotaxime**, **ceftriaxone**). Gram-positive bacilli suggest *L. monocytogenes* and require the use of **penicillin G** or **ampicillin**. Some experts would also add **gentamicin** for synergistic killing. In all cases, therapy should be adjusted accordingly once susceptibility results are available.

Table 19-3 Specific Antimicrobial Therapy for Acute Bacterial Meningitis (Based on Gram Stain of Cerebral Spinal Fluid)

Antibiotic Class	Antibiotic
Streptococcus pneumoniae	
• Third-generation cephalosporin	Cefotaxime, ceftriaxone
plus	
Glycopeptide	Vancomycin
Neisseria meningitidis	
• Natural penicillin	Penicillin G
or	
• Aminopenicillin	Ampicillin
Haemophilus influenzae	
• Third-generation cephalosporin	Cefotaxime, ceftriaxone
Listeria monocytogenes	
• Natural penicillin	Penicillin G
or	
• Aminopenicillin	Ampicillin
with or without	
Aminoglycoside	Gentamicin
Streptococcus agalactiae	
• Aminopenicillin	Ampicillin
plus	
Aminoglycoside	Gentamicin
Escherichia coli	
• Third-generation cephalosporin	Cefotaxime, ceftriaxone

QUESTIONS

1. In adults, the most common bacterial causes of acute meningitis are ____________, ____________, and ____________.
2. Appropriate empiric therapy for a 65-year-old patient with acute bacterial meningitis and a nondiagnostic Gram stain specimen of the cerebral spinal fluid is a ____________ plus ____________ plus ____________.
3. Appropriate therapy for a 19-year-old college student with acute meningitis and gram-negative diplococci in her cerebral spinal fluid is ____________ or ____________.
4. Appropriate therapy for a 2-month-old infant with acute meningitis and *Streptococcus agalactiae* growing from her cerebral spinal fluid sample is ____________ plus ____________.

ADDITIONAL READINGS

Brouwer MC, McIntyre P, de Gans J, et al. Corticosteroids for acute bacterial meningitis. *Cochrane Database Syst Rev*. 2010:CD004405.

Brouwer MC, Tunkel AR, van de Beek D. Epidemiology, diagnosis, and antimicrobial treatment of acute bacterial meningitis. *Clin Microbiol Rev*. 2010;23:467–492.

Tunkel AR, Hartman BJ, Kaplan SL, et al. Practice guidelines for the management of bacterial meningitis. *Clin Infect Dis*. 2004;39:1267–1284.

van de Beek D, de Gans J, Tunkel AR, et al. Community-acquired bacterial meningitis in adults. *N Engl J Med*. 2006;354:44–53.

CHAPTER 20

Cellulitis

Just as medieval castles had formidable walls designed to keep attackers out, our bodies are covered with a protective layer of skin that is deceptively effective in preventing bacteria from gaining access to the vulnerable deeper tissues. That the environment is filled with microorganisms held at bay by this barrier is evidenced by the high rates of infections associated with breaches in our skin, such as burn injuries or surgical wounds. One common type of infection that occurs when bacteria gain access to the dermis and subcutaneous tissues under the skin is cellulitis.

Individuals with cellulitis usually present with fever and local findings, such as a tender, warm, erythematous, swollen, and indurated area of skin, often surrounding the wound or abrasion that served as the portal of entry. In some cases, the disease may be severe, and signs of systemic toxicity including tachycardia and hypotension may be present.

The bacterial etiology of cellulitis depends on the location of the infection and any special exposures associated with its cause. For example, cellulitis following exposure of a wound to salt water suggests *Vibrio vulnificus* as an etiology. Cellulitis associated with foot ulcers in diabetic patients is caused by a mixture of aerobic gram-positive, aerobic gram-negative, and anaerobic bacteria. However, most cellulitis cases in immunocompetent hosts result from inoculation of skin organisms through breaks or disruption in the epidermis. Thus, uncomplicated cellulitis in an immunocompetent patient without a history of unusual exposures is usually caused by *Staphylococcus aureus*, *Streptococcus pyogenes*, or other streptococci (Table 20-1).

Because it is difficult to determine the specific bacterial etiology of cellulitis in individual patients, treatment is usually empiric and consists of agents with potent activity against gram-positive bacteria (Table 20-2 and Fig. 20-1). The increasing resistance of *Staphylococcus aureus* and *Streptococcus pyogenes* to antibiotics, however, has complicated treatment choices. In general, severe infections should be treated in the hospital with intravenous antibiotics, whereas mild-to-moderate infections may be treated with oral antibiotics in the outpatient setting. In regions where methicillin-resistant *Staphylococcus aureus* (MRSA) is common or when other risk factors for this pathogen are present (e.g., previous MRSA infection, recent antibiotic therapy), parenteral options include glycopeptides (**vancomycin**, **telavancin**), **linezolid**, **daptomycin**, **tigecycline**, and **ceftaroline**. **Doxycycline**, **trimethoprim-sulfamethoxazole**, **linezolid**, and **clindamycin** are oral agents that can be used. If the likelihood of MRSA is low, suitable choices for parenteral therapy include antistaphylococcal penicillins (**nafcillin**, **oxacillin**), first-generation cephalosporins (**cefazolin**), or **clindamycin**. Oral agents include **dicloxacillin**, oral first-generation cephalosporins (**cephalexin**, **cefadroxil**), **clindamycin**, or a macrolide (**azithromycin**, **clarithromycin**, **erythromycin**). In all situations, the actual choice should be guided by local resistance patterns.

Table 20-1 Bacterial Causes of Cellulitis

Bacterium	Incidence
Staphylococcus aureus	13%–37%
Streptococcus pyogenes	4%–17%
Other streptococci	1%–8%

Duvanel T, Auckenthaler R, Rohner P, et al. Quantitative cultures of biopsy specimens from cutaneous cellulitis. *Arch Intern Med.* 1989;149:293–296; Hook EW III, Hooton TM, Hortoon CA, et al. Microbiologic evaluation of cutaneous cellulitis in adults. *Arch Intern Med.* 1986;146:295–297; Kielhofner MA, Brown B, Dall L. Influence of underlying disease process on the utility of cellulitis needle aspirates. *Arch Intern Med.* 1988;148:2451–2452; Sigurdsson AF, Gudmundsson S. The etiology of bacterial cellulitis as determined by fine-needle aspiration. *Scand J Infect Dis.* 1989;21:537–542.

Table 20-2 Empiric Antimicrobial Therapy for Cellulitis

Antibiotic Class	Antibiotic
If methicillin-resistant *Staphylococcus aureus* is suspected	
Mild-to-moderate disease (oral formulations)	
• Tetracycline	Doxycycline
• Clindamycin	
• Sulfa drugs	Trimethoprim-sulfamethoxazole
• Linezolid	
Severe disease (intravenous formulations)	
• Glycopeptides	Vancomycin, telavancin
• Linezolid	
• Daptomycin	
• Tetracycline-like agents	Tigecycline, doxycycline
• Fifth-generation cephalosporin	Ceftaroline
If methicillin-resistant *Staphylococcus aureus* is not suspected	
Mild-to-moderate disease (oral formulations)	
• Antistaphylococcal penicillins	Dicloxacillin
• First-generation cephalosporins	Cephalexin, cefadroxil
• Clindamycin	
• Macrolides	Azithromycin, clarithromycin, erythromycin
Severe disease (intravenous formulations)	
• Antistaphylococcal penicillins	Nafcillin, oxacillin
• First-generation cephalosporins	Cefazolin
• Clindamycin	

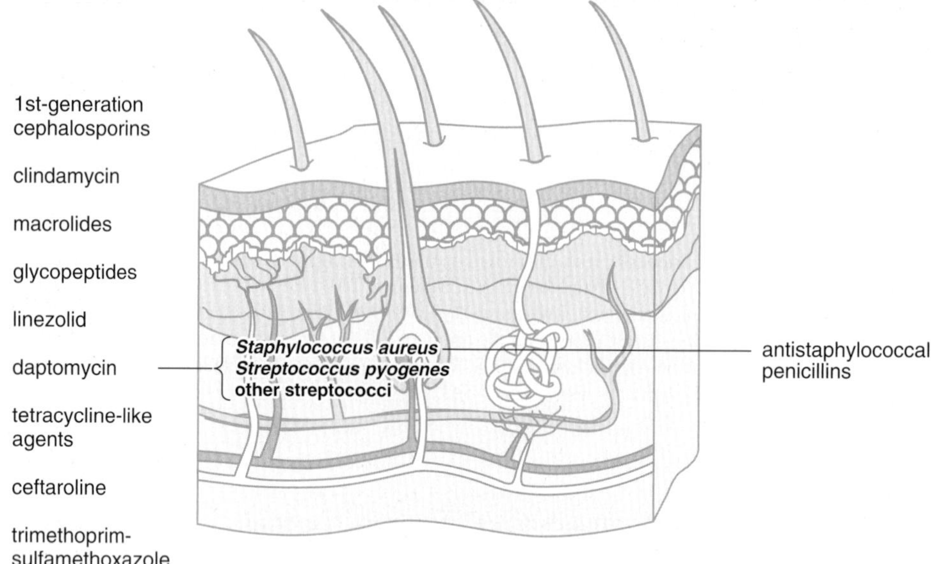

FIGURE 20-1. Activities of agents used to treat cellulitis.

QUESTIONS

1. In immunocompetent individuals without unusual exposures, the most common causes of cellulitis are ________________, ________________, and other ________________.
2. Appropriate empiric oral therapy for an otherwise healthy 48-year-old roofer who develops cellulitis on his arm at the site of an abrasion, who is not seriously ill, and who is at low risk for MRSA would be ________________, ________________, a ________________-generation cephalosporin, or a ________________.
3. In a patient at low risk for MRSA, appropriate parental therapy for cellulitis would be ________________, ________________, ________________, or ________________.
4. Appropriate therapy for a 72-year-old woman known to be colonized with methicillin-resistant *Staphylococcus aureus* and who is now hypotensive and has cellulitis involving her left leg at the site where a saphenous vein had been harvested several years earlier would be a ________________, ________________, ________________, ________________, or ________________.

ADDITIONAL READINGS

Dryden MS. Complicated skin and soft tissue infection. *J Antimicrob Chemother*. 2010;65(suppl 3): iii35–iii44.

Stevens DL, Bisno AL, Chambers HF, et al. Practice guidelines for the diagnosis and management of skin and soft-tissue infections. *Clin Infect Dis*. 2005;41:1373–1406.

Swartz MN. Clinical practice. Cellulitis. *N Engl J Med*. 2004;350:904–912.

CHAPTER 21

Otitis Media

Among children in the United States, acute otitis media is the most common illness for which antibacterial agents are prescribed. The pathogenesis of this infection reflects the continuity of the middle ear with the upper respiratory tract via the eustachian tube. Typically, an antecedent event such as an upper respiratory infection or allergies causes congestion of the respiratory mucosa and blockage of the eustachian tube. As a result, fluid accumulates in the middle ear and subsequently becomes infected by organisms of the upper respiratory tract.

Children with acute otitis media may present with the rapid onset of otalgia (ear pain), hearing loss, irritability, anorexia, apathy, fever, swelling around the ear, and otorrhea (discharge from the affected ear). On otoscopic examination, findings include middle ear effusion and inflammatory changes.

Because the fluid of the middle ear is seeded by organisms of the upper respiratory tract, it is not surprising that the bacteria that commonly cause acute otitis media are *Streptococcus pneumoniae*, *Haemophilus influenzae*, and *Moraxella catarrhalis* (Table 21-1). Each of these bacteria has a mechanism by which it resists the action of penicillin. An increasing number of *S. pneumoniae* strains produce altered penicillin-binding proteins (PBPs) that do not bind penicillins. Approximately one-third to one-half of *H. influenzae* strains that cause acute otitis media produce β-lactamases, as do nearly all strains of *M. catarrhalis*. These mechanisms must be taken into account when treating acute otitis media.

Currently, controversy exists regarding whether all children with acute otitis media should receive antimicrobial therapy. Some experts feel that children 2 years of age and older without severe symptoms at presentation may be treated symptomatically for 48 to 72 hours. If improvement occurs, these children may not require antibiotics. Other experts suggest that all children with acute otitis media should receive antibiotics. When treatment is indicated, it is empiric because cultures of middle ear fluid are infrequently obtained in uncomplicated acute otitis media.

Table 21-1 Bacterial Causes of Acute Otitis Media

Bacteria	Incidence
Streptococcus pneumoniae	25%–50%
Haemophilus influenzae	15%–30%
Moraxella catarrhalis	3%–20%

Klein JO. Otitis media. *Clin Infect Dis.* 1994;19:823–833.

Table 21-2 Empiric Antimicrobial Therapy for Acute Otitis Media

Antibiotic Class	Antibiotic
First-line therapy	
• Aminopenicillin	High-dose amoxicillin
If risk factors for amoxicillin resistance	
• Aminopenicillin/β-lactamase inhibitor	Amoxicillin/clavulanate
If mild allergy to penicillin	
• Oral cephalosporin	Cefdinir, cefpodoxime, cefuroxime
If type I hypersensitivity allergic reaction	
• Macrolide	Azithromycin, clarithromycin

High-dose **amoxicillin** is first-line therapy for acute otitis media (Table 21-2 and Fig. 21-1). At first glance, this agent appears to be an odd choice for the treatment of an infection caused by bacteria that are often penicillin resistant. When given in high doses, however, amoxicillin achieves levels in the middle ear fluid that exceed the minimal inhibitory concentrations of all but the most highly penicillin-resistant *S. pneumoniae* strains. Although many strains of *H. influenzae* and *M. catarrhalis* produce β-lactamases that degrade amoxicillin, clinical studies have demonstrated resolution in many cases of amoxicillin-treated otitis media caused by these two pathogens. Some experts recommend that patients at risk for infection caused by amoxicillin-resistant bacteria (e.g., children recently treated with β-lactam antibiotics; children with purulent conjunctivitis, which is usually caused by β-lactam-resistant *H. influenzae*) be treated with **amoxicillin/clavulanate**. In patients who have mild (non–type I hypersensitivity) allergic responses to amoxicillin, oral cephalosporins (**cefdinir**, **cefpodoxime**, **cefuroxime**) may be used. In those with type I hypersensitivity reactions (urticaria or anaphylaxis) to penicillins, macrolides (**azithromycin**, **clarithromycin**) are recommended.

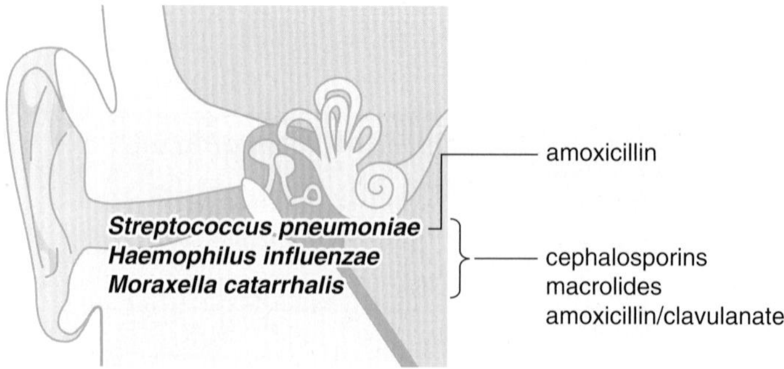

FIGURE 21-1. Activities of agents used to treat otitis media.

HISTORY

Antibiotics such as amoxicillin are used so commonly today that we have grown accustomed to their healing power. In contrast, health care providers who witnessed the early injections of penicillin were astounded by what they saw. Charles Grossman's description of the first person in the United States to be treated with penicillin is such an example. The patient was a severely ill 33-year-old woman who was dying of β-hemolytic streptococcal bacteremia (most likely *Streptococcus pyogenes*) in 1941. She had had fevers of 103° to 106° F for 4 weeks. Fortunately, her physician was also treating Dr. John F. Fulton. Dr. Fulton was a friend of Dr. Howard Florey, who had pioneered the use of penicillin in Great Britain. In fact, Dr. Florey's children were staying in the Fulton household to avoid the bombing of London. Dr. Fulton and his associates were able to use their influence to obtain a small quantity of penicillin, and treatment of the patient was begun on a Saturday. Already by Monday, the patient was improving and "eating hearty meals." She recovered and lived to the age of 90 years.

Grossman CM. The first use of penicillin in the United States. *Ann Intern Med.* 2008;149:135–136.

QUESTIONS

1. The most common bacterial causes of acute otitis media are ________________, ________________, and ________________.
2. The antibiotic treatment of choice for acute otitis media is high-dose ________________.
3. This agent is thought to be effective against penicillin-resistant ________________ because at high doses it achieves levels in the middle ear fluid that exceed the minimal inhibitory concentrations of all but the most highly penicillin-resistant strains.
4. You are asked to prescribe antibiotic therapy for a penicillin-allergic 5-year-old girl with acute otitis media that has failed to improve after 72 hours without antibiotics. Her mother states that the last time she received penicillin, she developed urticaria. Appropriate antibiotic therapy would be a ________________, such as ________________ or ________________.

ADDITIONAL READINGS

American Academy of Pediatrics Subcommittee on Management of Acute Otitis Media. Diagnosis and management of acute otitis media. *Pediatrics*. 2004;113:1451–1465.

Coker TR, Chan LS, Newberry SJ, et al. Diagnosis, microbial epidemiology, and antibiotic treatment of acute otitis media in children. *JAMA*. 2010;304:2161–2169.

Dowell SF, Butler JC, Giebink GS, et al. Acute otitis media: management and surveillance in an era of pneumococcal resistance—a report from the Drug-resistant Streptococcus pneumoniae Therapeutic Working Group. *Pediatr Infect Dis J*. 1999;18:1–9.

Klein JO. Is acute otitis media a treatable disease? *N Engl J Med*. 2011;364:168–169.

Paradise JL. A 15-month-old child with recurrent otitis media. *JAMA*. 2002;288:2589–2598.

CHAPTER 22

Infective Endocarditis

It has long been asserted that the heart is the most important organ in the human body. Our language is full of clichés that reflect this, for example, "get to the heart of the matter" and "heart-to-heart talk." If the heart falters for even a few minutes, life ceases. For this reason, a microbial attack on the heart has dire consequences. Such attacks may take the form of infective endocarditis, an infection of the endocardial surface of the heart, particularly the heart valves.

The etiology of infective endocarditis is straightforward. Typically, bacteria gain access to the bloodstream by various mechanisms, including inoculation during dental procedures, via a colonized intravenous catheter, or from injection of illicit drugs. The bacteria then attach to the surface of a heart valve, usually at a site of disrupted endothelium from anomalous blood flow patterns. Such patterns are often the consequence of valvular abnormalities caused by rheumatic fever or congenital defects. Vegetations—masses of fibrin, platelets, and bacteria attached to the endocardium—often form at the site of infection and provide a protected haven in which bacteria persist and multiply. The result of this process is the gradual destruction of the heart valve.

Although infective endocarditis has been recognized as a disease entity since the 1500s, its diagnosis remains difficult. Patients present with nonspecific complaints such as fatigue, malaise, weakness, weight loss, fever, chills, night sweats, and dyspnea upon exertion. Physical examination findings may also be nonspecific and include fever and hematuria. Signs that are more suggestive of infective endocarditis such as Osler nodes, Janeway lesions, Roth spots, and splinter hemorrhages are less common. However, one clear clue to the presence of infective endocarditis is a new heart murmur, which should make the attentive clinician suspect the diagnosis. Laboratory evaluation may show an elevated erythrocyte sedimentation rate and C-reactive protein level, mild anemia, and an abnormal urinalysis with hematuria, pyuria, or proteinuria.

The most common etiologic agents of infective endocarditis vary somewhat with the population being studied, but in general, viridans group streptococci, *Staphylococcus aureus*, and enterococci cause most cases of native valve endocarditis, whereas coagulase-negative staphylococci and *Staphylococcus aureus* are the major pathogens cultured from patients with prosthetic valve endocarditis (Table 22-1). Among the viridans group streptococci, *Streptococcus sanguinis*, *Streptococcus mutans*, and *Streptococcus mitis* are common. A small proportion of endocarditis cases are caused by a relatively obscure group of gram-negative bacilli referred to by the acronym HACEK: ***H**aemophilus parainfluenzae*, ***A**ggregatibacter aphrophilus*, ***A**ggregatibacter actinomycetemcomitans*, ***C**ardiobacterium hominis*, ***E**ikenella corrodens*, and ***K**ingella kingae*.

The protective environment provided by the vegetation makes bacterial endocarditis difficult to treat. Bactericidal, not bacteriostatic, antibiotics must be given in

Table 22-1 Causes of Bacterial Endocarditis

Bacteria	Incidence
Viridans group streptococci	18%–48%
Staphylococcus aureus	22%–32%
Enterococci	7%–11%
Coagulase-negative staphylococci	7%–11%
HACEK organisms	2%–7%

HACEK, ***Haemophilus parainfluenzae***, ***Aggregatibacter aphrophilus***, ***Aggregatibacter actinomycetemcomitans***, ***Cardiobacterium hominis***, ***Eikenella corrodens***, and ***Kingella kingae***. Fowler VG Jr, Miro JM, Hoen B, et al. Staphylococcus aureus endocarditis: a consequence of medical progress. *JAMA*. 2005;293:3012–3021; Tleyjeh IM, Steckelberg JM, Murad HS, et al. Temporal trends in infective endocarditis: a population-based study in Olmsted County, Minnesota. *JAMA*. 2005;293:3022–3028.

high doses for prolonged periods. Because the predominant causes of endocarditis are gram-positive bacteria, β-lactam agents are often used with synergistic doses of gentamicin to enhance killing. Even intensive therapy, however, is not always sufficient, and surgical intervention is often required, so management of patients with endocarditis should include surgical consultation. Given the difficulty in treating these infections and the prolonged courses of antibiotics that are required, identifying the causative organism by obtaining multiple blood cultures is critical for defining optimal therapy.

Not infrequently, patients with bacterial endocarditis present with blood cultures that have been sterilized by prior use of antibiotics. In these situations, **vancomycin** plus synergistic doses of **gentamicin** are recommended along with ciprofloxacin for empiric treatment of native valve endocarditis (Table 22-2 and Fig. 22-1). Vancomycin is effective against *S. aureus* and viridans group streptococci and is bactericidal against

Table 22-2 Empiric Antimicrobial Therapy for Infective Endocarditis

Native valve endocarditis • Vancomycin **plus** Gentamicin **plus** Ciprofloxacin
Prosthetic valve endocarditis • Vancomycin **plus** Gentamicin **plus** Rifampin or ciprofloxacin

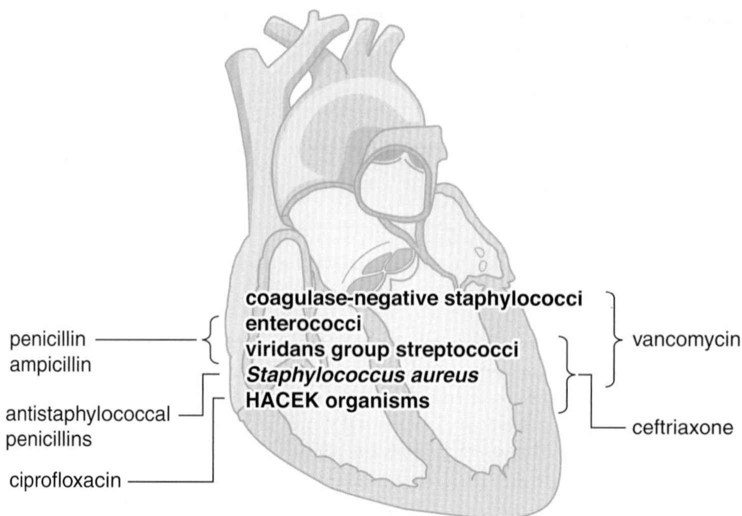

FIGURE 22-1. Activities of agents used to treat bacterial endocarditis.

most enterococcal strains when used in combination with gentamicin. Ciprofloxacin has activity against HACEK organisms. Empiric treatment of prosthetic valve endocarditis is complex but usually consists of **vancomycin** plus synergistic doses of **gentamicin** plus **rifampin** for optimal coverage of staphylococci. Rifampin is added because it may enhance clearance of staphylococci from prosthetic material. Some experts recommend adding ciprofloxacin to effectively treat other possible causative bacteria such as the HACEK organisms.

Ideally, blood cultures will eventually yield the bacterium responsible for the infection, allowing more focused treatment of patients with endocarditis. The antibiotic regimens described here follow logically from what is known about the susceptibility of the bacteria that commonly cause infective endocarditis but also have been shown to be efficacious in numerous clinical trials.

Treatment of native valve endocarditis caused by viridans group streptococci depends on the susceptibility of the causative strain to penicillins (Table 22-3 and Fig. 22-1). Infections that are caused by highly penicillin-susceptible (minimum inhibitory concentration [MIC] ≤0.12 μg/mL) strains should be treated with **penicillin G** or **ceftriaxone** for 4 weeks. Therapy can be shortened to 2 weeks if synergistic doses of **gentamicin** are used in conjunction with one of these two drugs because of synergistic killing that occurs when these agents are used together. For viridans group streptococci that have an intermediate level of susceptibility to penicillin (MIC >0.12 μg/mL and ≤0.5 μg/mL), **penicillin G** or **ceftriaxone** should be given for 4 weeks along with **gentamicin** for the first 2 weeks. Infections caused by highly penicillin-resistant (MIC >0.5 μg/mL) strains of viridans group streptococci should be treated with either **penicillin G** or **ampicillin** for 4 to 6 weeks, in conjunction with **gentamicin** for the entire duration of therapy. It is more difficult to eradicate bacteria from prosthetic material than from native valves, so in prosthetic valve endocarditis, **penicillin G** or **ceftriaxone** is given for 6 weeks instead of 4 weeks. **Gentamicin** is also given for 6 weeks unless the strain is fully susceptible (MIC ≤0.12 μg/mL) to penicillin. In these cases, gentamicin may be given for 2 weeks or not at all.

Table 22-3 Specific Antimicrobial Therapy for Infective Endocarditis Caused by Viridans Group Streptococci

Antibiotic	Duration
Native valve	
Highly penicillin-susceptible strains (MIC ≤0.12 μg/mL)	
• Penicillin G or ceftriaxone	4 weeks
• Penicillin G or ceftriaxone	2 weeks
+ Gentamicin	2 weeks
Intermediate penicillin-resistance strains (MIC >0.12 μg/mL and ≤0.5 μm/mL)	
• Penicillin G or ceftriaxone	4 weeks
+ Gentamicin	2 weeks
Highly penicillin-resistant strains (MIC >0.5 μg/mL)	
• Penicillin G or ampicillin	4–6 weeks
+ Gentamicin	4–6 weeks
Prosthetic valve	
Highly penicillin-susceptible strains (MIC ≤0.12 μg/mL)	
• Penicillin G or ceftriaxone	6 weeks
± Gentamicin	2 weeks
Intermediate or highly penicillin-resistant strains (MIC >0.12 μg/mL)	
• Penicillin G or ceftriaxone	6 weeks
+ Gentamicin	6 weeks

MIC, minimum inhibitory concentration.

Native valve and prosthetic valve endocarditis caused by susceptible enterococci are treated the same as highly resistant viridans group streptococcal endocarditis (Table 22-4 and Fig. 22-1). Either **penicillin G** or **ampicillin** is given in conjunction with **gentamicin** for 4 to 6 weeks. The gentamicin works synergistically with antibiotics active against the enterococcal cell wall and results in bactericidal activity against this bacterium. Infections caused by enterococci resistant to penicillin are treated with **vancomycin** plus **gentamicin** for 6 weeks. For strains resistant to gentamicin but susceptible to **streptomycin**, the latter may be substituted for the former in treatment regimens. Treatment of enterococcal endocarditis caused by strains resistant to all aminoglycosides or both penicillin and vancomycin is problematic and should be done in consultation with an expert.

Native valve endocarditis caused by *S. aureus* is treated with **nafcillin** or **oxacillin** for 6 weeks (Table 22-5 and Fig. 22-1). **Gentamicin** may be added in synergistic doses for the first 3 to 5 days; synergy between this agent and the antistaphylococcal penicillins causes more rapid clearance of the bacteria from the bloodstream. In infections caused by methicillin-resistant *S. aureus* (MRSA), **vancomycin** is used in place of the antistaphylococcal penicillin. In prosthetic valve endocarditis caused by *S. aureus* or *Staphylococcus epidermidis*, treatment is with either **nafcillin** or **oxacillin** in conjunction with

Table 22-4 Specific Antimicrobial Therapy for Infective Endocarditis Caused by Enterococci

Antibiotic	Duration
Native valve	
Penicillin-susceptible and aminoglycoside-susceptible strains	
• Penicillin G or ampicillin	4–6 weeks
+ Gentamicin	4–6 weeks
Penicillin-resistant and aminoglycoside-susceptible strains	
• Vancomycin	6 weeks
+ Gentamicin	6 weeks
Prosthetic valve	
Penicillin-susceptible and aminoglycoside-susceptible strains	
• Penicillin G or ampicillin	6 weeks
+ Gentamicin	6 weeks
Penicillin-resistant and aminoglycoside-susceptible strains	
• Vancomycin	6 weeks
+ Gentamicin	6 weeks

Infections caused by highly aminoglycoside-resistant strains should be treated in consultation with an expert.

Table 22-5 Specific Antimicrobial Therapy for Infective Endocarditis Caused by Staphylococci

Antibiotic	Duration
Native valve	
Methicillin-susceptible strains	
• Nafcillin or oxacillin	6 weeks
± Gentamicin	3–5 days
Methicillin-resistant strains	
• Vancomycin	6 weeks
Prosthetic valve	
Methicillin-susceptible strains	
• Nafcillin or oxacillin	≥6 weeks
+ Rifampin	≥6 weeks
+ Gentamicin	2 weeks
Methicillin-resistant strains	
• Vancomycin	≥6 weeks
+ Rifampin	≥6 weeks
+ Gentamicin	2 weeks

HISTORY

Despite appropriate antibiotic therapy, the mortality associated with infective endocarditis remains high (20% to 25%). Yet, these statistics are a vast improvement over outcomes in the preantibiotic era, when the diagnosis of infective endocarditis was a death sentence. This was poignantly documented in 1931 by the Harvard medical student Alfred S. Reinhart who had aortic insufficiency following a bout of rheumatic fever as a child. One night, Reinhart noted the presence of petechiae on his left arm and immediately self-diagnosed infective endocarditis.

> No sooner had I removed the left arm of my coat, than there was on the ventral aspect of my left wrist a sight which I shall never forget until I die. There greeted my eyes about fifteen or twenty bright red, slightly raised, hemorrhagic spots about 1 millimeter in diameter which did not fade on pressure and which stood defiant as if they were challenging the very gods of Olympus. . . . I took one glance at the pretty little collection of spots and turned to my sister-in-law, who was standing nearby, and calmly said: "I shall be dead within six months."

Weiss S. Self-observations and psychologic reactions of medical student A. S. R. to the onset and symptoms of subacute bacterial endocarditis. *J Mt Sinai Hosp.* 1942;8:1079–1094.

gentamicin and **rifampin** for methicillin-susceptible strains. Again, gentamicin acts to synergistically enhance eradication of the bacteria, and rifampin is thought to facilitate clearance of the staphylococci from prosthetic material. In infections caused by strains resistant to antistaphylococcal penicillins, **vancomycin** is substituted for nafcillin or oxacillin. Nafcillin, oxacillin, or vancomycin is continued for 6 weeks or longer if necessary. Rifampin is continued for 6 weeks, and gentamicin is used for only the first 2 weeks.

Native and prosthetic valve endocarditis caused by one of the HACEK bacteria are treated with **ceftriaxone** or **ampicillin-sulbactam** or **ciprofloxacin** for 4–6 weeks (Table 22-6 and Fig. 22-1).

Table 22-6 Specific Antimicrobial Therapy for Infective Endocarditis Caused by HACEK Organisms

Antibiotic	Duration
Native valve	
• Ceftriaxone	4 weeks
• Ampicillin-sulbactam	4 weeks
• Ciprofloxacin	4 weeks
Prosthetic valve	
• Ceftriaxone	6 weeks
• Ampicillin-sulbactam	6 weeks
• Ciprofloxacin	6 weeks

Questions

1. The three most common bacterial causes of native valve infectious endocarditis are ________________, ________________, and other ________________.
2. The two most common bacterial causes of prosthetic valve infectious endocarditis are ________________ and ________________.
3. The antibiotics used to treat endocarditis caused by viridans group streptococci with intermediate resistance to penicillin are either ________________ or ________________ in conjunction with ________________.
4. The antibiotics used to treat endocarditis caused by enterococci resistant to penicillin are ________________ and ________________.
5. The antibiotics used to treat prosthetic valve endocarditis caused by *Staphylococcus epidermidis* resistant to methicillin are ________________ plus ________________ plus ________________.
6. The antibiotics used to treat native valve endocarditis caused by *Staphylococcus aureus* susceptible to methicillin are ________________ or ________________ with or without a short course of ________________.
7. The antibiotic used to treat endocarditis caused by *Eikenella corrodens* is ________________ or ________________ or ________________.

Additional Readings

Baddour LM, Wilson WR, Bayer AS, et al. Infective endocarditis: diagnosis, antimicrobial therapy, and management of complications: a statement for healthcare professionals from the Committee on Rheumatic Fever, Endocarditis, and Kawasaki Disease, Council on Cardiovascular Disease in the Young, and the Councils on Clinical Cardiology, Stroke, and Cardiovascular Surgery and Anesthesia, American Heart Association: endorsed by the Infectious Diseases Society of America. *Circulation*. 2005;111:e394–e434.

Chopra T, Kaatz GW. Treatment strategies for infective endocarditis. *Expert Opin Pharmacother*. 2010;11:345–360.

Horstkotte D, Follath F, Gutschik E, et al. Guidelines on prevention, diagnosis and treatment of infective endocarditis executive summary; the Task Force on Infective Endocarditis of the European Society of Cardiology. *Eur Heart J*. 2004;25:267–276.

Mylonakis E, Calderwood SB. Infective endocarditis in adults. *N Engl J Med*. 2001;345:1318–1330.

CHAPTER 23

Intravascular-Related Catheter Infections

If skin is the human body's equivalent of a castle wall, then intravascular catheters are battering rams that breach this defense, allowing bacteria access to the vulnerable underlying bloodstream. Because intravascular catheters are an essential component of modern hospital care, catheter-related infections are quite common, occurring at a rate of 200,000 per year in the United States. Obviously, recognizing and appropriately treating these infections are crucial.

Diagnosis of intravascular-related catheter infections is problematic in that confirmation usually requires removal and culture of the catheter. Nonetheless, these infections should be suspected in anyone with an intravascular catheter and a fever of unclear etiology. Inflammation or purulence at the exit site of the catheter is specific but not sensitive for catheter infections. Growth of bacteria from blood cultures should increase suspicion for these infections.

Most bacterial intravascular-related catheter infections are caused by skin flora that contaminate the catheter during placement or migrate down the catheter after placement. Thus, it is not surprising that coagulase-negative staphylococci (especially *Staphylococcus epidermidis*) and *Staphylococcus aureus* are the pathogens most often associated with catheter infections (Table 23-1). In immunocompromised or severely ill patients, aerobic gram-negative bacilli also cause a significant percentage of these infections.

Table 23-1 Bacterial Causes of Community-Acquired Pneumonia

Bacteria	Incidence
Coagulase-negative staphylococci	32%–41%
Staphylococcus aureus	5%–14%
Enteric gram-negative bacilli	5%–11%
Pseudomonas aeruginosa	4%–7%

Haslett TM, Isenberg HD, Hilton E, et al. Microbiology of indwelling central intravascular catheters. *J Clin Microbiol.* 1988;26:696–701; and Jarvis WR. Epidemiology and control of Pseudomonas aeruginosa infections in the intensive care unit. In: Hauser AR, Rello J, eds. *Severe Infections Caused by Pseudomonas Aeruginosa.* Boston, MA: Kluwer Academic Publishers; 2003:153–168.

Table 23-2 Empiric Antimicrobial Therapy for Intravascular-Related Catheter Infections

Antibiotic Class	Antibiotic
Methicillin-resistance uncommon	
• Antistaphylococcal penicillin	Nafcillin, oxacillin
Methicillin-resistance common	
• Glycopeptide	Vancomycin
Immunocompromised or severely ill patient	
Add cephalosporin	Ceftazidime, cefepime

Empiric treatment of intravascular-related catheter infections is focused on staphylococci. **Vancomycin** has become the agent of choice in many locations (Table 23-2 and Fig. 23-1). In regions and hospitals where methicillin-resistant staphylococci are rare, **oxacillin** or **nafcillin** may be used. In severely ill or immunocompromised patients, a third- or fourth-generation cephalosporin (**ceftazidime, cefepime**) should be added to cover enteric gram-negative bacilli and *Pseudomonas aeruginosa*. Once a causative organism is identified from cultures of blood or the catheter itself, the antibiotic regimen should be focused on the identified bacterium. Antibiotic therapy alone, however, is not sufficient in most situations; catheter removal is usually required.

QUESTIONS

1. Bacterial pathogens that typically cause intravascular-related catheter infections are ________________, ________________, and ________________.
2. In settings where methicillin-resistant staphylococci are uncommon, ________________ and ________________ are the empiric antibiotics of choice for these infections.

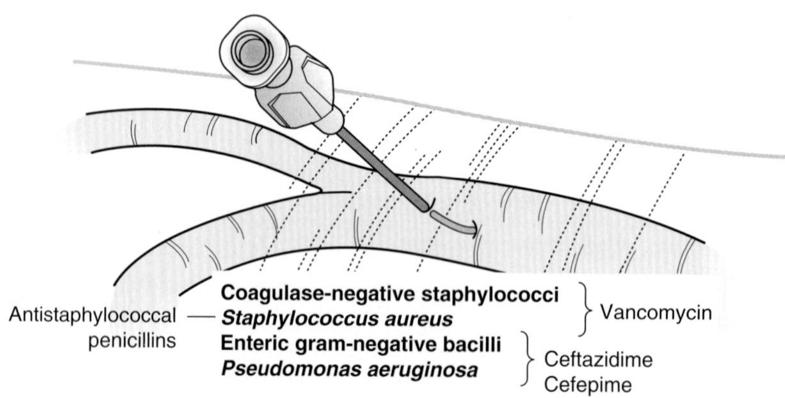

FIGURE 23-1. Activities of agents used to treat intravascular-related catheter infections.

3. In settings where methicillin-resistant staphylococci are common, ___________ is the empiric antibiotic of choice for these infections.

4. In immunocompromised or severely ill patients, ________________ or ________________ should be added to the antibiotic treatment regimens for intravascular-related catheter infections to cover enteric gram-negative bacilli and *Pseudomonas aeruginosa*.

ADDITIONAL READINGS

Fätkenheuer G, Cornely O, Seifert H. Clinical management of catheter-related infections. *Clin Microbiol Infect*. 2002;8:545–550.

Mermel LA, Farr BM, Sherertz RJ, et al. Guidelines for the management of intravascular catheter-related infections. *Clin Infect Dis*. 2001;32:1249–1272.

CHAPTER 24

Intra-abdominal Infections

Intra-abdominal infections include peritonitis, biliary tract infections, splenic abscesses, appendicitis, diverticulitis, and infections following loss of bowel integrity from trauma or surgery. Most of these syndromes have in common the contamination of a normally sterile abdominal site with microbial flora of the bowel. Thus, they are often polymicrobial in nature and are caused by aerobic and facultative gram-negative bacilli, anaerobic bacteria, and gram-positive aerobic cocci (Table 24-1). These infections can be quite severe and frequently lead to sepsis and death.

Table 24-1 Bacterial Causes of Complicated Intra-abdominal Infection

Bacteria	% of Patients
Escherichia coli	71
Klebsiella spp.	14
Pseudomonas aeruginosa	14
Proteus mirabilis	5
Enterobacter spp.	5
Anaerobic bacteria	
Bacteroides fragilis	35
Other *Bacteroides* spp.	71
Clostridium spp.	29
Peptostreptococcus spp.	17
Eubacterium spp.	17
Prevotella spp.	12
Fusobacterium spp.	9
Gram-positive aerobic cocci	
Streptococcus spp.	38
Enterococcus faecalis	12
Enterococcus faecium	3
Other *Enterococcus* spp.	8
Staphylococcus aureus	4

Solomkin JS, Mazuski JE, Bradley JS, et al. Diagnosis and management of complicated intra-abdominal infection in adults and children: guidelines by the Surgical Infection Society and the Infectious Disease Society of America. *Clin Infect Dis*. 2010;50:133–164.

The presentations of patients with intra-abdominal infections vary depending on the site and type of the infection but often include abdominal pain with tenderness, rebound, guarding on examination, fever, chills, nausea, and vomiting. Laboratory examination is often remarkable for a peripheral blood leukocytosis. Abdominal imaging studies may show evidence of an ileus, obstruction, or abdominal abscess or fluid collection.

As mentioned, the bacteria most often responsible for intra-abdominal infections are the flora of the bowel. This flora can vary markedly depending on whether the illness is community acquired or health care associated. In community-acquired infections, enteric gram-negative facultative and aerobic bacilli, gram-positive cocci, and anaerobic bacilli are most frequently isolated. Recommended treatment depends on the severity of the infection and may include a single agent or a combination of agents (Fig. 24-1 and Table 24-2). Antibiotics used in these regimens include carbapenems (**ertapenem**, **imipenem**, **meropenem**, **doripenem**), β-lactam/β-lactamase inhibitor combinations (**ticarcillin/clavulanate**, **piperacillin/tazobactam**), cephalosporins (**cefazolin**, **cefoxitin**, **cefuroxime**, **ceftriaxone**, **cefotaxime**, **ceftazidime**, **cefepime**), quinolones (**ciprofloxacin**, **levofloxacin**, **moxifloxacin**), **tigecycline**, and **metronidazole**.

In health care–associated infections, antibiotic-resistant bacteria are more common, including *Pseudomonas aeruginosa*, penicillin- or vancomycin-resistant enterococci, and methicillin-resistant *Staphylococcus aureus*. Recommended regimens include the following: **piperacillin/tazobactam** alone, a carbapenem alone (**imipenem**, **meropenem**, **doripenem**), or a cephalosporin (**ceftazidime**, **cefepime**) plus metronidazole (Table 24-2). When risk factors for methicillin-resistant *S. aureus* are present, **vancomycin** should be added. Aminoglycosides (**gentamicin**, **tobramycin**, **amikacin**) should be added if there is a concern for resistant aerobic or facultative gram-negative bacilli.

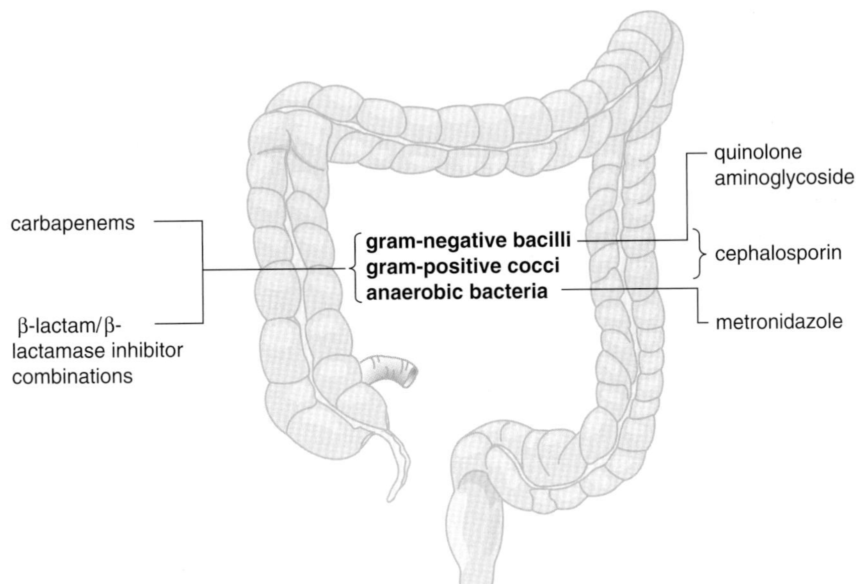

FIGURE 24-1. Activities of agents used to treat intra-abdominal infections.

Table 24-2 Empiric Antimicrobial Therapy for Intra-abdominal Infections

Antibiotic Class	Antibiotic
Community acquired	
For mild-to-moderate infections	
Cefoxitin, ertapenem, moxifloxacin, tigecycline, ticarcillin/clavulanate or (cefazolin, cefuroxime, ceftriaxone, cefotaxime, ciprofloxacin, or levofloxacin) + metronidazole	
For severe infections	
Imipenem, meropenem, doripenem, piperacillin/tazobactam or (cefepime, ceftazidime, ciprofloxacin, or levofloxacin) + metronidazole	
Health care associated	
• β-Lactam/β-lactamase inhibitor combination	Piperacillin/tazobactam
or	
• Carbapenems	Imipenem, meropenem, doripenem
or	
• Third- or fourth-generation cephalosporin	Ceftazidime, cefepime
plus	
Metronidazole	

QUESTIONS

1. Intra-abdominal infections are usually polymicrobial and are caused by the three main groups of bacteria found in the bowel: ________________, ________________, and ________________.
2. The facultative gram-negative bacillus most commonly isolated from intra-abdominal infections is ________________.
3. The following classes of antibiotics can be used as single agents to treat severe community-acquired intra-abdominal infections because they have broad activity against the three different groups of bacteria that cause these infections: ________________ and ________________.
4. Intra-abdominal infections acquired in a health care setting can be treated with ceftazidime or cefepime, but because these agents lack activity against anaerobes, it is recommended that they be used in conjunction with ________________.

ADDITIONAL READINGS

Blot S, De Waele JJ. Critical issues in the clinical management of complicated intra-abdominal infections. *Drugs*. 2005;65:1611–1620.

Montravers P, Gauzit R, Muller C, et al. Emergence of antibiotic-resistant bacteria in cases of peritonitis after intraabdominal surgery affects the efficacy of empirical antimicrobial therapy. *Clin Infect Dis*. 1996;23:486–494.

Solomkin JS, Mazuski JE, Bradley JS, et al. Diagnosis and management of complicated intra-abdominal infection in adults and children: guidelines by the Surgical Infection Society and the Infectious Diseases Society of America. *Clin Infect Dis*. 2010;50:133–164.

PART V

Clinical Cases

"All things, at first try, are difficult to handle. The bow is difficult to draw and the halberd is difficult to wield. When you grow accustomed to a weapon it gets to be easy to handle."

—THE BOOK OF FIVE RINGS, MIYAMOTO MUSASHI

The acquisition of any skill requires practice, and prescribing appropriate antibiotics is no exception. In this section, a series of clinical cases is presented to help you assimilate the information from the previous sections. The answers to the clinical case questions are at the end of this section.

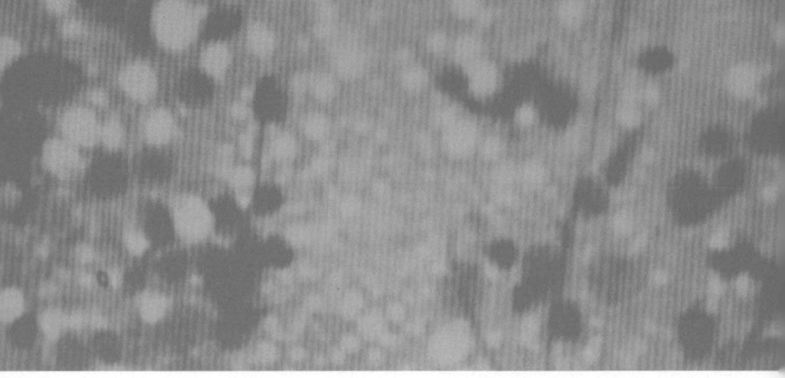

Case 1

A 62-year-old man presents with a 4-day history of fevers, chills, malaise, and a cough productive of purulent sputum. He also states that his right chest hurts when he coughs or takes a deep breath. Although he feels ill, his oral intake has been near his normal level. His past medical and surgical history is remarkable for hypertension and arthroscopic surgery on the left knee 10 years prior to admission. He has not been hospitalized since his knee surgery. His only medication is lisinopril. He has not taken any antibiotics over the past 3 months. He works as an accountant and drinks socially and does not smoke. He denies any recent travel or exposure to birds or animals other than his pet dog.

The patient is a mildly obese man with a temperature of 38.5°C, blood pressure of 152/84, pulse of 74, respiratory rate of 16, and oxygen saturation of 98% on room air. Examination is otherwise remarkable for dullness to percussion of the chest wall, bronchial breath sounds, and splinting on the right side of the chest. His neck is supple, and no heart murmurs are heard.

Laboratory analysis is remarkable for a peripheral blood leukocyte count of 16,600 cells/mm^3 with 75% neutrophils and 10% band forms. Electrolytes are within normal limits, and glucose is 155 mg/dL. A chest radiograph shows lobar consolidation with a questionable effusion on the right side.

Questions

a. What is your diagnosis?

b. What are the bacteria that most commonly cause this syndrome?

c. Which antibiotic(s) would you use to empirically treat this patient?

d. Which antibiotic(s) would you use to empirically treat this patient if he became hypoxemic and required admission to a medical ward?

e. Which antibiotic(s) would you use to empirically treat this patient if he became hypotensive, required vasopressor support, and was admitted to the intensive care unit?

f. If a blood culture later grows *Streptococcus pneumoniae*, which antibiotic(s) would you then use to treat this patient?

g. If instead a urinary antigen test result for *Legionella pneumophila* was reported as positive, which antibiotic(s) would you use to treat this patient?

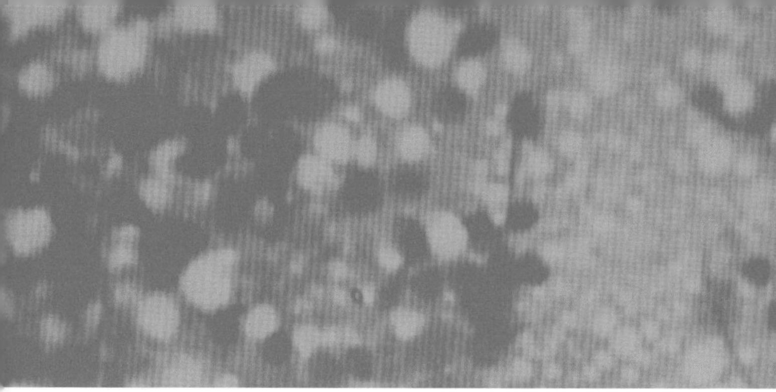

Case 2

A 68-year-old woman is admitted to the surgical service for colectomy following the diagnosis of nonmetastatic colon cancer. The colectomy is performed on the second day of hospitalization. Her postoperative course is complicated by poor respiratory function due to underlying chronic obstructive pulmonary disease. As a result, she remains mechanically ventilated. On postoperative day 6, she is noted to have a fever and a marked increase in the purulence and quantity of her respiratory secretions. Her pulmonary examination is remarkable for bilateral rhonchi. Her peripheral leukocyte count has risen to 18,200 cells/mm^3 with 81% neutrophils. A chest radiograph shows the development of bilateral patchy infiltrates. Preliminary examination of a tracheal aspirate sample shows many neutrophils and gram-negative bacilli.

QUESTIONS

a. What is your diagnosis?

b. What are the bacteria that most commonly cause this syndrome?

c. Which antibiotic(s) would you use to empirically treat this patient?

d. Which antibiotic(s) would you use to empirically treat this patient if the tracheal aspirate had shown a mixture of gram-negative bacilli and gram-positive cocci?

e. If a tracheal aspirate subsequently grows many colonies of *Pseudomonas aeruginosa*, which antibiotic(s) would you use?

f. If a tracheal aspirate subsequently grows many colonies of *Staphylococcus aureus*, which antibiotic(s) would you use?

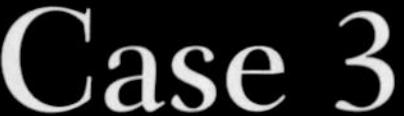

Case 3

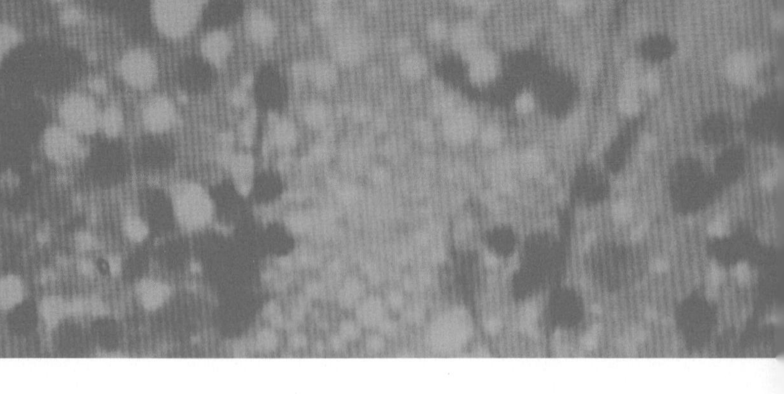

A 23-year-old sexually active woman presents with a 3-day history of dysuria, frequency, and hematuria. She denies fever, chills, nausea, vomiting, or flank pain and states that she is not pregnant. Her past medical history is remarkable for a "bladder infection" 1 year ago. Examination reveals no fevers or costovertebral angle tenderness. A urine dipstick is positive for leukocyte esterase.

QUESTIONS

a. What is your diagnosis?

b. Is this a "complicated" or "uncomplicated" infection?

c. Which antibiotic(s) would you use to empirically treat this patient?

d. Which antibiotic(s) would you use to empirically treat this patient if she resided in a region where 40% of community-acquired *Escherichia coli* are resistant to trimethoprim-sulfamethoxazole?

e. Which antibiotic(s) would you use to empirically treat this patient if she were diabetic and a urine Gram stain showed many gram-negative bacilli?

Case 4

A 26-year-old sexually active woman presents with a 6-day history of fevers, chills, dysuria, frequency, and flank pain. She also reports nausea and has repeatedly vomited and been unable to maintain oral intake. Her past medical history is remarkable only for the normal vaginal delivery of a daughter 3 years ago. She states that she is not currently pregnant. Vital signs are as follows: a temperature of 38.7°C, a recumbent blood pressure of 98/66 and pulse of 88, a standing blood pressure of 88/55 and pulse of 101, and a respiratory rate of 13. Physical examination is otherwise remarkable for costovertebral angle tenderness to palpation on the left side. Laboratory analysis shows a peripheral blood leukocyte count of 26,200 cells/mm^3 with 82% neutrophils and 15% band forms. Electrolytes are within normal limits, and glucose is 93 mg/dL. A urine sample shows pyuria and >100,000 bacteria.

QUESTIONS

- **a.** What is your diagnosis?
- **b.** Is this a "complicated" or "uncomplicated" infection?
- **c.** Which antibiotic(s) would you use to empirically treat this patient?

Case 5

A 17-year-old sexually active woman presents with a 1-week history of fevers, chills, lower abdominal pain, and vaginal discharge. She denies nausea, vomiting, and diarrhea. Her past medical history is remarkable for two episodes of *Chlamydia* infections during the past 2 years. Vital signs are as follows: temperature of 37.4°C, blood pressure of 126/78, pulse of 72, and respiratory rate of 11. Physical examination is otherwise remarkable for bilateral lower abdominal tenderness without evidence of a mass. On pelvic examination, cervical motion tenderness, bilateral adnexal tenderness, and mucopurulent cervical discharge are noted. Laboratory analysis shows a peripheral blood leukocyte count of 8,300 cells/mm^3 with 60% neutrophils and no band forms. Electrolytes and glucose are within normal limits.

Questions

a. What is your diagnosis?

b. What are the likely causes of this patient's infection?

c. Which antibiotic(s) would you use to empirically treat this patient?

d. If her sexual partner is subsequently found to be infected with *Chlamydia trachomatis*, which antibiotic(s) would you use to treat him?

e. If her sexual partner is subsequently found to be infected with *Neisseria gonorrhoeae*, which antibiotic(s) would you use to treat him?

Case 6

A 62-year-old man complains of fever, chills, nausea, vomiting, headache, confusion, and a stiff neck for the past 24 hours. He states that he has had nasal congestion and a cough for the past week but has otherwise been healthy. His past medical history is remarkable for hypertension and alcohol abuse. His examination is remarkable for a temperature of 38.7°C, pain on flexion of the neck, questionable papilledema, and orientation to self and place but not year. Because of concerns about the presence of a central nervous system mass, it is decided that a head computed tomography (CT) scan will be obtained prior to performing a lumbar puncture.

QUESTIONS

a. What infection should you be concerned about?

b. Which bacteria frequently cause this infection?

c. Should this patient receive antibiotics prior to being sent for his head CT scan?

d. If it is decided that antibiotics are appropriate, which agents should be given?

A head CT is performed and shows no evidence of a central nervous system mass lesion. A lumbar puncture is performed, which yields cerebrospinal fluid (CSF) with the following parameters: white cells, 412 cells/mm^3 (96% neutrophils); protein, 110 mg/dL; glucose, 23 mg/dL (simultaneous serum glucose of 98 mg/dL). Gram stain examination reveals gram-positive cocci in pairs.

QUESTIONS

e. Which organism is the likely cause of this patient's illness?

f. What changes would you now make to this patient's antibiotic regimen?

Several days later, the microbiology laboratory reports that *S. pneumoniae* susceptible to penicillin is growing from the CSF.

QUESTIONS

g. What changes would you now make to this patient's antibiotic regimen?

h. Which antibiotics would you choose if the Gram stain results show gram-negative cocci in pairs?

i. Which antibiotics would you choose if the Gram stain results show gram-positive bacilli?

Case 7

A 56-year-old woman complains of a painful rash on her right foot. Five days ago, she developed a blister on her foot after wearing a new pair of shoes. Three days ago, the skin around the blister became red and tender. Over the following days, the redness spread and now involves most of her foot and ankle, and she now has difficulty putting weight on the foot because of pain. She has also noted fever, chills, and rigors over the past 24 hours. Her past medical history is remarkable for hypertension, hyperlipidemia, and hypothyroidism. Her medications are hydrochlorothiazide, lovastatin, and levothyroxine. She resides in a city where there is a high incidence of methicillin-resistant *Staphylococcus aureus* (MRSA) infections acquired in the community. Her vital signs are as follows: temperature, 39.1°C; pulse, 96 beats per minute; respiratory rate, 16 breaths per minute; blood pressure, 123/74 mm Hg. On physical examination, an erythematous, warm, somewhat tender, swollen region is noted over her right foot and extending halfway up her calf. No bullae are noted. Pedal pulses are intact, as is sensation over the region of the rash. She is able to move her foot with minimal pain.

QUESTIONS

- **a.** What is your diagnosis?
- **b.** Which bacteria frequently cause this infection?
- **c.** Which antibiotic(s) would you use to empirically treat this patient?
- **d.** If a blood culture later grows *Streptococcus pyogenes*, which antibiotic(s) would you then use to treat this patient?
- **e.** If a blood culture later grows *S. aureus* susceptible to methicillin, which antibiotic(s) would you then use to treat this patient?

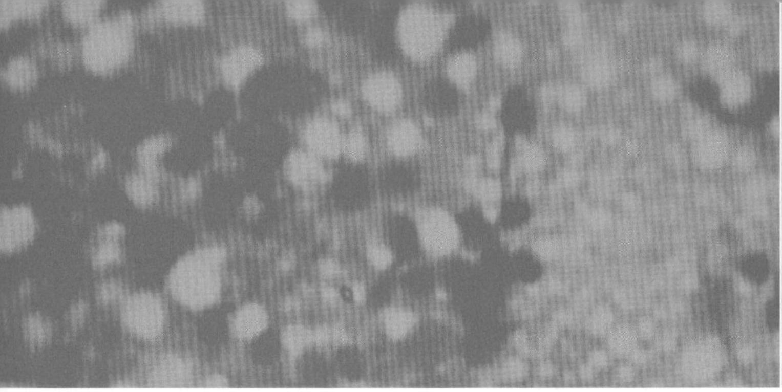

Case 8

A mother brings her 5-year-old daughter to be seen for complaints of right ear pain for the last 72 hours. One of your partners saw the patient 2 days ago and diagnosed acute otitis media at that time. He had told the patient's mother to watch her carefully and to return if her symptoms did not resolve over the next 2 days. Since that time, her ear pain has persisted and she now has a fever. Her past medical history is remarkable for one prior ear infection, which occurred 24 months earlier. On examination, her temperature is 38.8° C; her other vital signs are within normal limits. The right tympanic membrane is bulging and inflamed. There is no evidence of conjunctivitis.

QUESTIONS

a. What is your diagnosis?

b. Which bacteria frequently cause this infection?

c. Which antibiotic would you use to empirically treat this patient?

Upon further questioning, the mother informs you that the patient received amoxicillin for her last ear infection but developed a rash shortly after starting the medication. She states that the rash did not itch, and she was told by her physician, who saw the rash, that it was not hives.

QUESTIONS

d. Which antibiotic would you use to treat this patient?

e. Which antibiotic would you use if the patient did have a history of hives (urticaria) associated with amoxicillin?

Case 9

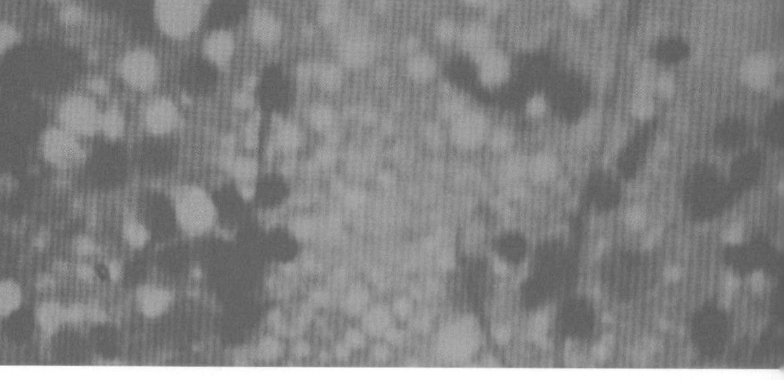

A 38-year-old woman presents with a 2-week history of fevers, chills, and malaise. Her past medical history is remarkable for poor dentition, which resulted in the extraction of several teeth 6 weeks prior to admission, and for rheumatic fever as a child, although she has neglected to take antibiotic prophylaxis before procedures. She works as an accountant and drinks socially and does not smoke or use recreational drugs.

The patient is a thin woman with a temperature of 38.2°C, blood pressure of 122/54, pulse of 83 and bounding, and respiratory rate of 12. Examination is otherwise remarkable for a III/VI early high-pitched diastolic murmur heard at the upper right sternal border that was not present at her last visit. Conjunctival petechiae are also noted. Laboratory evaluation is remarkable for a peripheral blood leukocyte count of 10,600 cells/mm^3 with 65% neutrophils and a hemoglobin content of 12 g/dL. Electrolytes are within normal limits and glucose is 95 mg/dL. Urinalysis is remarkable for hematuria. Echocardiography shows aortic regurgitation with a vegetation on a leaflet of the aortic valve.

Questions

a. What is your diagnosis?

b. What are the bacteria that most commonly cause this syndrome?

c. Blood cultures are drawn and a decision is made to empirically treat the patient while awaiting their results. Which antibiotic(s) would you use to empirically treat this patient?

d. If blood cultures subsequently grow viridans group streptococci fully susceptible to penicillin (minimum inhibitory concentration $\leq$0.12 μg/mL), which antibiotic(s) would you use to treat this patient?

e. If blood cultures subsequently grow *S. aureus* resistant to methicillin, which antibiotic(s) would you use to treat this patient?

f. If blood cultures subsequently grow enterococci susceptible to penicillin and aminoglycosides, which antibiotic(s) would you use to treat this patient?

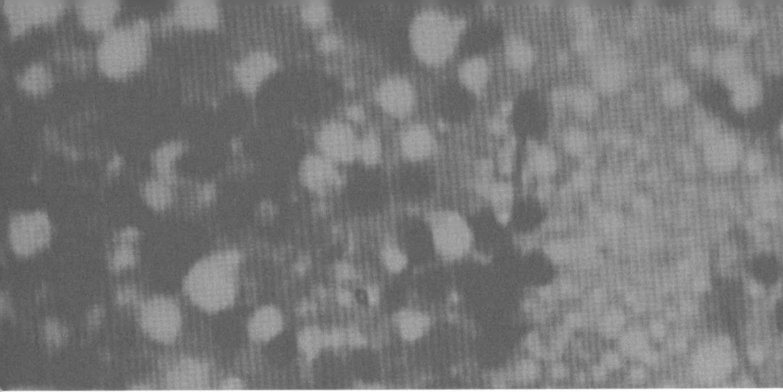

Case 10

A 74-year-old man presents with a 1-week history of fevers, chills, and increasing shortness of breath. His past medical history is remarkable for placement of a prosthetic mitral valve 5 months prior to admission. He is a retired banking executive. He reports moderate alcohol consumption and smokes one pack of cigarettes per day.

Vital signs are as follows: temperature of 38.4°C, blood pressure of 112/75, pulse of 92, and respiratory rate of 19. Examination is otherwise remarkable for venous jugular distension, crackles at the bases of both lungs, and a low-pitched early diastolic murmur. Laboratory evaluation is remarkable for a peripheral blood leukocyte count of 12,400 cells/mm^3 with 70% neutrophils and a hemoglobin content of 13.2 g/dL. Electrolytes are within normal limits and glucose is 89 mg/dL. Echocardiography shows a malfunctioning prosthetic valve with vegetations.

QUESTIONS

a. What is your diagnosis?

b. What are the bacteria that most commonly cause this syndrome?

c. Blood cultures are drawn and a decision is made to empirically treat the patient while awaiting their results. Which antibiotic(s) would you use to empirically treat this patient?

d. If blood cultures subsequently grow *Staphylococcus epidermidis* resistant to methicillin, which antibiotic(s) would you use to treat this patient?

e. If blood cultures subsequently grow *S. aureus* susceptible to methicillin, which antibiotic(s) would you use to treat this patient?

f. If blood cultures subsequently grow *Haemophilus aphrophilus*, which antibiotic(s) would you use to treat this patient?

Case 11

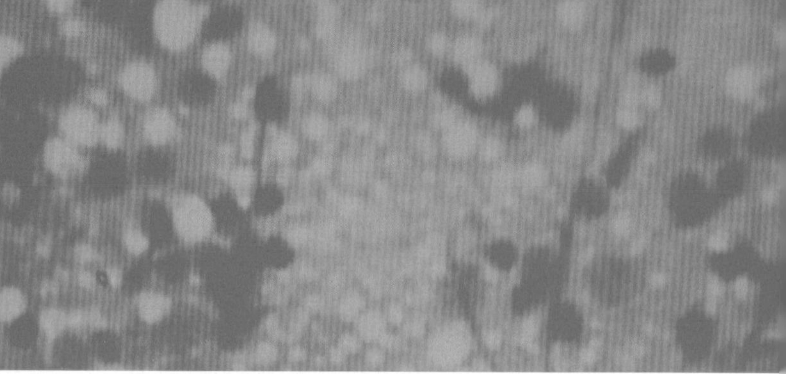

An 85-year-old woman is in the intensive care unit following resection of her colon for colon cancer. On postoperative day 3, you are asked to see her because she has developed a fever.

The patient is mechanically ventilated and sedated. Her temperature is 38.6°C, blood pressure of 128/75, and pulse of 96. She is receiving minimal respiratory support, and the nurse reports scant respiratory secretions on suctioning. On examination, her lungs are clear and her abdomen is soft. The surgical wound is only minimally erythematous without purulence or drainage, and stool is present in the colostomy bag. A Foley catheter is in place. She has no rash, but there is purulent drainage from the exit site of her femoral triple-lumen catheter. Laboratory evaluation is remarkable for a peripheral blood leukocyte count of 13,400 cells/mm^3 with 85% neutrophils. Electrolytes, glucose, and urinalysis are within normal limits. Chest radiograph shows no evidence of an infiltrate.

QUESTIONS

a. What diagnosis do you suspect?

b. What are the bacteria that most commonly cause this infection?

c. You ask that blood cultures be obtained, the catheter be removed, and the catheter tip sent for culture. While awaiting culture results, you wish to empirically start antibiotics. Which antibiotic(s) would you use to empirically treat this patient?

d. Upon further review of the patient's chart, you find that she has a history of systemic lupus erythematosus and has been on high doses of steroids for some time. Which antibiotic(s) would you use to empirically treat this patient?

e. If blood cultures subsequently grow *S. aureus* susceptible to methicillin, which antibiotic(s) would you use to treat this patient?

f. If blood cultures subsequently grow *S. aureus* susceptible to methicillin but the patient has a history of an anaphylactic reaction to amoxicillin, which antibiotic(s) would you use?

Case 12

A 21-year-old man presents with a 4-day history of severe abdominal pain that initially was centered in his right lower quadrant but is now more diffuse. He also reports fevers, chills, nausea, and vomiting. His past medical history is unremarkable and he is not taking any medications.

The patient's temperature is 38.5°C, blood pressure is 90/53, and pulse is 121. His physical examination is remarkable for diffuse abdominal tenderness with rigidity, rebound, and guarding. Bowel sounds are absent. Laboratory evaluation shows a peripheral blood leukocyte count of 23,100 cells/mm^3 with 95% neutrophils. Electrolytes, glucose, and urinalysis are within normal limits. Abdominal radiograph shows an ileus with air–fluid levels and free air. Ultrasound examination is consistent with appendicitis with rupture. The patient is immediately prepared for surgery.

QUESTIONS

a. The patient now has secondary peritonitis and a ruptured appendix. What are the bacteria that most commonly cause this syndrome?

b. Which antibiotic(s) would you use to empirically treat this patient?

c. If this patient had cystic fibrosis and had recently been hospitalized and had in the past received multiple courses of antibiotics for respiratory infections, which antibiotic(s) would you use to empirically treat him?

ANSWERS TO CLINICAL CASES

Case 1

a. This patient has pneumonia, as evidenced by the recent onset of fevers, chills, a productive cough, an elevated peripheral blood leukocyte count, and an infiltrate on his chest radiograph. The pneumonia is classified as community acquired because the patient has not recently been hospitalized or otherwise exposed to the health care environment or taken antibiotics.

b. The most common bacterial causes of community-acquired pneumonia in adults are *Streptococcus pneumoniae*, *Haemophilus influenzae*, *Legionella* spp., *Mycoplasma pneumoniae*, other aerobic gram-negative bacteria, *Chlamydophila pneumoniae*, and *Staphylococcus aureus*. The age of the patient, the productive cough, and the lobar consolidation would make one suspicious of a "typical" organism, as opposed to an "atypical" organism. However, these clinical distinctions have been shown to be unreliable, and the choice of therapy should not be based on them.

c. This patient's pneumonia is mild and can be treated in the outpatient setting. He has no risk factors for penicillin-resistant *S. pneumoniae*. Appropriate antibiotic choices include an oral macrolide (azithromycin, clarithromycin, erythromycin) or doxycycline.

d. If the patient's pneumonia was severe enough to require admission to a medical ward, treatment should be given intravenously and include both a macrolide (azithromycin, clarithromycin, erythromycin) and a β-lactam (cefotaxime, ceftriaxone, high-dose ampicillin). An intravenous quinolone with antistreptococcal activity (moxifloxacin, levofloxacin) would also be appropriate.

e. If the patient's illness was severe and required admission to an intensive care unit, treatment would be given intravenously using a β-lactam (cefotaxime, ceftriaxone, high-dose ampicillin/sulbactam) in combination with either a macrolide (azithromycin) or a quinolone with antistreptococcal activity (moxifloxacin, levofloxacin). Note that this patient does not have risk factors for *Pseudomonas aeruginosa* or MRSA infection, so antipseudomonal or anti-MRSA antibiotics are not indicated.

f. The presence of *S. pneumoniae* in the patient's blood indicates that his pneumonia is caused by this bacterium. If this is the case, the treatment regimen can be narrowed and focused on this pathogen. Appropriate antibiotic therapy would be high-dose penicillin G. A second- or third-generation cephalosporin would also be appropriate. Note that there have been several reports suggesting that patients with bacteremic pneumococcal pneumonia have better outcomes with combination therapy consisting of a β-lactam plus a macrolide (azithromycin) compared to β-lactams alone, so combination therapy could be considered.

g. If diagnostic testing indicated that this patient's pneumonia is caused by *Legionella* spp., therapy should be targeted against this bacterium. Appropriate antibiotics would be azithromycin or a quinolone (either levofloxacin or moxifloxacin).

Case 2

a. This patient has pneumonia, as evidenced by the new onset of fever, increased production of purulent respiratory secretions, an elevated peripheral blood leukocyte count, and an infiltrate on her chest radiograph. The pneumonia is classified as hospital acquired because it developed after the patient was in the hospital.

b. This patient's pneumonia developed after she had been in the hospital for 8 days. It is thus a late-onset hospital-acquired pneumonia. In such a patient, one must be especially concerned about *Pseudomonas aeruginosa*, *Acinetobacter* spp., antibiotic-resistant enteric gram-negative bacilli, and MRSA. The presence of many gram-negative bacilli in the endotracheal aspirate suggests *P. aeruginosa* or antibiotic-resistant enteric gram-negative bacilli.

c. Appropriate therapy would include one agent from each of the two groups of antibiotics. Group 1 includes antipseudomonal cephalosporins (ceftazidime, cefepime), carbapenems (imipenem, meropenem), and extended-spectrum penicillin/β-lactamase inhibitor combinations (piperacillin/tazobactam). Group 2 includes quinolones (ciprofloxacin, levofloxacin) and aminoglycosides (gentamicin, tobramycin, amikacin).

d. The presence of gram-positive cocci in the tracheal aspirate suggests *Staphylococcus aureus*. Because the incidence of MRSA is high in an intensive care unit, antibiotics effective against this organism should be given. Thus, an appropriate regimen would be the combination of antibiotics described in "c" with the addition of linezolid or vancomycin.

e. Growth of *P. aeruginosa* from the tracheal aspirate suggests that this bacterium is the cause of the pneumonia. Appropriate therapy would include two agents with antipseudomonal activity, such as an antipseudomonal cephalosporin (ceftazidime, cefepime) or piperacillin in combination with either ciprofloxacin or an aminoglycoside (gentamicin, tobramycin, amikacin). Actual choices should be guided by local resistance patterns and the previous antibiotic exposure of this patient. Note that piperacillin would be used instead of piperacillin/tazobactam because tazobactam is not active against the β-lactamases of *P. aeruginosa*. Also, recall that ciprofloxacin has the best antipseudomonal activity of the quinolones.

f. Growth of *S. aureus* from the tracheal aspirate suggests that this bacterium is the cause of the pneumonia. Appropriate therapy would be linezolid or vancomycin.

Case 3

a. This patient has acute cystitis, as evidenced by the symptoms of dysuria, frequency, and a positive urine dipstick. The absence of fever, chills, nausea, vomiting, or flank pain make pyelonephritis unlikely.

b. This urinary tract infection would be classified as "uncomplicated" acute cystitis because the patient is young, healthy, not pregnant, not hospitalized, and without evidence of structural abnormalities of her urinary tract.

c. Appropriate therapy for this patient would be a 5-day course of nitrofurantoin or possibly a 3-day course of oral trimethoprim-sulfamethoxazole if she lives in a region in which the prevalence of uropathogens resistant to this agent is less than 20%.

d. If this patient resided in a region in which resistance to trimethoprim-sulfamethoxazole was common, nitrofurantoin would be appropriate therapy.

e. A past diagnosis of diabetes would predispose this patient to infection by a broader range of bacteria and would cause her urinary tract infection to be classified as a "complicated" acute cystitis. Because her infection is mild, she could be treated with oral antibiotics. Ciprofloxacin would be a good choice because it is effective against many of the gram-negative bacilli that might cause this infection, including *Pseudomonas aeruginosa* and many Enterobacteriaceae.

Case 4

a. This patient has acute pyelonephritis, as evidenced by symptoms of fever, chills, dysuria, frequency, and flank pain.

b. This case of acute pyelonephritis would be classified as uncomplicated because the patient is young, healthy, not pregnant, not hospitalized, and without evidence of structural abnormalities of her urinary tract.

c. Because this patient is dehydrated and unable to tolerate oral intake, she should be hospitalized and receive intravenous antibiotics as well as hydration. Appropriate empiric antibiotic therapy would be a quinolone (ciprofloxacin, levofloxacin); an aminoglycoside (gentamicin, tobramycin, amikacin) with or without ampicillin; an extended-spectrum penicillin (piperacillin) with or without an aminoglycoside; a third-generation cephalosporin (ceftriaxone, cefotaxime) with or without an aminoglycoside; or a carbapenem (imipenem, meropenem, doripenem, ertapenem).

Case 5

a. This patient has pelvic inflammatory disease (PID), as evidenced by symptoms of fever, chills, lower abdominal pain, and findings of cervical motion tenderness, bilateral adnexal tenderness, and mucopurulent cervical discharge.

b. The sexually transmitted bacteria that are most often implicated are *Neisseria gonorrhoeae* and *Chlamydia trachomatis*. Many other bacteria are frequently isolated from PID lesions, including *Bacteroides* and *Peptostreptococcus* spp. as well as *Escherichia coli*, *Gardnerella vaginalis*, *Haemophilus influenzae*, and group B streptococci. Of these, anaerobic bacteria are most likely to play a significant role in the pathogenesis of PID, and many experts feel that antibiotics effective against anaerobic bacteria should be included in PID treatment regimens.

c. Because this patient's illness is relatively mild, she is a candidate for outpatient therapy. An appropriate antibiotic regimen would be a single intramuscular dose of a cephalosporin (ceftriaxone, cefotaxime, cefoxitin + probenecid) plus oral doxycycline. The addition of oral metronidazole would also be reasonable.

d. Uncomplicated *C. trachomatis* urethritis is treated with doxycycline, azithromycin, ofloxacin, or levofloxacin.

e. Gonorrhea is treated with ceftriaxone or cefixime. All patients with gonorrhea should also be treated for *Chlamydia*.

Case 6

a. This patient may have acute bacterial meningitis, as evidenced by the acute onset of fever, chills, nausea, vomiting, headache, confusion, and a stiff neck. Examination of the cerebrospinal fluid is necessary to definitively make the diagnosis.

b. In an adult patient, acute bacterial meningitis is most frequently caused by *Streptococcus pneumoniae* or *Neisseria meningitidis*. In an older individual such as this patient, *Listeria monocytogenes* and aerobic gram-negative bacilli are also a concern.

c. Even a delay of several hours can have a detrimental effect on the outcomes of patients with acute bacterial meningitis. For this reason, antibiotic therapy should not be withheld while awaiting the results of neuroimaging studies. Note that most experts would also initiate steroid therapy prior to or at the same time as starting antibiotics.

d. Empiric therapy in this patient would include a third-generation cephalosporin (ceftriaxone or cefotaxime) to cover *N. meningitidis* and most strains of *S. pneumoniae*, as well as aerobic gram-negative bacilli. Vancomycin should be added to cover highly penicillin-resistant strains of *S. pneumoniae*. Because this patient is older than 50 years, ampicillin should also be added to cover *L. monocytogenes*.

e. The lumbar puncture results confirm the diagnosis of acute bacterial meningitis. The gram-positive cocci in pairs seen on Gram stain of the cerebrospinal fluid indicate that *S. pneumoniae* is the likely cause. If the patient were an infant, one would also be concerned about *Streptococcus agalactiae*, but meningitis caused by this bacterium is rare in adults.

f. Acute bacterial meningitis caused by *S. pneumoniae* is treated with a third-generation cephalosporin plus vancomycin, so the ampicillin should be discontinued.

g. Meningitis caused by penicillin-susceptible *S. pneumoniae* can be treated with either penicillin or a third-generation cephalosporin.

h. Cerebrospinal fluid containing gram-negative cocci in pairs indicates that *N. meningitidis* is the cause of the meningitis. The patient should be treated with penicillin G or a third-generation cephalosporin (ceftriaxone, cefotaxime).

i. Cerebrospinal fluid containing gram-positive bacilli indicates that *L. monocytogenes* is the cause of the meningitis. The patient should be treated with ampicillin plus gentamicin.

Case 7

a. This patient has cellulitis, as evidenced by an erythematous and tender skin rash, fevers, chills, and rigors. One would also be concerned about deeper infections, such as necrotizing fasciitis, but she does not have bullae, violaceous skin discoloration, or paresthesia, making these more serious infections less likely.

b. This patient is not immunocompromised, and the infection did not result from an unusual exposure, such as to seawater. Therefore, her cellulitis is most likely caused by skin bacteria, such as *Staphylococcus aureus*, *Streptococcus pyogenes*, or other streptococci.

c. Given her high fever and decreased mobility, this patient should be admitted to the hospital and treated with intravenous antibiotics. Because she lives in a region where community-acquired MRSA infections are common, agents should be chosen that are effective against this organism as well as streptococci. A glycopeptide (vancomycin, telavancin), linezolid, daptomycin, tigecycline, or ceftaroline would be appropriate choices.

d. The presence of *S. pyogenes* in the blood indicates that this bacterium is the cause of the cellulitis. The antibiotic regimen can therefore be changed to penicillin G, which has excellent activity against this organism.

e. The presence of methicillin-susceptible *S. aureus* in the blood indicates that this bacterium is the cause of the cellulitis. The antibiotic regimen can therefore be changed to an antistaphylococcal penicillin, such as nafcillin or oxacillin, because MRSA is no longer a concern.

Case 8

a. This patient has acute otitis media, as evidenced by ear pain, fever, and an inflamed tympanic membrane.

b. Acute otitis media is most commonly caused by *Streptococcus pneumoniae*, *Haemophilus influenzae*, or *Moraxella catarrhalis*.

c. This patient's ear infection has not resolved over 72 hours, and she now has a fever, so antibiotic therapy is definitely indicated. There are no risk factors for β-lactamase-producing bacteria, so high-dose amoxicillin is the treatment of choice.

d. The patient has a mild allergy to penicillin, so an oral cephalosporin (cefdinir, cefpodoxime, cefuroxime) should be used to treat the ear infection.

e. When there is a history of a type I hypersensitivity allergic reaction to a penicillin, a macrolide (azithromycin, clarithromycin) should be used to treat otitis media.

Case 9

a. This patient has infective endocarditis, as evidenced by a fever and a new murmur in a patient with a history of rheumatic fever and a recent dental procedure during which she did not receive antibiotic prophylaxis. Other supporting features include conjunctival petechiae, mild anemia, and hematuria. The finding of a vegetation by echocardiography confirms the diagnosis.

b. Native valve endocarditis is most frequently caused by viridans group streptococci, *Staphylococcus aureus*, enterococci, and the HACEK organisms.

c. Vancomycin plus gentamicin plus ciprofloxacin is appropriate empiric therapy. This regimen will cover most viridans group streptococci, staphylococci, enterococci, and HACEK organisms.

d. Appropriate antimicrobial therapy for endocarditis caused by penicillin-susceptible viridans group streptococci is penicillin G or ceftriaxone for 4 weeks. Alternatively, if penicillin G or ceftriaxone is given in conjunction with gentamicin, the treatment course may be shortened to 2 weeks.

e. Appropriate antimicrobial therapy for endocarditis caused by MRSA is vancomycin for 6 weeks.

f. Appropriate antimicrobial therapy for endocarditis caused by penicillin- and gentamicin-susceptible enterococci is penicillin G or ampicillin for 4 to 6 weeks. Gentamicin should also be given for 4 to 6 weeks to allow for synergistic bactericidal killing of the enterococci.

Case 10

a. This patient has prosthetic valve endocarditis, as evidenced by a fever and a new murmur in a patient with a history of mitral valve replacement. Infection of the prosthetic valve has caused it to malfunction, resulting in the signs and symptoms of congestive heart failure. The finding of a vegetation and malfunctioning prosthetic valve by echocardiography confirms the diagnosis.

b. Prosthetic valve endocarditis is most frequently caused by coagulase-negative staphylococci and *Staphylococcus aureus*.

c. Vancomycin plus gentamicin plus rifampin is appropriate empiric therapy. This regimen will cover staphylococci.

d. Appropriate antimicrobial therapy for prosthetic valve endocarditis caused by methicillin-resistant *Staphylococcus epidermidis* is vancomycin plus rifampin for 6 or more weeks. Gentamicin should be given for the first 2 weeks.

e. Appropriate antimicrobial therapy for prosthetic valve endocarditis caused by methicillin-susceptible *S. aureus* is nafcillin or oxacillin for 6 or more weeks. Rifampin should also be given for 6 or more weeks, and gentamicin should be added for the first 2 weeks.

f. Appropriate antimicrobial therapy for endocarditis caused by one of the HACEK organisms is ceftriaxone or ampicillin-sulbactam or ciprofloxacin for 6 weeks.

Case 11

a. This patient likely has an intravascular catheter infection, as evidenced by a fever, purulent drainage from the catheter exit site, and lack of evidence to support an alternative diagnosis.

b. Intravascular-related catheter infections are most commonly caused by coagulase-negative staphylococci and *Staphylococcus aureus*.

c. If methicillin-resistant staphylococci are rarely isolated in this hospital, one could use nafcillin or oxacillin. Otherwise, vancomycin would be the antibiotic of choice.

d. Appropriate empiric antimicrobial therapy for intravascular-related catheter infections in an immunocompromised host would be vancomycin to cover staphylococci plus either ceftazidime or cefepime to cover enteric gram-negative bacilli and *Pseudomonas aeruginosa*.

e. Nafcillin or oxacillin would be appropriate antimicrobial therapy for an intravascular catheter infection caused by methicillin-susceptible *S. aureus*.

f. Antistaphylococcal penicillins should not be given to a patient with a history of an anaphylactic reaction to penicillins. Likewise, cephalosporins should be avoided. Vancomycin would be the agent of choice in this situation.

Case 12

a. The bacteria that most commonly cause secondary peritonitis are enteric gram-negative bacilli, such as *Escherichia coli*; gram-positive cocci, such as enterococci and streptococci; and anaerobic bacteria, such as *Bacteroides* spp.

b. This patient has a community-acquired infection and is severely ill, so appropriate single-agent antimicrobial therapy would be a carbapenem (imipenem, meropenem, doripenem) or piperacillin/tazobactam. Combination regimens would include metronidazole together with cefepime, ceftazidime, ciprofloxacin, or levofloxacin.

c. If this patient's intra-abdominal infection were health care-associated, antibiotics with activity against resistant bacteria, including *Pseudomonas aeruginosa* and resistant Enterobacteriaceae, would be preferred. Such regimens would be piperacillin/tazobactam, imipenem, meropenem, doripenem, cefepime plus metronidazole, or ceftazidime plus metronidazole. The actual regimen chosen would depend on the antibiotics to which this patient had been previously exposed, the bacteria with which he is colonized, and regional antibiotic resistance patterns.

PART VI

Review Questions and Answers

1. Which of the following antibiotics is NOT a β-lactam?
   a. ampicillin
   b. meropenem
   c. ceftriaxone
   d. vancomycin
   e. aztreonam

2. Which of the following antibiotics has little activity against anaerobic bacteria?
   a. imipenem
   b. metronidazole
   c. ceftriaxone
   d. clindamycin
   e. amoxicillin/clavulanate

3. Which of the following antibiotics could you use in someone who has a history of developing anaphylaxis after taking penicillin?
   a. aztreonam
   b. ertapenem
   c. cefazolin
   d. piperacillin/tazobactam
   e. cefotetan

4. Which of the following agents is NOT useful in the treatment of enterococcal infections?
   a. penicillin
   b. cefazolin
   c. ampicillin
   d. gentamicin
   e. vancomycin

5. Which of the following quinolones has the greatest activity against *Pseudomonas aeruginosa*?
   a. levofloxacin
   b. moxifloxacin
   c. gatifloxacin
   d. gemifloxacin
   e. ciprofloxacin

6. Rifampin is useful in treatment or prophylaxis against all of the following bacteria EXCEPT:
   a. *Staphylococcus aureus*
   b. *Staphylococcus epidermidis*
   c. *Bacteroides fragilis*
   d. *Neisseria meningitidis*
   e. *Mycobacterium tuberculosis*

7. Severe infections caused by which of the following bacteria are routinely treated with a single antibiotic?
   a. *Treponema pallidum*
   b. *Brucella melitensis*
   c. *Pseudomonas aeruginosa*
   d. *Mycobacterium tuberculosis*
   e. *Helicobacter pylori*

8. Which of the following agents is NOT useful in treating infections caused by *Mycobacterium avium* complex?
   a. clarithromycin
   b. isoniazid
   c. ethambutol
   d. rifabutin
   e. ciprofloxacin

9. Which of the following agents is useful in the treatment of infections caused by *Clostridium difficile*?
   a. clindamycin
   b. imipenem
   c. penicillin
   d. metronidazole
   e. piperacillin/tazobactam

10. Which of the following agents would be useful in the treatment of an infection caused by an *Escherichia coli* strain that produces an extended-spectrum β-lactamase?
    a. ceftriaxone
    b. ceftazidime
    c. meropenem
    d. aztreonam
    e. piperacillin

11. Which of the following agents does NOT inhibit bacterial cell wall synthesis?
    a. gentamicin
    b. aztreonam
    c. imipenem
    d. vancomycin
    e. ampicillin

12. Penicillin is still commonly used to treat all of the following bacteria EXCEPT:
    a. *Treponema pallidum*
    b. *Streptococcus pyogenes*
    c. *Clostridium perfringens*
    d. *Neisseria meningitidis*
    e. *Staphylococcus aureus*

13. Which of the following bacteria is susceptible to vancomycin?
    a. *Bordetella pertussis*
    b. *Clostridium difficile*
    c. *Pseudomonas aeruginosa*
    d. *Haemophilus influenzae*
    e. *Enterobacter aerogenes*

14. All of the following would be appropriate treatment for an infection caused by *Haemophilus influenzae* EXCEPT:
    a. amoxicillin/clavulanate
    b. cefuroxime
    c. ampicillin
    d. doxycycline
    e. cefotaxime

15. Which of the following antibiotics can be safely used in small children?
    a. ciprofloxacin
    b. azithromycin
    c. tetracycline
    d. gemifloxacin
    e. doxycycline

16. All of the following are relatively common adverse reactions to aminoglycosides EXCEPT:
    a. auditory impairment
    b. nephrotoxicity
    c. vestibular toxicity
    d. biliary sludging
    e. decreased renal function

17. Pyrazinamide is used to treat infections caused by which of the following?
    a. *Mycobacterium tuberculosis*
    b. *Mycobacterium avium* complex
    c. *Mycobacterium leprae*
    d. *Rickettsia rickettsii*
    e. *Legionella pneumophila*

18. The sexually transmitted disease chlamydia may be treated with each of the following agents EXCEPT:
    a. doxycycline
    b. azithromycin
    c. ofloxacin
    d. levofloxacin
    e. ceftriaxone

19. Empiric use of vancomycin in a patient with infective endocarditis would fail to cover which of the following organisms?
    a. *Staphylococcus aureus*
    b. *Staphylococcus epidermidis*
    c. viridans group streptococci
    d. enterococci
    e. HACEK organisms

20. Which of the following antibiotics targets the bacterial ribosome?
    a. isoniazid
    b. vancomycin
    c. tetracycline
    d. levofloxacin
    e. trimethoprim-sulfamethoxazole

21. Which of the following antibiotics would NOT be used to treat a patient infected with *Borrelia burgdorferi*?
    a. doxycycline
    b. clindamycin
    c. amoxicillin
    d. cefuroxime
    e. ceftriaxone

22. Doxycycline is useful in treating infections caused by all of the following bacteria EXCEPT:
    a. *Leptospira interrogans*
    b. *Brucella abortus*
    c. *Chlamydia trachomatis*
    d. *Pseudomonas aeruginosa*
    e. *Rickettsia rickettsii*

23. Which of the following antibiotics targets bacterial RNA polymerase?
    a. cefotetan
    b. amikacin
    c. rifampin

d. azithromycin
e. daptomycin

24. Which of the following agents does NOT have activity against vancomycin-resistant *Enterococcus faecium*?
a. quinupristin/dalfopristin
b. linezolid
c. daptomycin
d. tigecycline
e. vancomycin

25. Which of the following antibiotic regimens would be appropriate for a patient with a severe infection caused by *Pseudomonas aeruginosa*?
a. ceftazidime + tobramycin
b. ceftriaxone + gentamicin
c. piperacillin + rifampin
d. ertapenem + amikacin
e. ampicillin + tobramycin

26. Vancomycin is added to ceftriaxone in the empiric treatment of community-acquired acute bacterial meningitis to allow for effective treatment of which organism?
a. *Neisseria meningitidis*
b. *Streptococcus pneumoniae*
c. *Staphylococcus aureus*
d. *Haemophilus influenzae*
e. *Enterococcus faecium*

27. Which of the following types of bacteria have acquired resistance to all β-lactam antibiotics by producing a special penicillin-binding protein that is not bound by these agents?
a. vancomycin-resistant enterococci
b. *Escherichia coli* strains that produce extended-spectrum β-lactamases
c. *Enterobacter aerogenes* strains that constitutively express AmpC β-lactamases
d. methicillin-resistant *Staphylococcus aureus*
e. multidrug-resistant *Pseudomonas aeruginosa*

28. The β-lactamase inhibitors clavulanate, sulbactam, and tazobactam effectively inhibit many of the β-lactamases of the following groups of bacteria EXCEPT:
a. *Pseudomonas aeruginosa*
b. *Bacteroides fragilis*
c. *Staphylococcus aureus*
d. *Haemophilus influenzae*
e. *Proteus mirabilis*

29. Accepted regimens for the treatment of *Helicobacter pylori* may contain each of the following agents EXCEPT:
a. amoxicillin
b. clarithromycin
c. cefotaxime
d. metronidazole
e. bismuth subsalicylate

30. Which of the following antibiotics is effective against bacteria that cause an atypical pneumonia?
a. amoxicillin
b. amoxicillin/clavulanate
c. cefotaxime
d. vancomycin
e. azithromycin

31. Streptomycin is used to treat infections caused by all of the following bacteria EXCEPT:
a. *Enterococcus faecalis*
b. *Borrelia burgdorferi*
c. *Francisella tularensis*
d. *Mycobacterium tuberculosis*
e. *Brucella abortus*

32. Which of the following bacteria frequently alters the composition of the peptide side chain of peptidoglycan to cause resistance to vancomycin?
a. *Staphylococcus aureus*
b. *Staphylococcus epidermidis*
c. *Enterococcus faecium*
d. *Streptococcus pneumoniae*
e. *Enterobacter aerogenes*

33. All of the following agents are used to treat patients with tuberculosis EXCEPT:
a. pyrazinamide
b. isoniazid

c. rifampin
d. dapsone
e. ethambutol

34. Which of the following would be considered appropriate therapy for an acute uncomplicated urinary tract infection?
a. nitrofurantoin
b. amoxicillin
c. ampicillin
d. ceftriaxone
e. meropenem

35. Which of the following antibiotics is effective against *Helicobacter pylori*, *Mycobacterium avium* complex, *Bordetella pertussis*, and some strains of *Staphylococcus aureus* and *Streptococcus pneumoniae*?
a. amoxicillin
b. amoxicillin/clavulanate
c. ceftriaxone
d. doxycycline
e. clarithromycin

36. Which of the following is NOT an aminoglycoside?
a. streptomycin
b. gentamicin
c. tobramycin
d. erythromycin
e. amikacin

37. All of the following are appropriate antimicrobial regimens for late-onset hospital-acquired pneumonia EXCEPT:
a. cefepime + levofloxacin
b. piperacillin/tazobactam + ceftazidime
c. imipenem + ciprofloxacin
d. ceftazidime + tobramycin
e. piperacillin/tazobactam + amikacin

38. Which of the following is appropriate therapy for infections caused by *Leptospira interrogans*?
a. amoxicillin
b. vancomycin
c. linezolid
d. streptomycin
e. metronidazole

39. Relatively common adverse reactions to the penicillin include all of the following EXCEPT:
a. diarrhea
b. rash
c. anaphylaxis
d. cartilage damage
e. serum sickness

40. Clindamycin predisposes to infection by which of the following bacteria?
a. *Clostridium perfringens*
b. *Clostridium difficile*
c. *Clostridium tetani*
d. *Clostridium botulinum*
e. *Clostridium septicum*

41. Third-generation cephalosporins should be used with caution in infections caused by certain bacteria that produce inducible chromosomal AmpC β-lactamases because resistance may develop during treatment. Each of the following is an example of such bacteria EXCEPT:
a. *Morganella* spp.
b. *Serratia* spp.
c. *Haemophilus* spp.
d. *Enterobacter* spp.
e. *Citrobacter* spp.

42. Which of the following antibiotics has clinically useful activity against anaerobic bacteria?
a. cefotetan
b. cefotaxime
c. cefuroxime
d. cefazolin
e. ceftazidime

43. Which of the following antibiotics has the least activity against *Pseudomonas aeruginosa*?
a. imipenem
b. meropenem
c. ertapenem
d. ceftazidime
e. piperacillin

44. Which of the following antibiotics does NOT have activity against *Legionella pneumophila*?
  a. azithromycin
  b. levofloxacin
  c. moxifloxacin
  d. telithromycin
  e. piperacillin/tazobactam

45. Which of the following antibiotics is used to treat leprosy?
  a. isoniazid
  b. ethambutol
  c. clofazimine
  d. streptomycin
  e. amoxicillin/clavulanate

46. Which of the following would be appropriate antibiotic therapy for a patient with native valve infective endocarditis caused by a highly penicillin-resistant (minimum inhibitory concentration >0.5 μg/mL) strain of viridans group streptococci?
  a. penicillin G
  b. ampicillin + streptomycin
  c. ceftriaxone
  d. ampicillin + gentamicin
  e. oxacillin + gentamicin

47. All of the following antibiotics are active against *Campylobacter jejuni* EXCEPT:
  a. erythromycin
  b. cefazolin
  c. azithromycin
  d. ciprofloxacin
  e. doxycycline

48. Each of the following might be appropriate empiric monotherapy for cellulitis EXCEPT:
  a. ceftazidime
  b. vancomycin
  c. oxacillin
  d. cefazolin
  e. clindamycin

49. Which of the following is a major toxicity of the antimycobacterial drug ethambutol?
  a. rash
  b. hepatotoxicity
  c. gout
  d. serum sickness
  e. optic neuritis

50. Optimal antibiotic therapy for a patient with prosthetic valve endocarditis caused by *Staphylococcus aureus* might include each of the following agents EXCEPT:
  a. nafcillin
  b. rifampin
  c. linezolid
  d. vancomycin
  e. gentamicin

ANSWERS TO REVIEW QUESTIONS

1. d. vancomycin. Like the β-lactams, vancomycin works by inhibiting cell wall synthesis. However, its structure lacks the β-lactam ring that is characteristic of β-lactam antibiotics, and it is therefore not included in this group. β-Lactam antibiotics include penicillins (e.g., ampicillin), cephalosporins (e.g., ceftriaxone), carbapenems (e.g., meropenem), and monobactams (e.g., aztreonam).

2. c. ceftriaxone. Whereas imipenem, metronidazole, clindamycin, and amoxicillin/clavulanate all have good or excellent activity against anaerobic bacteria, ceftriaxone has limited activity against them.

3. a. aztreonam. All β-lactam antibiotics should be avoided in someone with a history of an immediate hypersensitivity response (e.g., urticaria or anaphylaxis) to penicillin with the exception of the monobactam aztreonam. There are few allergic cross-reactions between aztreonam and other β-lactam agents.

4. b. cefazolin. Enterococcal infections are usually treated with a penicillin (e.g., penicillin, ampicillin, or piperacillin) in conjunction with an aminoglycoside (gentamicin or streptomycin). Vancomycin is often used for penicillin-resistant strains. All enterococci are resistant to cephalosporins.

5. e. ciprofloxacin. Of the commercially available quinolones, ciprofloxacin has the greatest activity against *Pseudomonas aeruginosa*.

6. c. *Bacteroides fragilis*. Rifampin is used in conjunction with an antistaphylococcal penicillin or vancomycin to treat infections involving prosthetic material caused by staphylococci. It is used as prophylaxis in individuals exposed to *Neisseria meningitidis* and is one of the major reagents used to treat *Mycobacterium tuberculosis* infections. It is not used in the treatment of anaerobic infections, such as those caused by *B. fragilis*.

7. a. *Treponema pallidum*. Infections caused by *T. pallidum*, the etiologic agent of syphilis, are usually treated with penicillin alone. *Brucella* infections are usually treated with doxycycline + rifampin, gentamicin, or streptomycin. Serious *Pseudomonas aeruginosa* infections are usually treated with two agents. Active infections caused by *Mycobacterium tuberculosis* and *Helicobacter pylori* are routinely treated with multiple drug regimens.

8. b. isoniazid. Although isoniazid is part of the core antibiotic regimen used to treat *Mycobacterium tuberculosis*, it is not active against *Mycobacterium avium* complex. Clarithromycin, ethambutol, rifabutin, and ciprofloxacin are active against *M. avium* complex.

9. d. metronidazole. *Clostridium difficile* infections are treated with metronidazole or vancomycin. Clindamycin, imipenem, penicillin, and piperacillin/tazobactam have no activity against this organism. Clindamycin, in particular, predisposes to disease by *C. difficile*.

10. c. meropenem. Extended-spectrum β-lactamase–producing bacteria are frequently resistant to all classes of antibiotics except the carbapenems. Thus, of the agents listed, only meropenem would reliably have activity against these bacteria.

11. a. gentamicin. Aztreonam, imipenem, and ampicillin are all β-lactam antibiotics that act by inhibiting penicillin-binding proteins, which are essential

for cell wall synthesis. Likewise, vancomycin prevents incorporation of new peptidoglycan subunits into the cell wall. Gentamicin, on the other hand, is an aminoglycoside and acts by inhibiting the bacterial ribosome.

12. e. *Staphylococcus aureus*. Although penicillin is still commonly used to treat infections caused by *Treponema pallidum* (syphilis), *Streptococcus pyogenes* (streptococcal pharyngitis), *Clostridium perfringens* (gas gangrene), and *Neisseria meningitidis* (meningococcemia), it is not active against almost all strains of *Staphylococcus aureus*.

13. b. *Clostridium difficile*. Vancomycin only has activity against gram-positive bacteria. *Bordetella pertussis*, *Pseudomonas aeruginosa*, *Haemophilus influenzae*, and *Enterobacter aerogenes* are all gram-negative bacteria.

14. c. ampicillin. A significant proportion of *Haemophilus influenzae* strains now produce β-lactamases that destroy ampicillin and amoxicillin. These β-lactamases, however, are inhibited by commercially available β-lactamase inhibitors, so amoxicillin/clavulanate is effective against strains that produce them. Cefuroxime and cefotaxime are resistant to degradation by these β-lactamases and are therefore also effective against these strains. Doxycycline is also active against most *Haemophilus influenzae* strains.

15. b. azithromycin. Quinolones, such as ciprofloxacin and gemifloxacin, should be used with caution in infants and children younger than 18 years of age because they have been associated with cartilage damage in juvenile animals. Tetracycline and doxycycline should usually be avoided in children younger than 8 years of age. Azithromycin is safe for use in children.

16. d. biliary sludging. Relatively common adverse effects associated with the use of aminoglycosides include nephrotoxicity (which results in decreased renal function), auditory impairment, and vestibular toxicity. Biliary sludging is associated with the use of ceftriaxone.

17. a. *Mycobacterium tuberculosis*. Pyrazinamide is a core component of the basic four-drug regimen used to treat tuberculosis: isoniazid, rifampin, pyrazinamide, and ethambutol. It does not have significant activity against *Mycobacterium avium* complex, *Mycobacterium leprae*, or nonmycobacterial organisms.

18. e. ceftriaxone. *Chlamydia trachomatis*, which causes chlamydia, is susceptible to doxycycline, azithromycin, ofloxacin, and levofloxacin but not ceftriaxone. Ceftriaxone is used to treat the sexually transmitted disease gonorrhea, caused by *Neisseria gonorrhoeae*.

19. e. HACEK organisms. The HACEK organisms (*Haemophilus parainfluenzae*, *Aggretibacter aphrophilus*, *Aggretibacter actinomycetemcomitans*, *Cardiobacterium hominis*, *Eikenella corrodens*, and *Kingella kingae*) are gram-negative bacteria and therefore not susceptible to vancomycin.

20. c. tetracycline. Tetracycline binds to the 30S subunit of the bacterial ribosome and prevents binding of tRNA loaded with an amino acid. Isoniazid inhibits the synthesis of mycolic acid. Vancomycin inhibits cell wall synthesis. Levofloxacin inhibits topoisomerases. Trimethoprim-sulfamethoxazole inhibits the synthesis of tetrahydrofolate, a precursor necessary for the production of DNA.

21. b. clindamycin. Clindamycin is active against many gram-positive bacteria and anaerobic bacteria but not spirochetes such as *Borrelia burgdorferi*. This bacterium, which causes Lyme disease, is susceptible to doxycycline, amoxicillin, cefuroxime, and ceftriaxone, as well as erythromycin and penicillin.

22. d. *Pseudomonas aeruginosa.* Doxycycline has excellent activity against *Leptospira interrogans*, *Brucella abortus*, *Chlamydia trachomatis*, and *Rickettsia rickettsii* but not *P. aeruginosa.*

23. c. rifampin. Rifampin targets bacterial RNA polymerase, whereas cefotetan prevents cell wall synthesis, amikacin and azithromycin target the bacterial ribosome, and daptomycin forms an ion-conducting channel in the bacterial cytoplasmic membrane.

24. e. vancomycin. Just checking if you were paying attention. The point is that quinupristin/dalfopristin, linezolid, daptomycin, and tigecycline each are effective against many strains of vancomycin-resistant *Enterococcus faecium*. Note that *Enterococcus faecalis* strains are resistant to quinupristin/dalfopristin.

25. a. ceftazidime + tobramycin. Both ceftazidime and tobramycin have antipseudomonal activity and would allow two agents to be targeted against *Pseudomonas aeruginosa*. In contrast, each of the remaining regimens contains only a single agent with activity against this bacterium. Ceftriaxone, rifampin, ertapenem, and ampicillin have poor or no antipseudomonal activity.

26. b. *Streptococcus pneumoniae.* Some strains of *Streptococcus pneumoniae* are resistant to ceftriaxone, so vancomycin is added to empirically cover for this possibility. *Neisseria meningitidis* and *Haemophilus influenzae* would be adequately covered with ceftriaxone alone. Vancomycin would be appropriate empiric therapy for *Staphylococcus aureus* and *Staphylococcus epidermidis*, but these bacteria rarely cause community-acquired acute bacterial meningitis.

27. d. methicillin-resistant *Staphylococcus aureus* (MRSA). MRSA produce PBP2, a penicillin-binding protein (PBP) that is not recognized by any β-lactam antibiotics. For this reason, MRSA cannot be treated with these agents.

28. a. *Pseudomonas aeruginosa*. The addition of clavulanate, sulbactam, or tazobactam to a penicillin increases activity against anaerobes such as *Bacteroides fragilis*; many gram-negative bacteria such as *Haemophilus influenzae* and *Proteus mirabilis*; and some staphylococci such as *Staphylococcus aureus*. These inhibitors, however, do not appreciably increase activity against *Pseudomonas aeruginosa*.

29. c. cefotaxime. Regimens used to treat *Helicobacter pylori* infections include amoxicillin + clarithromycin + proton pump inhibitor; metronidazole + clarithromycin + proton pump inhibitor; and bismuth subsalicylate + metronidazole + tetracycline + proton pump inhibitor. Cefotaxime has not been used to treat this bacterium.

30. e. azithromycin. The common bacterial causes of atypical pneumonia are *Mycoplasma pneumoniae*, *Chlamydophila pneumoniae*, and *Legionella pneumophila*. Antibiotics that target the cell wall, such as β-lactams (amoxicillin, amoxicillin/clavulanate, and cefotaxime) and vancomycin, are not effective against these bacteria. They are, however, susceptible to the macrolides, such as azithromycin.

31. b. *Borrelia burgdorferi.* Streptomycin is used to treat enterococcal infections, tularemia, tuberculosis, and brucellosis. It is not a component of recommended regimens for Lyme disease (*Borrelia burgdorferi*).

32. c. *Enterococcus faecium*. Some *E. faecium* strains substitute D-alanine–D-lactate for the terminal D-alanine–D-alanine residues of the peptide side chain of peptidoglycan. This prevents binding of vancomycin, resulting in resistance. Although some *Staphylococcus aureus* strains that also have this capability have recently been identified, this mode of resistance to vancomycin is most common among the enterococci.

33. d. dapsone. Isoniazid, rifampin, pyrazinamide, and ethambutol are commonly used to treat tuberculosis. Dapsone is used to treat leprosy.

34. a. nitrofurantoin. Nitrofurantoin or trimethoprim-sulfamethoxazole is the recommended antibiotic for acute uncomplicated urinary tract infections.

35. e. clarithromycin. Clarithromycin is routinely used to treat infections caused by *Helicobacter pylori*, *Mycobacterium avium* complex, and *Bordetella pertussis*. In addition, some strains of *Staphylococcus aureus* and *Streptococcus pneumoniae* remain susceptible to it. Amoxicillin is not active against *Staphylococcus aureus*, *M. avium* complex, or *B. pertussis*. Amoxicillin/clavulanate is not used to treat infections caused by *M. avium* complex or *B. pertussis*. Ceftriaxone is not used to treat infections caused by *H. pylori*, *M. avium* complex, or *B. pertussis*. Doxycycline is not routinely used to treat infections caused by *M. avium* complex or *Staphylococcus aureus*.

36. d. erythromycin. Erythromycin is a macrolide, whereas streptomycin, gentamicin, tobramycin, and amikacin are all aminoglycosides.

37. b. piperacillin/tazobactam + ceftazidime. Recommended therapy for late-onset hospital-acquired pneumonia includes two agents with activity against resistant gram-negative bacteria. The first agent should be an antipseudomonal cephalosporin, antipseudomonal carbapenem, or piperacillin/tazobactam. The second agent should be either an aminoglycoside or an antipseudomonal quinolone. If there is suspicion of methicillin-resistant *Staphylococcus aureus*, linezolid or vancomycin should be added.

38. a. amoxicillin. Amoxicillin is appropriate therapy for mild leptospirosis. Vancomycin, linezolid, streptomycin, and metronidazole are not recommended for these infections.

39. d. cartilage damage. Penicillins have been associated with diarrhea, rash, anaphylaxis, and serum sickness. Cartilage damage, however, has occurred in juvenile animals exposed to quinolones.

40. b. *Clostridium difficile*. Use of clindamycin is associated with the development of diarrhea and pseudomembranous colitis caused by *C. difficile*.

41. c. *Haemophilus* spp. Whereas *Morganella*, *Serratia*, *Enterobacter*, and *Citrobacter* (and *Providencia*) spp. each produce an inducible chromosomally encoded AmpC β-lactamase that may lead to treatment failures with third-generation cephalosporins, *Haemophilus* spp. do not produce this β-lactamase.

42. a. cefotetan. Of the commercially available cephalosporins, only cefotetan and cefoxitin have appreciable activity against anaerobic bacteria.

43. c. ertapenem. Unlike the carbapenems imipenem and meropenem, ertapenem has relatively weak antipseudomonal activity. Ceftazidime and piperacillin have potent antipseudomonal activity.

44. e. piperacillin/tazobactam. First-line agents for infections caused by *Legionella pneumophila* include azithromycin, levofloxacin, and moxifloxacin.

Telithromycin is a second-line agent. Piperacillin/tazobactam does not have activity against this bacterium, presumably because it does not penetrate as well into macrophages, where the *Legionella* bacteria reside.

45. c. clofazimine. The recommended antibiotic regimen for the treatment of leprosy is dapsone + rifampin with or without clofazimine. Isoniazid, ethambutol, and streptomycin are used to treat tuberculosis but do not have activity against *Mycobacterium leprae*. Amoxicillin/clavulanate also does not have activity against this bacterium.

46. d. ampicillin + gentamicin. Ampicillin + gentamicin or penicillin G + gentamicin is the recommended antibiotic regimen for patients with native valve endocarditis caused by highly penicillin-resistant strains of viridans group streptococci. Penicillin G or ceftriaxone would be appropriate for infections caused by penicillin-susceptible strains. Oxacillin would be used for infective endocarditis caused by susceptible strains of *Staphylococcus aureus*. Ampicillin + streptomycin might be used to treat infective endocarditis caused by susceptible strains of enterococci but not viridans group streptococci.

47. b. cefazolin. Cefazolin is not effective in the treatment of patients with *Campylobacter jejuni* diarrhea. Erythromycin, azithromycin, and ciprofloxacin are each first-line agents for these infections. Doxycycline is an alternative.

48. a. ceftazidime. Appropriate empiric therapy for cellulitis should include agents with potent activity against gram-positive cocci, which cause most of these infections. Vancomycin, oxacillin, cefazolin, and clindamycin each are highly active against gram-positive cocci, but ceftazidime has poor activity against these bacteria.

49. e. optic neuritis. Use of ethambutol is associated with the development of optic neuritis, which may lead to decreased visual acuity and loss of red–green discrimination.

50. c. linezolid. Recommended antimicrobial therapy for patients with prosthetic valve endocarditis caused by methicillin-susceptible *Staphylococcus aureus* is an antistaphylococcal penicillin (nafcillin or oxacillin) + rifampin + gentamicin. Recommended therapy for methicillin-resistant *S. aureus* infections is vancomycin + rifampin + gentamicin. Linezolid is a bacteriostatic agent and would not be optimal for the treatment of infective endocarditis.

APPENDIX 1

Dosing of Antibacterial Agents in Adults

AGENT	USUAL ADULT DOSAGE WITH NORMAL RENAL FUNCTION
Natural penicillins	
Penicillin G	2–30 million units/day in divided doses IV/IM q4–6h (Note: IM route should not be used for concentrations >10 million units/mL)
Penicillin V	125–500 mg PO q6–8h
Antistaphylococcal penicillins	
Nafcillin	0.5–2 g IV/IM q4–6h
Oxacillin	Mild-to-moderate infections: 250–500 mg IV/IM q4–6h Severe infections: 1–2 g IV q4–6h
Dicloxacillin	125–500 mg PO q6h
Aminopenicillins	
Ampicillin	Mild-to-moderate infections: 250–1,000 mg PO, IM, or IV q6h Severe infections: 150–200 mg/kg/day IV/IM in divided doses q3–4h (usual dose: 2 g IV q4h)
Amoxicillin	250–500 mg PO q8h or 500–875 mg PO q12h (1 g PO q8h for *Streptococcus pneumoniae* pneumonia)
Aminopenicillins + β-lactamase inhibitors	
Ampicillin-sulbactam	1.5–3 g IV/IM q6h (maximum: 12 g/day)
Amoxicillin-clavulanate	250 mg amoxicillin/125 mg clavulanate, 1 tab PO q8h 500 mg amoxicillin/125 mg clavulanate, 1 tab PO q8–12h or 875 mg amoxicillin/125 mg clavulanate, 1 tab PO q12h
Amoxicillin-clavulanate extended release	1,000 mg amoxicillin/62.5 mg clavulanate, 2 tabs PO q12h (use extended-release formulation for *S. pneumoniae* pneumonia)
Extended-spectrum penicillin	
Piperacillin	3–4 g IV/IM q4–6h (maximum: 24 g/day) (IM route should not be used for doses exceeding 3 g)

(continued)

AGENT	USUAL ADULT DOSAGE WITH NORMAL RENAL FUNCTION
Extended-spectrum penicillins + β-lactamase inhibitors	
Piperacillin-tazobactam	3.375 g q6h or 4.5 g IV q8h (4.5 g IV q6h for *Pseudomonas aeruginosa*)
Ticarcillin-clavulanate	3.1 g IV q4–6h
First-generation cephalosporins	
Cefazolin	0.5–2 g IV/IM q6–8h (maximum: 12 g/day)
Cefadroxil	1–2 g PO in divided doses q12–24h
Cephalexin	0.25–1 g PO q6h (maximum: 4 g/day)
Second-generation cephalosporins	
Cefotetan	1–3 g IV/IM q12h (maximum: 6 g/day)
Cefoxitin	1–2 g IV/IM q4–8h or 1–2 g IV q4h (maximum: 12 g/day)
Cefuroxime	0.75–1.5 g IV/IM q8h Meningitis: 3 g IV q8h
Cefuroxime axetil	250–500 mg PO q12h
Cefprozil	250 mg PO q12h or 500 mg PO q12–24h
Cefaclor	250–500 mg PO q8h
Loracarbef	200–400 mg PO q12h
Third-generation cephalosporins	
Cefotaxime	1 g IV q8–12h to 2 g IV q4h
Ceftazidime	1–2 g IV q8–12h
Ceftriaxone	1–2 g IV q12–24h
Cefdinir	300 mg PO q12h or 600 mg PO q24h
Cefditoren	200–400 mg PO q12h
Cefpodoxime	100–400 mg PO q12h
Ceftibuten	400 mg PO q24h
Cefixime	400 mg/day PO in divided doses q12–24h
Fourth-generation cephalosporin	
Cefepime	1–2 g IV q8–12h
Fifth-generation cephalosporin	
Ceftaroline	600 mg IV q12h

(continued)

AGENT	USUAL ADULT DOSAGE WITH NORMAL RENAL FUNCTION
Carbapenems	
Imipenem/cilastatin	0.5–1 g (imipenem component) IV q6–8h (maximum: 50 mg [imipenem component]/kg or 4 g [imipenem component]/day, whichever is lower) or 500–750 mg IM q12h
Meropenem	0.5–2 g IV q8h
Ertapenem	1 g IV/IM q24h
Doripenem	0.5 g IV q8h
Monobactam	
Aztreonam	1–2 g IV/IM q8–12h up to 2 g q6–8h (maximum: 8 g/day)
Glycopeptides	
Vancomycin	15 mg/kg IV q12h 0.5–2 g/day PO in divided doses q6–8h (PO should not be used for systemic infections; dose should be adjusted based on serum levels when appropriate.)
Telavancin	10 mg/kg IV q24h
Daptomycin	4–6 mg/kg IV q24h
Colistin (colistimethate)	2.5–5 mg/kg/day IM/IV in 2–4 divided doses
Rifamycins	
Rifampin	Tuberculosis therapy: 10 mg/kg PO/IV q24h (maximum: 600 mg/day) Synergy for staphylococcal infections: 300–600 mg PO/IV q8–12h with other antibiotics
Rifabutin	*Mycobacterium avium*–intracellulare complex therapy: initial phase: 5 mg/kg PO q24h (maximum: 300 mg/day); second phase: 5 mg/kg PO daily or twice weekly; may need to adjust dose in patients receiving concomitant protease inhibitor therapy
Rifapentine	Tuberculosis therapy: 600 mg PO given twice weekly (q72h) during first 2 months of treatment, once weekly thereafter
Rifaximin	200 mg PO q8h
Aminoglycosides	(Doses should be adjusted based on peak and trough concentrations.)
Streptomycin	1–2 g/day IM in divided doses q6–12h Tuberculosis therapy: 15 mg/kg IM q24h (maximum: 1 g/day)

(continued)

AGENT	USUAL ADULT DOSAGE WITH NORMAL RENAL FUNCTION
Gentamicin	2 mg/kg IV/IM load, then 5.1 mg/kg/day IV/IM in divided doses q8h; once-per-day dosing: 4–7 mg/kg IV q24h
Tobramycin	2 mg/kg IV load, then 5.1 mg/kg/day IV in divided doses q8h; once-per-day dosing: 4–7 mg/kg IV q24h
Amikacin	15 mg/kg IV in divided doses q8–12h; once-per-day dosing: 15 mg/kg IV q24h
Macrolides and ketolides	
Erythromycin	Base, estolate, stearate preparations: 250–500 mg PO q6–12h (maximum: 4 g/day) Ethylsuccinate preparation: 400–800 mg PO q6h (maximum: 3.2 g/day) Lactobionate preparation: 15–20 mg/kg/day IV in divided doses q6h or 0.5–1 g IV q6h (maximum: 4 g/day)
Azithromycin	500 mg in a single loading dose PO on day 1, followed by 250 mg/day as a single dose on days 2–5 or 500 mg/day PO for a total of 3 days Extended-release suspension: 2 g PO as a single dose 500 mg IV q24h
Clarithromycin	250–500 mg PO q12h Extended-release formulation: 1 g PO q24h
Telithromycin	800 mg PO q24h
Tetracyclines and glycylcyclines	
Tetracycline	250–500 mg PO q6h
Doxycycline	100–200 mg/day PO/IV in divided doses q12–24h
Minocycline	200 mg PO first dose, then 100 mg PO q12h
Tigecycline	100 mg IV first dose, followed by 50 mg IV q12h
Chloramphenicol	50–100 mg/kg/day in divided doses PO/IV q6h (maximum: 4 g/day)
Clindamycin	150–450 mg PO q6–8h (maximum: 1.8 g/day) 0.6–2.7 g IV/IM in divided doses q6–12h
Streptogramin	
Quinupristin/dalfopristin	7.5 mg/kg IV q8–12h
Linezolid	600 mg PO/IV q12h
Nitrofurantoin	Furadantin, Macrodantin: 50–100 mg PO q6h Macrobid: 100 mg q12h

(continued)

AGENT	USUAL ADULT DOSAGE WITH NORMAL RENAL FUNCTION
Trimethoprim-sulfamethoxazole	1 DS tablet PO q12h 8–10 mg (trimethoprim component)/kg/day IV in divided doses q6–12h up to 15–20 mg (trimethoprim component)/kg/day in divided doses q6–8h
Quinolones	
Ofloxacin	200–400 mg PO q12h
Ciprofloxacin	250–750 mg PO q12h Cipro XR 500–1,000 mg PO q24h 200–400 mg IV q8–12h
Levofloxacin	250–750 mg PO/IV q24h
Moxifloxacin	400 mg PO/IV q24h
Gemifloxacin	320 mg PO q24h
Metronidazole	250–750 mg PO/IV q6–8h
Antimycobacterial agents	(Doses are those recommended for once-daily regimens)
Isoniazid	5 mg/kg PO/IM q24h (maximum: 300 mg/day)
Rifampin	Tuberculosis therapy: 10 mg/kg PO/IV q24h (maximum: 600 mg/day)
Pyrazinamide	25–30 mg/kg/day PO q24h (maximum: 2 g/day)
Ethambutol	15–25 mg/kg/day PO q24h

Adapted from Gilbert DN, Moellering RC Jr, Eliopoulos GM, et al. *The Sanford Guide to Antimicrobial Therapy, 2011.* 41st ed. Sperryville, VA: Antimicrobial Therapy, Inc.; 2011; Rose BD. *UptoDate.* Available at: http://www.uptodate.com. Accessed February 2011; Micromedex Healthcare Series (http://www.micromedex.com). Greenwood Village, CO: Thomson Micromedex; 2006; Clinical Pharmacology. Tampa, FL: Gold Standard, Inc., 2006. Available at: http://www.clinicalpharmacology.com. Accessed September 2006; American Society of Health-System Pharmacists. *AHFS Drug Information 2011.* Bethesda, MD: American Society of Health-System Pharmacists; 2011.

APPENDIX 2

Dosing of Antibacterial Agents in Children

AGENT	USUAL PEDIATRIC DOSAGE WITH NORMAL RENAL FUNCTION*
Natural penicillins	
Penicillin G	Infants and children: Mild-to-moderate infections: 25,000–50,000 units/kg/day IV/IM in divided doses q4h Severe infections: 250,000–400,000 units/kg/day IV/IM in divided doses q4–6h (maximum: 24 million units/day)
Penicillin V	Children <12 years: 25–50 mg/kg/day PO in divided doses q6–8h (maximum: 3 g/day) Children ≥12 years: 125–500 mg PO q6–8h
Antistaphylococcal penicillins	
Nafcillin	Infants and children: Mild-to-moderate infections: 50–100 mg/kg/day IV/IM in divided doses q6h Severe infections: 100–200 mg/kg/day IV in divided doses q4–6h (maximum: 12 g/day)
Oxacillin	Mild-to-moderate infections: 100–150 mg/kg/day IV/IM in divided doses q6h (maximum: 4 g/day) Severe infections: 150–200 mg/kg/day IV in divided doses q6h (maximum: 12 g/day)
Dicloxacillin	Children <40 kg: 25–50 mg/kg/day PO in divided doses q6h Children >40 kg: 125–500 mg PO q6h (maximum: 2 g/day)
Aminopenicillins	
Ampicillin	Infants and children: 100–400 mg/kg/day IM/IV in divided doses q6h (maximum: 12 g/day) 50–100 mg/kg/day PO in divided doses q6h (maximum: 2–4 g/day)
Amoxicillin	Infants ≤3 months: 20–30 mg/kg/day PO in divided doses q12h Infants and children >3 months: 20–90 mg/kg/day PO in divided doses q8–12h

(continued)

AGENT	USUAL PEDIATRIC DOSAGE WITH NORMAL RENAL FUNCTION*
Aminopenicillins + β-lactamase inhibitors	
Ampicillin-sulbactam	Infants >1 month: 100–300 mg (ampicillin component)/kg/day IV/IM in divided doses q6h Children ≥1 year: 100–400 mg (ampicillin component)/kg/day IV/IM in divided doses q6h (maximum: 8 g ampicillin/day)
Amoxicillin-clavulanate	Infants <3 months: 30 mg (amoxicillin component)/kg/day PO in divided doses q12h using the 125 mg/5 mL suspension Children <40 kg: 20–40 mg (amoxicillin component)/kg/day PO in divided doses q8h, or 25–45 mg (amoxicillin component)/kg/day in divided doses q12h using either 200 mg/5 mL or 400 mg/5 mL suspension, or 200- or 400-mg (amoxicillin component) chewable tablet formulation (multidrug-resistant *Streptococcus pneumoniae* otitis media: 90 mg [amoxicillin component]/kg/day in divided doses q12h; use 7:1 BID formulation or Augmentin ES-600). Children <40 kg should not receive the 250-mg film-coated tablets
Extended-spectrum penicillin	
Piperacillin	Infants and children: 200–300 mg/kg/day IV/IM in divided doses q4–6h (maximum: 24 g/day)
Extended-spectrum penicillins + β-lactamase inhibitors	
Piperacillin-tazobactam	Safety and efficacy in children <12 years has not been established. Infants and children: 200–300 mg/kg/day in divided doses q6–8h
Ticarcillin-clavulanate	Infants and children ≥3 months: 200–300 mg (ticarcillin component)/kg/day IV in divided doses q4–6h (maximum: 18–24 g/day)
First-generation cephalosporins	
Cefazolin	Infants and children: 25–100 mg/kg/day IV/IM in divided doses q6–8h (maximum: 6 g/day)
Cefadroxil	Infants and children: 30 mg/kg/day PO in divided doses q12h (maximum: 2 g/day)
Cephalexin	Children >1 year: 25–100 mg/kg/day PO in divided doses q6–8h (maximum: 4 g/day)
Second-generation cephalosporins	
Cefotetan	Children: 40–80 mg/kg/day IV/IM in divided doses q12h (maximum: 6 g/day)

(continued)

AGENT	USUAL PEDIATRIC DOSAGE WITH NORMAL RENAL FUNCTION*
Cefoxitin	Infants ≥3 months and children: 80–160 mg/kg/day IV/IM in divided doses q4–6h (maximum: 12 g/day)
Cefuroxime	Infants ≥3 months to children 12 years: 75–150 mg/kg/day IV/IM in divided doses q8h up to 200–240 mg/kg/day in divided doses q6–8h (maximum: 9 g/day) Children ≥13 years: 0.75–1.5 g IV/IM q8h
Cefuroxime axetil	Infants ≥3 months to children 12 years: Suspension: 20–30 mg/kg/day PO in divided doses q12h (maximum: 1 g/day) Tablet: 125–250 mg PO q12h Children ≥13 years: 250–500 mg PO q12h
Cefprozil	Children >6 months to 12 years: 7.5 mg/kg PO q12h or 20 mg/kg PO q24h (maximum: 1 g/day) Children >12 years: 250–500 mg PO q12h or 500 mg PO q24h
Cefaclor	Infants >1 month and children: 20–40 mg/kg/day PO in divided doses q8–12h (maximum: 1 g/day)
Loracarbef	Children >6 months to <12 years: 15–30 mg/kg/day PO in divided doses q12h Children >12 years: 200–400 mg PO q12h
Third-generation cephalosporins	
Cefotaxime	Children 1 month to 12 years: <50 kg: 75–100 mg/kg/day up to 150–300 mg/kg/day in divided doses q6–8h Children >12 years: 1–2 g IV q6–8h
Ceftazidime	Children 1 month to 12 years: 100–150 mg/kg/day IV/IM q8h (maximum: 6 g/day) Children >12 years: 1–2 g IV/IM q8–12h
Ceftriaxone	Infants and children: 50–100 mg/kg/day IV/IM in divided doses q12–24h (maximum: 4 g/day)
Cefdinir	Children 6 months to 12 years: 14 mg/kg/day PO in divided doses q12–24h (maximum: 600 mg/day) Children >12 years: 300 mg PO q12h or 600 mg PO q24h
Cefditoren	Children ≥12 years: 200–400 mg PO q12h
Cefpodoxime	Children 2 months to 12 years: 10 mg/kg/day PO in divided dose q12h (maximum: 200 mg/dose and 400 mg/day) Children >12 years: 100–400 mg PO q12h
Ceftibuten	Children <12 years: 9 mg/kg PO q24h (maximum: 400 mg/day) Children ≥12 years: 400 mg PO q24h

(continued)

AGENT	USUAL PEDIATRIC DOSAGE WITH NORMAL RENAL FUNCTION*
Cefixime	Infants and children: 8 mg/kg/day PO in divided doses q12–24h (maximum: 400 mg/day)
Fourth-generation cephalosporin	
Cefepime	Children 2 months to 16 years, ≤40 kg in weight: 50 mg/kg IV/IM q8–12h
Carbapenems	
Imipenem/cilastatin	Infants 4 weeks to 3 months: 100 mg/kg/day IV in divided doses q6h Infants ≥3 months and children: 60–100 mg/kg/day IV in divided doses q6h (maximum: 4 g/day)
Meropenem	Children >3 months (<50 kg): 10–40 mg/kg/day IV q8h (maximum: 1–2 g q8h) Children >50 kg: 1–2 g IV q8h
Ertapenem	Children 3 months to 12 years: 30 mg/kg/day IV/IM in divided doses q12h (maximum: 1 g/day)
Monobactam	
Aztreonam	Children >1 month: 30 mg/kg/dose IV/IM q6–8h up to 50 mg/kg/dose IV q6–8h (maximum: 120 mg/kg/day or 8 g/day)
Glycopeptide	
Vancomycin	Infants >1 month and children: 40–60 mg/kg/day IV in divided doses q6–8h (maximum: 2 g/day)
Colistin (colistimethate)	2.5–5 mg/kg/day IV/IM in 2–4 divided doses
Rifamycins	
Rifabutin	Children ≥6 years: 300 mg PO q24h
Rifampin	Tuberculosis therapy: Infants and children: 10–20 mg/kg PO/IV q24h (maximum: 600 mg PO q24h)
Rifaximin	Children ≥12 years: 200 mg PO q8h
Aminoglycosides	(Doses should be adjusted based on peak and trough concentrations.)
Streptomycin	20–30 mg/kg/day IM in divided doses q12h Tuberculosis therapy: 20–40 mg/kg IM q24h (maximum: 1 g/day)
Gentamicin	Children <5 years: 7.5 mg/kg/day IV/IM in divided doses q8h Children ≥5 years: 6–7.5 mg/kg/day IV/IM q8h Once-daily dosing: 5 mg/kg IV/IM q24h

(continued)

AGENT	USUAL PEDIATRIC DOSAGE WITH NORMAL RENAL FUNCTION*
Tobramycin	Infants and children: 6–7.5 mg/kg/day IV/IM q6–8h
Amikacin	Infants and children: 15–22.5 mg/kg/day IV/IM in divided doses q8h
Macrolides	
Erythromycin	Infants and children: Base, estolate, and stearate preparations: 30–50 mg/kg/day PO in divided doses q6–8h (maximum: 2 g/day) Ethylsuccinate preparation: 30–50 mg/kg/day PO in divided doses q6–8h (maximum: 3.2 g/day) Lactobionate preparation: 15–50 mg/kg/day IV in divided doses q6h (maximum: 4 g/day)
Azithromycin	Children ≥6 months: Respiratory tract infections: 10 mg/kg PO on day 1 (maximum: 500 mg/day) followed by 5 mg/kg PO q24h on days 2–5 (maximum: 250 mg/day) Otitis media: 30 mg/kg PO as a single dose (maximum: 1,500 mg) 3-day regimen: 10 mg/kg PO q24h for 3 days (maximum: 500 mg/day) 5-day regimen: 10 mg/kg PO on day 1 (maximum: 500 mg), followed by 5 mg/kg PO q24h on days 2–5 (maximum: 250 mg/day)
Clarithromycin	Infants and children: 15 mg/kg/day PO in divided doses q12h
Tetracyclines	
Tetracycline	Children >8 years: 25–50 mg/kg/day PO in divided doses q6–12h (maximum: 3 g/day)
Doxycycline	Children ≥8 years: 2.2–4.4 mg/kg/day PO/IV in divided doses q12–24h (maximum: 200 mg/day)
Minocycline	Children >8 years: 4 mg/kg PO first dose followed by 4 mg/kg/day PO in divided doses q12h
Chloramphenicol	Infants >30 days and children: 50–100 mg/kg/day PO/IV in divided doses q6h (maximum: 4 g/day)
Clindamycin	Infants and children: 8–20 mg/kg/day PO as hydrochloride; 8–25 mg/kg/day PO as palmitate in divided doses q6–8h Children >1 month: 20–40 mg/kg/day IV/IM in divided doses q6–8h

(continued)

AGENT	USUAL PEDIATRIC DOSAGE WITH NORMAL RENAL FUNCTION*
Streptogramin	
Quinupristin/dalfopristin	7.5 mg/kg IV q8–12h
Linezolid	Infants and children: 30 mg/kg/day PO/IV in divided doses q8h
Nitrofurantoin	Children >1 month (Furadantin, Macrodantin): 5–7 mg/kg/day PO in divided doses q6h (maximum: 400 mg/day) Children >12 years (Macrobid): 100 mg PO q12h
Trimethoprim-sulfamethoxazole	Children >2 months: Mild-to-moderate infections: 6–10 mg (trimethoprim component)/kg/day PO/IV in divided doses q12h up to 15–20 mg (trimethoprim component)/kg/day PO/IV in divided doses q6–8h
Quinolones	Quinolones are not approved for use in children <16 years.
Metronidazole	Infants and children: 30–50 mg/kg/day PO/IV in divided doses q6–8h (maximum: 4 g/day)
Antimycobacterial agents	(Doses are those recommended for once-daily regimens.)
Isoniazid	Infants and children: 10–15 mg/kg PO/IM q24h (maximum: 300 mg/day)
Rifampin	Tuberculosis therapy: Infants and children: 10–20 mg/kg/day PO/IV q24h
Pyrazinamide	Infants and children: 15–30 mg/kg/day PO q24h (maximum: 2 g/day)
Ethambutol	Infants and children: 15–25 mg/kg/day PO q24h (maximum: 2.5 g/day) (use cautiously in children <13 years)

*Note: These dosing recommendations do not apply to neonates.

Adapted from Gilbert DN, Moellering RC Jr, Eliopoulos GM, et al. *The Sanford Guide to Antimicrobial Therapy, 2011.* 41st ed. Sperryville, VA: Antimicrobial Therapy, Inc.; 2011; Rose BD. *UptoDate.* Available at: http://www.uptodate.com. Accessed February 2011; Micromedex Healthcare Series (http://www.micromedex.com). Greenwood Village, CO: Thomson Micromedex; 2006; Clinical Pharmacology. Tampa, FL: Gold Standard, Inc., 2006. Available at: http://www.clinicalpharmacology.com. Accessed September 2006; American Society of Health-System Pharmacists. *AHFS Drug Information 2011.* Bethesda, MD: American Society of Health-System Pharmacists; 2011.

APPENDIX 3

Dosing of Antibacterial Agents in Adults with Renal Insufficiency

AGENT	CREATININE CLEARANCE (CrCl) (mL/min)	TYPICAL DOSE*#$
Natural penicillins		
Penicillin G	>50 10–50 <10	2–4 million units IV q4h 2–4 million units IV q6h 1–2 million units IV q6h
Penicillin V	>10 <10	500 mg PO q6h 500 mg PO q8h
Antistaphylococcal penicillins		
Nafcillin	Not renally dosed	2 g IV q4h
Oxacillin	<10	Adjustment to the lower range of the usual dosage
Dicloxacillin	Not renally dosed	500 mg PO q6h
Aminopenicillins		
Ampicillin	>50 10–50 <10	2 g IV q6h 2 g IV q6–12h 2 g IV q12h
Amoxicillin	>30 10–30 <10	500 mg PO q8h 500 mg PO q12h 500 mg PO q24h
Aminopenicillins + β-lactamase inhibitors		
Ampicillin-sulbactam	>30 15–30 <15	2 g (ampicillin component) IV q6h 2 g IV q12h 2 g IV q24h
Amoxicillin-clavulanate	>30 10–30 <10	500 mg (amoxicillin component) PO q8h 500 mg (amoxicillin component) PO q12h (875 mg tablet should not be used with CrCl <30) 500 mg (amoxicillin component) PO q24h

(continued)

AGENT	CREATININE CLEARANCE (CrCl) (mL/min)	TYPICAL DOSE*#$
Amoxicillin-clavulanate extended release	>30	2 g PO q12h
	<30	Do not use
Extended-spectrum penicillin		
Piperacillin	>40	4 g IV q8h
	20–40	3–4 g IV q8h
	<20	3–4 g IV q12h
Extended-spectrum penicillins + β-lactamase inhibitors		
Piperacillin-tazobactam	>40	3.375 g (piperacillin component) IV q6h or 4.5 g IV q6h
	20–40	2.25 g IV q6h or 3.375 g IV q6h
	<20	2.25 g IV q8h or 2.25 g IV q6h
Ticarcillin-clavulanate	>60	3.1 g IV q4h
	30–60	2 g IV q4h
	10–30	2 g IV q8h
	<10	2 g IV q12h
First-generation cephalosporins		
Cefazolin	>55	1 g IV q6–8h
	35–54	1 g IV q8h
	11–34	1 g IV q12h
	<10	1 g IV q24h
Cefadroxil	>25	500 mg PO q12h
	10–25	500 mg PO q24h
	<10	500 mg PO q36h
Cephalexin	>40	500 mg PO q6h
	10–40	250 mg PO q8h
	<10	250 mg PO q12h
Second-generation cephalosporins		
Cefotetan	>30	1–2 g IV q12h
	10–30	1–2 g IV q24h or 1 g IV q12h
	<10	1–2 g IV q48h or 500 mg IV q12h
Cefoxitin	>50	1–2 g IV q6h
	30–50	1–2 g IV q8–12h
	10–30	1–2 g IV q12–24h
	5–10	0.5–1 g IV q12–24h
	<5	0.5–1 g IV q24–48h
Cefuroxime	>20	750 mg IV q8h
	10–20	750 mg IV q12h
	<10	750 mg IV q24h

(continued)

AGENT	CREATININE CLEARANCE (CrCl) (mL/min)	TYPICAL DOSE*#$
Cefuroxime axetil	Not renally dosed	250 mg PO q12h
Cefprozil	>30	500 mg PO q12h
	<30	250 mg PO q12h
Cefaclor	>10	500 mg PO q8h
	<10	250 mg PO q8h
Loracarbef	>50	400 mg PO q12h
	10–50	200 mg PO q12h or 400 mg PO q24h
	<10	200–400 mg PO q3–5d
Third-generation cephalosporins		
Cefotaxime	>20	1–2 g IV q8h
	<20	1 g IV q8h
Ceftazidime	>50	1–2 g IV q8h
	30–50	1–2 g IV q12h
	15–30	1–2 g IV q24h
	6–15	1 g IV q24h
	<6	1 g IV q24–48h
Ceftriaxone	Not renally dosed	1 g IV q24h
Cefdinir	>30	600 mg PO q24h
	<30	300 mg PO q24h
Cefditoren	>50	400 mg PO q12h
	30–50	200 mg PO q12h
	<30	200 mg PO q24h
Cefpodoxime	>30	200 mg PO q12h
	<30	200 mg PO q24h
Ceftibuten	>50	400 mg PO q24h
	30–50	200 mg PO q24h
	<30	100 mg PO q24h
Cefixime	>60	400 mg PO q24h
	20–60	300 mg PO q24h
	<20	200 mg PO q24h
Fourth-generation cephalosporin		
Cefepime	>60	1–2 g IV q12h
	30–60	1–2 g IV q24h
	10–30	1 g IV q24h
	<10	500 mg IV q24h
Fifth-generation cephalosporin		
Ceftaroline	>50	600 mg IV q12h
	30–50	400 mg IV q12h

(continued)

AGENT	CREATININE CLEARANCE (CrCl) (mL/min)	TYPICAL DOSE[*#$]
Carbapenems		
Imipenem/cilastatin	>70	(All doses are imipenem component and based on weight ≥70 kg.) 500 mg IV q6h
	40–70	500 mg IV q8h
	20–40	250 mg IV q6h
	6–20	250 mg IV q12h
	<6	Do not use
Meropenem	>50	1 g IV q8h
	25–50	1 g IV q12h
	10–25	500 mg IV q12h
	<10	500 mg IV q24h
Ertapenem	>30	1 g IV q24h
	<30	500 mg IV q24h
Doripenem	>50	500 mg IV q8h
	30–50	250 mg IV q8h
	10–30	250 mg IV q12h
Monobactam		
Aztreonam	>30	2 g IV q8h
	10–30	1 g IV q8h
	<10	500 mg IV q8h
Glycopeptides		
Vancomycin	>70	1 g (15 mg/kg) IV q12h
	50–70	1 g (15 mg/kg) IV q24h
	<50	1 g (15 mg/kg) IV with interval determined by serum levels
Telavancin	>50	10 mg/kg IV q24h
	30–50	7.5 mg/kg IV q24h
	10–30	10 mg/kg IV q48h
Daptomycin	>30	4–6 mg/kg IV q24h
	<30	4–6 mg/kg IV q48h
Rifamycins		
Rifampin	Not renally dosed	600 mg PO q24h
Rifabutin	Not renally dosed	300 mg PO q24h
Rifapentine	Not renally dosed	600 mg PO q72h
Rifaximin	Not renally dosed	200 mg PO q8h
Aminoglycosides	(Doses should be adjusted based on peak and trough concentrations.)	

(continued)

AGENT	CREATININE CLEARANCE (CrCl) (mL/min)	TYPICAL DOSE[*#$]
Streptomycin	>80	15 mg/kg IM q24h
	50–80	7.5 mg/kg IM q24h
	10–50	7.5 mg/kg IM q24–72h
	<10	7.5 mg/kg IM q72–96h
Gentamicin	>60	Conventional dosing: 1.7 mg/kg IV q8h; once-daily dosing: 4–7 mg/kg IV q24h
	40–60	Conventional dosing: 1.7 mg/kg IV q12h; once-daily dosing: 4–7 mg/kg IV q36h
	20–40	Conventional dosing: 1.7 mg/kg IV q24h; once-daily dosing: 4–7 mg/kg IV q48h
	<20	Based on serum levels
Tobramycin	>60	Conventional dosing: 1.7 mg/kg IV q8h; once-daily dosing: 4–7 mg/kg IV q24h
	40–60	Conventional dosing: 1.7 mg/kg IV q12h; once-daily dosing: 4–7 mg/kg IV q36h
	20–40	Conventional dosing: 1.7 mg/kg IV q24h; once-daily dosing: 4–7 mg/kg IV q48h
	<20	Based on serum levels
Amikacin	>60	Conventional dosing: 15 mg/kg/day IV in divided doses q8–12h; once-daily dosing: 15 mg/kg IV q24h
	40–60	Conventional dosing: 7.5 mg/kg IV q12h; once-daily dosing: 15 mg/kg IV q36h
	20–40	Conventional dosing: 7.5 mg/kg IV q24h; once-daily dosing: 15 mg/kg IV q48h
	<20	Based on serum levels
Macrolides and ketolides		
Erythromycin	Not renally dosed	1 g IV q6h 500 mg PO q6h
Azithromycin	Not renally dosed	500 mg IV q24h 500 mg PO × 1, then 250 mg PO q24h
Clarithromycin	>30	500 mg PO q12h
	<30	250 mg PO q12h or 500 mg PO q24h
Telithromycin	>30	800 mg PO q24h
	<30	600 mg PO q24h

(continued)

AGENT	CREATININE CLEARANCE (CrCl) (mL/min)	TYPICAL DOSE*#$
Tetracyclines and glycylcyclines		
Tetracycline	>80 50–80 10–50 <10	500 mg PO q6h 500 mg PO q8–12h 500 mg PO q12–24h Do not use
Doxycycline	Not renally dosed	100 mg IV/PO q12h
Minocycline	Not renally dosed	100 mg PO q12h
Tigecycline	Not renally dosed	100 mg IV first dose, followed by 50 mg IV q12h
Chloramphenicol	Not renally dosed	500 mg IV/PO q6h
Clindamycin	Not renally dosed	600–900 mg IV q8h 150–450 mg PO q6h
Streptogramin		
Quinupristin/dalfopristin	Not renally dosed	7.5 mg/kg IV q8h
Linezolid	Not renally dosed	600 mg IV/PO q12h
Nitrofurantoin	>60 <60	Furadantin, Macrodantin: 50–100 mg PO q6h Macrobid: 100 mg q12h contraindicated
Trimethoprim-sulfamethoxazole	>30 15–30 <15	2.5 mg/kg IV q6h 1 DS tablet PO q12h 1.25 mg/kg IV q6h 1 SS tablet PO q12h Not recommended
Quinolones		
Ofloxacin	>50 20–50 <20	400 mg PO q12h 400 mg PO q24h 200 mg PO q24h
Ciprofloxacin	>50 30–50 5–30 <5	400 mg IV q12h 500 mg PO q12h 400 mg IV q12h 250–500 mg PO q12h 200–400 mg IV q18–24h 250–500 mg PO q18h 200 mg IV q24h 250 mg PO q24h

(continued)

AGENT	CREATININE CLEARANCE (CrCl) (mL/min)	TYPICAL DOSE*#$
Levofloxacin	>50 20–50 10–20	500–750 mg IV/PO q24h 250 mg IV/PO q24h or 750 mg IV/PO q48h 250 mg IV/PO q48h or 500 mg IV/PO q48h
Moxifloxacin	Not renally dosed	400 mg IV/PO q24h
Gemifloxacin	>40 <40	320 mg PO q24h 160 mg PO q24h
Metronidazole	>10 <10	500 mg IV/PO q6h 250 mg IV/PO q6h
Antimycobacterial agents		
Isoniazid	Not renally dosed	300 mg PO q24h
Rifampin	Not renally dosed	600 mg PO q24h
Pyrazinamide	>30 <30	25–35 mg/kg PO q24h 25–35 mg/kg PO three times per week
Ethambutol	>50 10–50 <10	15–25 mg/kg PO q24h 15–25 mg/kg PO q24–36h 15–25 mg/kg PO q48h

*Actual dose may vary depending on indication, severity of infection, and patient characteristics.

#These recommendations do not apply to individuals receiving dialysis.

$Loading doses may be required for some agents.

Adapted from Blumberg HM, Burman WJ, Chaisson RE, et al. American Thoracic Society/Centers for Disease Control and Prevention/Infectious Diseases Society of America: treatment of tuberculosis. *Am J Respir Crit Care Med.* 2003;167:603–662; Cunha BA. *Antibiotic Essentials.* Royal Oak, MI: Physicians' Press; 2004; Gilbert DN, Moellering RC Jr, Eliopoulos GM, et al. *The Sanford Guide to Antimicrobial Therapy, 2011.* 41st ed. Sperryville, VA: Antimicrobial Therapy, Inc.; 2011; Rose BD. *UptoDate.* Available at: http://www.uptodate.com. Accessed February 2011; Micromedex Healthcare Series (http://www.micromedex.com). Greenwood Village, CO: Thomson Micromedex; 2006; Clinical Pharmacology. Tampa, FL: Gold Standard, Inc., 2006. Available at: http://www.clinicalpharmacology.com. Accessed September 2006; American Society of Health-System Pharmacists. *AHFS Drug Information 2011.* Bethesda, MD: American Society of Health-System Pharmacists; 2011.

APPENDIX 4

Antibacterial Agents in Pregnancy

Antibiotics vary in their safety in pregnancy as well as in how well their use in pregnancy has been studied. As a result, the U.S. Food and Drug Administration places these agents into five categories with regard to use in pregnant women:

Category A: Adequate, well-controlled studies in pregnant women have not shown an increased risk of fetal abnormalities.

Category B: Either

(1) animal studies have revealed no evidence of harm to the fetus; however, there are no adequate studies in pregnant women; or

(2) animal studies have shown an adverse effect, but adequate studies in pregnant women have failed to demonstrate a risk to the fetus.

Category C: Either

(1) animal studies have shown an adverse effect and there are no adequate studies in pregnant women; or

(2) no animal studies have been conducted and there are no adequate studies in pregnant women.

Category D: Studies in pregnant women have demonstrated a risk to the fetus, but the benefits of therapy may outweigh the potential risk.

Category X: Studies in animals or pregnant women have demonstrated positive evidence of fetal abnormalities or risks. As a result, the use of the product is contraindicated in women who are or may become pregnant.

AGENT	PREGNANCY RISK CATEGORY
Natural penicillins	
Penicillin G	B
Penicillin V	B
Antistaphylococcal penicillins	
Nafcillin	B
Oxacillin	B
Dicloxacillin	B
Aminopenicillins	
Ampicillin	B
Amoxicillin	B

(continued)

AGENT	PREGNANCY RISK CATEGORY
Aminopenicillins + β-lactamase inhibitors	
Ampicillin-sulbactam	B
Amoxicillin-clavulanate	B
Extended-spectrum penicillin	
Piperacillin	B
Extended-spectrum penicillins + β-lactamase inhibitors	
Piperacillin-tazobactam	B
Ticarcillin-clavulanate	B
First-generation cephalosporins	
Cefazolin	B
Cefadroxil	B
Cephalexin	B
Second-generation cephalosporins	
Cefotetan	B
Cefoxitin	B
Cefuroxime	B
Cefuroxime axetil	B
Cefprozil	B
Cefaclor	B
Loracarbef	B
Third-generation cephalosporins	
Cefotaxime	B
Ceftazidime	B
Ceftriaxone	B
Cefdinir	B
Cefditoren	B
Cefpodoxime	B
Ceftibuten	B
Cefixime	B
Fourth-generation cephalosporin	
Cefepime	B

(continued)

AGENT	PREGNANCY RISK CATEGORY
Carbapenems	
Imipenem/cilastatin	C
Meropenem	B
Ertapenem	B
Doripenem	B
Monobactam	
Aztreonam	B
Glycopeptides	
Vancomycin	C
Telavancin	C
Daptomycin	B
Colistin	C
Rifamycins	
Rifampin	C
Rifaximin	C
Rifabutin	B
Aminoglycosides	
Streptomycin	D
Gentamicin	D
Tobramycin	D
Amikacin	D
Macrolides and ketolides	
Erythromycin	B
Azithromycin	B
Clarithromycin	C
Telithromycin	C
Tetracyclines and glycylcyclines	
Tetracycline	D
Doxycycline	D
Minocycline	D
Tigecycline	D

(continued)

AGENT	PREGNANCY RISK CATEGORY
Chloramphenicol	C
Clindamycin	B
Linezolid	C
Nitrofurantoin	B
Trimethoprim-sulfamethoxazole	C
Quinolones	
Ofloxacin	C
Ciprofloxacin	C
Levofloxacin	C
Moxifloxacin	C
Gemifloxacin	C
Metronidazole	B
Antimycobacterial agents	
Isoniazid	C
Rifampin	C
Pyrazinamide	C
Ethambutol	B

Adapted from Gilbert DN, Moellering RC Jr, Eliopoulos GM, et al. *The Sanford Guide to Antimicrobial Therapy, 2011.* 41st ed. Sperryville, VA: Antimicrobial Therapy, Inc.; 2011; Briggs GG, Freeman RK, Yaffe SJ. *Drugs in Lactation and Pregnancy.* 7th ed. Philadelphia, PA: Lippincott Williams & Wilkins; 2005.

5

Generic and Trade Names of Commonly Used Antibacterial Agents

Trade Name	Generic Name
Amikin	amikacin
Amoxil	amoxicillin
Ancef	cefazolin
Augmentin	amoxicillin-clavulanate
Avelox	moxifloxacin
Azactam	aztreonam
Bactrim	trimethoprim-sulfamethoxazole
Biaxin, Biaxin XL	clarithromycin
Ceclor	cefaclor
Cedax	ceftibuten
Cefotan	cefotetan
Ceftin	cefuroxime axetil
Cefzil	cefprozil
Cipro, Cipro XR	ciprofloxacin
Claforan	cefotaxime
Cleocin	clindamycin
Coly-Mycin M	colistin
Cubicin	daptomycin
Doribax	doripenem
Duricef	cefadroxil
Dynapen	dicloxacillin
E.E.S.	erythromycin ethylsuccinate
Eryc	erythromycin
Ery-Ped	erythromycin ethylsuccinate
Ery-Tab	erythromycin
Erythrocin	erythromycin lactobionate
Factive	gemifloxacin
Flagyl	metronidazole
Floxin	ofloxacin
Fortaz	ceftazidime
Furadantin	nitrofurantoin
Garamycin	gentamicin
Geocillin	carbenicillin
Ilosone	erythromycin estolate
Ilotycin	erythromycin
Invanz	ertapenem
Keflex	cephalexin
Kefurox	cefuroxime
Ketek	telithromycin
Lamprene	clofazimine
Levaquin	levofloxacin
Lorabid	loracarbef
Macrobid	nitrofurantoin
Macrodantin	nitrofurantoin
Maxipime	cefepime
Mefoxin	cefoxitin
Merrem	meropenem

(continued)

Trade Name	Generic Name
Minocin	minocycline
Myambutol	ethambutol
Mycobutin	rifabutin
My-E	erythromycin stearate
Nafcil	nafcillin
Nebcin	tobramycin
Omnicef	cefdinir
Omnipen	ampicillin
Pediamycin	erythromycin ethylsuccinate
Pfizerpen	penicillin G
Pipracil	piperacillin
Polycillin	ampicillin
Polymox	amoxicillin
Priftin	rifapentine
Primaxin	imipenem-cilastatin
Principen	ampicillin
Prostaphlin	oxacillin
Rifadin	rifampin
Rimactane	rifampin
Rocephin	ceftriaxone
Septra	trimethoprim-sulfamethoxazole
Spectracef	cefditoren pivoxil
Suprax	cefixime
Synercid	quinupristin/dalfopristin
Tazicef	ceftazidime
Teflaro	ceftaroline
Ticar	ticarcillin
Timentin	ticarcillin-clavulanate
Tygacil	tigecycline
Unasyn	ampicillin-sulbactam
Unipen	nafcillin
Vancocin	vancomycin
Vantin	cefpodoxime proxetil
Veetids	penicillin V
Vibativ	telavancin
Vibramycin	doxycycline
Xifaxan	rifaximin
Zinacef	cefuroxime
Zithromax	azithromycin
Zmax	azithromycin ER
Zosyn	piperacillin-tazobactam
Zyvox	linezolid

Generic Name	Trade Name
amikacin	Amikin
amoxicillin	Amoxil, Polymox
amoxicillin-clavulanate	Augmentin
ampicillin	Omnipen, Polycillin, Principen
ampicillin-sulbactam	Unasyn
azithromycin	Zithromax
azithromycin ER	Zmax
aztreonam	Azactam
carbenicillin	Geocillin
cefaclor	Ceclor
cefadroxil	Duricef
cefazolin	Ancef
cefdinir	Omnicef
cefditoren pivoxil	Spectracef
cefepime	Maxipime
cefixime	Suprax
cefotaxime	Claforan
cefotetan	Cefotan
cefoxitin	Mefoxin
cefpodoxime proxetil	Vantin
cefprozil	Cefzil
ceftaroline	Teflaro
ceftazidime	Fortaz, Tazicef
ceftibuten	Cedax
ceftriaxone	Rocephin
cefuroxime	Kefurox, Zinacef
cefuroxime axetil	Ceftin
cephalexin	Keflex
ciprofloxacin	Cipro, Cipro XR
clarithromycin	Biaxin, Biaxin XL
clindamycin	Cleocin
clofazimine	Lamprene
colistin	Coly-Mycin M
daptomycin	Cubicin
dicloxacillin	Dynapen
doripenem	Doribax
doxycycline	Vibramycin
ertapenem	Invanz
erythromycin	Ery-Tab, Eryc
erythromycin estolate	Ilosone
erythromycin ethylsuccinate	E.E.S., Ery-Ped, Pediamycin
erythromycin lactobionate	Erythrocin
erythromycin stearate	My-E
ethambutol	Myambutol
gemifloxacin	Factive
gentamicin	Garamycin
imipenem-cilastatin	Primaxin
levofloxacin	Levaquin
linezolid	Zyvox
loracarbef	Lorabid
meropenem	Merrem
metronidazole	Flagyl
minocycline	Minocin
moxifloxacin	Avelox
nafcillin	Nafcil, Unipen
nitrofurantoin	Furadantin, Macrobid, Macrodantin
ofloxacin	Floxin
oxacillin	Prostaphlin

(continued)

Generic Name	Trade Name
penicillin G	Pfizerpen
penicillin V	Veetids
piperacillin	Pipracil
piperacillin-tazobactam	Zosyn
quinupristin/dalfopristin	Synercid
rifabutin	Mycobutin
rifampin	Rifadin, Rimactane
rifapentine	Priftin
rifaximin	Xifaxan
telavancin	Vibativ
telithromycin	Ketek
ticarcillin	Ticar
ticarcillin-clavulanate	Timentin
tigecycline	Tygacil
tobramycin	Nebcin
trimethoprim-sulfamethoxazole	Bactrim, Septra
vancomycin	Vancocin

Adapted from Gilbert DN, Moellering RC Jr, Eliopoulos GM, et al. *The Sanford Guide to Antimicrobial Therapy, 2011.* 41st ed. Sperryville, VA: Antimicrobial Therapy, Inc.; 2011; Rose BD. *UptoDate.* Available at: http://www.uptodate.com. Accessed February 2011.

APPENDIX 6

Treatment of Infections Caused by Bacterial Agents of Bioterrorism

Certain microbes or microbial toxins have properties that make them especially conducive for use as agents of bioterrorism. These microbes have been divided into three categories: A, B, and C. Agents in category A are deemed to pose the highest risk to the public because they are easily spread and have the potential to cause high mortality rates. Six microbes are currently designated as category A agents: (1) *Bacillus anthracis* (anthrax), (2) *Clostridium botulinum* (botulism), (3) *Yersinia pestis* (plague), (4) *Francisella tularensis* (tularemia), (5) smallpox virus, and (6) viruses that cause hemorrhagic fever such as Ebola and Marburg viruses. Of these six, the first four are bacteria; recommended treatments of bioterrorism-related infections for these are listed in the following table.

TREATMENT OF INFECTIONS CAUSED BY BACTERIAL AGENTS OF BIOTERRORISM
Bacillus anthracis **(inhalational anthrax)**
• Ciprofloxacin or doxycycline
plus one of the following:
rifampin, vancomycin, penicillin, ampicillin, chloramphenicol, imipenem, clindamycin, clarithromycin
Clostridium botulinum **(botulinum toxin)**
• Supportive care
• Trivalent antitoxin
• Antibiotics are not routinely indicated
Francisella tularensis
• Streptomycin or gentamicin
Alternatives: doxycycline, ciprofloxacin, chloramphenicol
Yersinia pestis **(pneumonic plague)**
• Streptomycin or gentamicin
Alternatives: doxycycline, ciprofloxacin, chloramphenicol

ADDITIONAL READINGS

Arnon SS, Schechter R, Inglesby TV, et al. Botulinum toxin as a biological weapon: medical and public health management. *JAMA*. 2001;285:1059–1070.

Dennis DT, Inglesby TV, Henderson DA, et al. Tularemia as a biological weapon: medical and public health management. *JAMA*. 2001;285:2763–2773.

Inglesby TV, Dennis DT, Henderson DA, et al. Plague as a biological weapon: medical and public health management. Working Group on Civilian Biodefense. *JAMA*. 2000;283:2281–2290.

Inglesby TV, O'Toole T, Henderson DA, et al. Anthrax as a biological weapon, 2002: updated recommendations for management. *JAMA*. 2002;287:2236–2252.

APPENDIX 7

Medical References

The information presented in this book was compiled from the following references in addition to those listed at the end of each chapter. The reader is referred to these sources for excellent overviews of clinical and microbiologic aspects of antibiotic therapy for infections caused by bacteria.

American Society of Health-System Pharmacists. *AHFS Drug Information 2011*. Bethesda, MD: American Society of Health-System Pharmacists; 2011.

Brunton LL, Chabner BA, Knollman BC, eds. *Goodman & Gilman's The Pharmacological Basis of Therapeutics*. 12th ed. New York, NY: McGraw-Hill; 2010.

Gilbert DN, Moellering RC Jr, Eliopoulos GM, et al. *The Sanford Guide to Antimicrobial Therapy, 2011*. 41st ed. Sperryville, VA: Antimicrobial Therapy, Inc.; 2011.

Mandell GL, Bennett JE, Dolin R. *Mandell, Douglas, and Bennett's Principles and Practice of Infectious Diseases*. 7th ed. Philadelphia, PA: Elsevier; 2009.

Mascaretti OA. *Bacteria versus Antibacterial Agents: An Integrated Approach*. Washington, DC: ASM Press; 2003.

Rose BD. *UptoDate*. Available at: http://www.uptodate.com. Accessed February 2011.

Walsh C. *Antibiotics: Actions, Origins, Resistance*. Washington, DC: ASM Press; 2003.

APPENDIX 8

Literary References

The quotations at the start of many of the chapters were taken from the following sources:

Anonymous. *The Anglo-Saxon Chronicle*. Swanton M, trans-ed. New York, NY: Routledge; 1998.
Anonymous. *Gesta Stephani*. Potter KR, trans-ed. Oxford, England: Clarendon Press; 1976.
Ceasar J. *The Battle for Gaul*. Boston, MA: David R. Godine, Publisher, Inc.; 1985.
Froissart J. *Chronicles*. London, England: Penguin Books; 1978.
Josephus. *The Jewish War*. Harmondsworth, England: Penguin Books; 1986.
Musashi M. *The Book of Five Rings*. New York, NY: Bantam Books; 1992.
Payne-Gallwey SR. *Crossbow*. New York, NY: Marlboro Books, Dorset Press; 1989.
Prestwich M. *Armies and Warfare in the Middle Ages. The English Experience*. New Haven, CT: Yale University Press; 1996.
Seward D. *The Hundred Years War. The English in France, 1337–1453*. New York, NY: Atheneum; 1978.
Tuchman BW. *A Distant Mirror*. New York, NY: Ballantine Books; 1979.
Tzu S. *The Art of War*. Oxford, England: Oxford University Press; 1971.
von Clausewitz C. *On War*. London, England: Penguin Books; 1982.
Warner P. *Sieges of the Middle Ages*. Barnsley, England: Pen & Sword Military Classics; 2004.

APPENDIX 9

Answers to Chapter Questions

Chapter 1

1. peptidoglycan
2. penicillin-binding proteins or PBPs
3. bacilli

Chapter 2

1. anaerobic
2. RNA polymerase
3. 50S, 30S, rRNA, proteins

Chapter 3

1. deoxynucleotides
2. circular
3. topoisomerases

Chapter 4

1. bactericidal
2. Kirby-Bauer
3. broth dilution

Chapter 5

1. peptidoglycan
2. penicillins, cephalosporins, carbapenems, monobactams
3. PBPs or penicillin-binding proteins
4. β-lactamases
5. β-lactam ring, side chain
6. penicillin-binding proteins or PBPs, peptidoglycan
7. gram-negative
8. staphylococci
9. gram-negative bacteria
10. staphylococci, gram-negative bacteria
11. gram-negative bacteria, *Pseudomonas aeruginosa*
12. gram-positive bacteria, gram-negative bacteria, anaerobic bacteria
13. generations, β-lactams
14. penicillin-binding proteins or PBPs
15. gram-positive
16. gram-negative, anaerobic
17. gram-negative
18. *Pseudomonas aeruginosa*, Enterobacteriaceae
19. methicillin-resistant
20. ceftriaxone
21. penicillins
22. cilastatin
23. gram-positive, gram-negative, anaerobic
24. *Pseudomonas aeruginosa*, *Acinetobacter* spp.
25. aztreonam
26. gram-negative, gram-positive, anaerobic
27. β-lactam
28. gram-positive
29. enterococci
30. peptidoglycan
31. lipoglycopeptide
32. cyclic lipopeptide
33. gram-positive
34. lipopolysaccharide
35. gram-negative

Chapter 6

1. RNA polymerase, mRNA
2. mycobacteria, staphylococci
3. resistance
4. gram-negative
5. gram-positive
6. nephrotoxicity, ototoxicity
7. azithromycin, *Haemophilus influenzae*
8. azithromycin, clarithromycin
9. anaerobic
10. ketolide
11. respiratory
12. ribosomes
13. atypical
14. pregnant women, children
15. glycylcyclines
16. gram-positive, gram-negative

17. ribosomes
18. anaerobic, atypical
19. acetylation, efflux pumps
20. toxicity, bone marrow, aplastic anemia
21. gram-positive, anaerobic
22. macrolides or erythromycin
23. pseudomembranous colitis
24. two
25. gram-positive
26. methicillin, penicillin, vancomycin
27. methicillin, vancomycin
28. ribosomes
29. intravenously, orally
30. gram-negative, gram-positive
31. blood
32. resistance

Chapter 7

1. tetrahydrofolate or THF
2. gram-positive, gram-negative
3. HIV
4. leprosy
5. gram-negative, gram-positive
6. ciprofloxacin
7. moxifloxacin
8. DNA gyrase, topoisomerase IV
9. cartilage
10. anaerobic
11. microaerophilic
12. reduce

Chapter 8

1. multiple
2. isoniazid, rifampin, pyrazinamide, ethambutol
3. hepatotoxicity

Chapter 10

1. oxacillin, nafcillin
2. methicillin-resistant *Staphylococcus aureus* or MRSA
3. β-lactams
4. vancomycin
5. penicillin, ampicillin
6. penicillin-binding proteins or PBPs
7. cephalosporins, quinolones, vancomycin, telithromycin
8. clindamycin, macrolides, tetracyclines, trimethoprim-sulfamethoxazole
9. penicillin
10. clindamycin
11. penicillin
12. aminoglycosides
13. penicillin G, ampicillin, piperacillin
14. vancomycin
15. bacteriostatic, bactericidal
16. linezolid, daptomycin, quinupristin/dalfopristin, tigecycline
17. ampicillin, gentamicin
18. cephalosporins
19. trimethoprim-sulfamethoxazole
20. ciprofloxacin, doxycycline
21. two

Chapter 11

1. community, health care
2. trimethoprim-sulfamethoxazole, quinolone
3. *Escherichia coli*, *Klebsiella* spp.
4. carbapenems, β-lactam/β-lactamase inhibitor combinations
5. carbapenems
6. aminoglycoside
7. gastroenteritis, quinolones, third-generation cephalosporins, azithromycin
8. ceftazidime, cefepime
9. piperacillin
10. two
11. antipseudomonal β-lactams + aminoglycosides, extended-spectrum penicillins + quinolones
12. penicillin
13. ceftriaxone, cefixime
14. *Chlamydia trachomatis*
15. not
16. macrolides, quinolones
17. multiple
18. antibiotic, acid-blocking
19. tetracycline, doxycycline
20. ciprofloxacin, erythromycin, azithromycin, trimethoprim-sulfamethoxazole
21. β-lactamase
22. aminopenicillin + β-lactamase inhibitor combinations, second-generation cephalosporins, third-generation cephalosporins, tetracyclines
23. azithromycin, clarithromycin, erythromycin

24. trimethoprim-sulfamethoxazole, quinolones, tetracyclines, telithromycin
25. β-lactamase
26. sulbactam

Chapter 12
1. anaerobic, spore, positive
2. penicillin, metronidazole
3. metronidazole, vancomycin
4. *Bacteroides*, *Prevotella*, *Porphyromonas*
5. β-lactam/β-lactamase inhibitor combinations, carbapenems, metronidazole, chloramphenicol
6. clindamycin, piperacillin, moxifloxacin, tigecycline, cephalosporins

Chapter 13
1. macrolides, tetracyclines, quinolones
2. β-lactams, amoxicillin
3. macrolides, tetracyclines, quinolones
4. β-lactams
5. azithromycin, levofloxacin, moxifloxacin
6. macrophages
7. doxycycline, gentamicin, streptomycin, rifampin
8. rifampin, gentamicin, streptomycin
9. rifampin, trimethoprim-sulfamethoxazole
10. streptomycin
11. gentamicin
12. tetracycline, doxycycline, chloramphenicol
13. doxycycline
14. tetracycline, chloramphenicol, ciprofloxacin

Chapter 14
1. penicillin
2. stage
3. benzathine penicillin
4. doxycycline
5. amoxicillin, cefuroxime, erythromycin
6. ceftriaxone, penicillin G
7. doxycycline
8. doxycycline, amoxicillin
9. penicillin, ampicillin, ceftriaxone

Chapter 15
1. four
2. isoniazid, rifampin, pyrazinamide, ethambutol
3. streptomycin, amikacin, cycloserine, ethionamide, capreomycin, *p*-aminosalicylic acid, quinolone
4. isoniazid
5. two, three
6. clarithromycin, ethambutol
7. azithromycin
8. multiple, prolonged
9. dapsone, rifampin
10. clofazimine

Chapter 16
1. *Mycoplasma pneumoniae*, *Chlamydophila pneumoniae*, *Legionella pneumophila*
2. macrolides, β-lactams, quinolones
3. β-lactam, azithromycin, quinolone
4. early-onset, late-onset
5. ceftriaxone, quinolone, ampicillin/sulbactam, ertapenem
6. cephalosporin, carbapenem, piperacillin/tazobactam, quinolone, aminoglycoside, linezolid, vancomycin

Chapter 17
1. *Escherichia coli*
2. nitrofurantoin, trimethoprim-sulfamethoxazole
3. enterococci
4. complicated
5. cefepime, quinolone, extended-spectrum penicillin/β-lactamase inhibitor combinations, carbapenem

Chapter 18
1. *Neisseria gonorrhoeae*, *Chlamydia trachomatis*, anaerobic
2. cephalosporin, doxycycline, metronidazole
3. cephalosporin, doxycycline, clindamycin, gentamicin
4. *Neisseria gonorrhoeae*, anaerobic, *Chlamydia trachomatis*

Chapter 19
1. *Streptococcus pneumoniae*, *Neisseria meningitidis*, *Listeria monocytogenes*
2. third-generation cephalosporin, vancomycin, ampicillin
3. penicillin G, ampicillin
4. ampicillin, gentamicin

Chapter 20

1. *Staphylococcus aureus*, *Streptococcus pyogenes*, streptococci
2. dicloxacillin, clindamycin, first, macrolide
3. nafcillin, oxacillin, cefazolin, clindamycin
4. glycopeptide, linezolid, daptomycin, tigecycline, ceftaroline

Chapter 21

1. *Streptococcus pneumoniae*, *Haemophilus influenzae*, *Moraxella catarrhalis*
2. amoxicillin
3. *Streptococcus pneumoniae*
4. macrolide, azithromycin, clarithromycin

Chapter 22

1. viridans group streptococci, *Staphylococcus aureus*, enterococci
2. coagulase-negative staphylococci, *Staphylococcus aureus*
3. penicillin G, ceftriaxone, gentamicin
4. vancomycin, gentamicin
5. vancomycin, rifampin, gentamicin
6. nafcillin, oxacillin, gentamicin
7. ceftriaxone, ampicillin-sulbactam, ciprofloxacin

Chapter 23

1. coagulase-negative staphylococci, *Staphylococcus aureus*, aerobic gram-negative bacilli
2. nafcillin, oxacillin
3. vancomycin
4. ceftazidime, cefepime

Chapter 24

1. facultative and aerobic gram-negative bacilli, gram-positive cocci, anaerobic bacilli
2. *Escherichia coli*
3. β-lactam/β-lactamase inhibitor combinations, carbapenems
4. metronidazole

INDEX

Page numbers in *italics* denote figures; those followed by t denote tables, those followed by b denote boxes.